Social History of Africa

BLACK DEATH, WHITE MEDICINE

**Recent Titles in
Social History of Africa Series**
Series Editors: Allen Isaacman and Jean Allman

Making Ethnic Ways: Communities and Their Transformations in Taita, Kenya, 1800–1950
Bill Bravman

Pride of Men: Ironworking in 19th Century West Central Africa
Colleen E. Kriger

Gender and the Making of a South African Bantustan:
A Social History of the Ciskei, 1945–1959
Anne Kelk Mager

The African Rank-and-File: Social Implications of Colonial Military Service in the King's African Rifles, 1902–1964
Timothy H. Parsons

Memoirs of the Maelstrom: A Senegalese Oral History of the First World War
Joe Lunn

"We Women Worked so Hard": Gender, Urbanization, and Social Reproduction in Colonial Harare, Zimbabwe, 1930–1956
Teresa A. Barnes

Bo-Tsotsi: The Youth Gangs of Soweto, 1935–1976
Clive Glaser

History and Memory in the Age of Enslavement: Becoming Merina in Highland Madagascar, 1770–1822
Pier M. Larson

"I Will Not Eat Stone": A Women's History of Colonial Asante
Jean Allman and Victoria B. Tashjian

Making the Town: Ga State and Society in Early Colonial Accra
John Parker

Chiefs Know Their Boundaries: Essays on Property, Power, and the Past in Asante, 1896–1996
Sara S. Berry

"Wicked" Women and the Reconfiguration of Gender in Africa
Dorothy L. Hodgson and Sheryl A. McCurdy, editors

BLACK DEATH, WHITE MEDICINE

BUBONIC PLAGUE AND THE POLITICS OF PUBLIC HEALTH IN COLONIAL SENEGAL, 1914–1945

Myron Echenberg

HEINEMANN
Portsmouth, NH

JAMES CURREY
Oxford

DAVID PHILIP
Cape Town

Heinemann
A division of Reed Elsevier Inc.
361 Hanover Street
Portsmouth, NH 03801-3912
USA
www.heinemann.com

James Currey Ltd.
73 Botley Road
Oxford OX2 0BS
United Kingdom

David Philip Publishers (Pty) Ltd.
208 Werdmuller Centre
Claremont 7708
Cape Town, South Africa

Offices and agents throughout the world

© 2002 by Myron Echenberg. All rights reserved. No part of this book may be reproduced in any form or by any electronic or mechanical means, including information storage and retrieval systems, without permission in writing from the publisher, except by a reviewer, who may quote brief passages in a review.

ISBN 0-325-07017-2 (Heinemann cloth)
ISBN 0-325-07016-4 (Heinemann paper)
ISBN 0-85255-696-9 (James Currey cloth)
ISBN 0-85255-646-2 (James Currey paper)

British Library Cataloguing in Publication Data

Echenberg, Myron J.
  Black death, white medicine : bubonic plague and the politics of public health in colonial Senegal, 1914–1945.— (Social history of Africa)
  1. Plague—Senegal—History—20th century 2. Plague—Social aspects—Senegal—History—20th century 3. Public health—Senegal—History—20th century 4. Public health—Political aspects—Senegal—History—20th century
  5. Imperialism—Health aspects—Senegal—History—20th century
  I. Title
  614.5'732'009663'09041
  ISBN 0-85255-646-2 (James Currey paper)
  ISBN 0-85255-696-9 (James Currey cloth)

Library of Congress Cataloging-in-Publication Data

Echenberg, Myron J.
  Black death, white medicine : bubonic plague and the politics of public health in colonial Senegal / Myron Echenberg.
    p. cm.—(Social history of Africa, ISSN 1099-8098)
  Includes bibliographical references and index.
  ISBN 0-325-07017-2 (alk. paper)—ISBN 0-325-07016-4 (pbk. : alk. paper)
  1. Black death—Social aspects—Senegal—History—20th century. 2. Plague—Social aspects—Senegal—History—20th century. 3. Public health—Political aspects—Senegal—History—20th century. 4. Imperialism—Health aspects—Senegal—History—20th century. I. Title. II. Series.
RC179.S38 E26 2002
614.5'732'009663—dc21   2001024564

Paperback cover photo: Women and men being dusted with DDT, Dakar Médina, 1944. Courtesy of the family of the late Milton H. Buehler. All rights reserved.

Printed in the United States of America on acid-free paper.

05 04 03 02 01 SB 1 2 3 4 5 6 7 8 9

For Eva

CONTENTS

Illustrations	ix
Acknowledgments	xi
Abbreviations	xv
Glossary	xvii
Introduction	**1**
1 Epidemics and French Colonial Medicine	3
2 Background to the Senegalese Bubonic Plague Epidemics, 1880–1914	15
Part I: "Take [a Job in Dakar] if You Want to Die": The Plague Epidemic of 1914	**49**
3 Outbreak, April–May 1914	51
4 Plague's Progress in Dakar, May–November 1914	58
5 The Medical Response	90
6 Measuring the Impact of the 1914 Epidemic	115
Part II: *Kooxa Dooma Ka*: "Acute Headaches," 1919–38	**137**
7 "The Plague Leaps out of the Ground": Plague Ecology in Senegal	139

8	Visions of the Plague: The Rural Impact	159
9	Plague in the City: Epidemics in Dakar, Rufisque, and Saint-Louis	184

Part III: "Merely a Disease of Natives": Plague, War, and Politics, 1939–45 **211**

10	The Dakar Plague Epidemic of 1944	213
11	The Plague's Retreat after 1945	255

Appendix: The Statistical Picture — 267

Sources — 273

Index — 295

ILLUSTRATIONS

MAPS

3.1	Streets of Dakar Infected by Plague, 1914	55
5.1	*Cordons Sanitaires* Established in 1914	93
5.2	Plague Zone in Dakar, 1914	94
7.1	Sereer Ndut and Their Neighbors	140
7.2	Sereer Ndut Region	143
A.1	Plague in Senegal, Overview, 1922–37	269

TABLES

6.1	1914 Plague Epidemic in Senegal	116
6.2	Plague Death Rates in Selected Cities, 1894–1914	117
10.1	1944 Plague Epidemic in Dakar	217
10.2	Population Growth of Dakar, 1936–45	219
10.3	Population of Dakar in 1941	220
A.1	Urban and Rural Plague Deaths, 1914–45	268

CHARTS

4.1	Dakar Plague of 1914, Monthly Mortality	59
4.2	Dakar Dwellings Burned or Disinfected, 1914	72

PHOTOGRAPHS

3.1	Vincens Street, Dakar, c. 1910	54
4.1	Village of Hock, c. 1910	70
5.1	Disinfection Crew, Dakar Health Service, c. 1908	100
5.2	Advertisement for the Antiseptic "Aniodol," Dakar, 1914	105
6.1	Fuulbe Pastoralists in Their Temporary Homes Northeast of Thiès, c. 1912	129
8.1	Rat Cage Distributed by the Health Service	170
9.1	African Laboratory Workers at the Pasteur Institute of Dakar Dissecting Rat Cadavers for Signs of Plague, 1920s	194
10.1	Crew Member Dusting a Médina Dwelling with DDT Powder, 1944	228
10.2	African Crew Members Preparing for DDT Dusting, Dakar Médina, 1944	229
10.3	African Crew Members Dusting Women and Children, Dakar Médina, 1944	230
10.4	Women and Men Being Dusted with DDT, Dakar Médina, 1944	231
10.5	Woman Being Dusted with DDT Powder under the Watchful Eye of a Policeman, Dakar Médina, 1944	232

ACKNOWLEDGMENTS

This book, like *Colonial Conscripts* before it, continues my investigation of the impact of French colonial rule on African society. Once again, I am seeking to understand those especially intrusive factors which transformed the lives of Africans politically and socially. The first book studied the impact of military service; this one examines the consequences of epidemic disease. Once again, I draw my inspiration from the lived experience of my African informants. In the initial study, the stories of African ex-servicemen helped me recognize the value of rendering their history on paper. This time, when I initially set out to do a study of a different epidemic in Senegal, the 1918 influenza outbreak, repeated interviews in rural Sereer districts made it clear to me that it was *pisty*, bubonic plague, which was the epidemic more vividly embedded within the region's collective memory, and the one meriting a full-length monograph.

As the Sereer term has it, endo-epidemic plague was indeed a "severe headache" for the thousands of Senegalese men, women, and children who suffered both from its ravages and from the harsh measures imposed upon them by the French colonial authorities in their efforts to control this terrible disease. Nor did the abrupt retreat of bubonic plague from Senegal after 1945 release people for long from the threat of infectious disease. After what must now seem like a brief interlude of one generation, Senegal, like other jurisdictions on the African continent, is confronted by the specter of human immunodeficiency virus (HIV) and acquired immune deficiency syndrome (AIDS). While HIV/AIDS is in many ways a more "severe headache" than was bubonic plague, both diseases symbolize the past and present inequalities of public health within the world economic system. In the twentieth century, bubonic plague has posed a serious threat to impoverished populations obliged to live in flea- and rat-infested housing. As for HIV/AIDS, treatments that are available and affordable in the Western world remain beyond the financial means of the overwhelming majority of African patients.

Generous assistance from several quarters made my research in Senegal enjoyable and productive. My interpreters Guedj Faye and Thomas Gana Diouf shared with me their knowledge of Sereer culture in general and the healing arts in particular. Thomas not only introduced me to my most eloquent informant, his remarkable mother, Marie-Anne Yaayo Diouf, but through his tireless efforts as president of the Association Njawor Ciss pour la Rénovation de Mont-Roland, Thomas has also helped to preserve social and cultural solidarity among Sereer Ndut brethren in a rapidly changing world.

During and after my visits to Senegal, I benefited from the valuable support and friendship of an extraordinary Franco-Senegalese couple, Charles and Angélique Becker, and their extended family. The foremost researcher working on the history and sociology of health and disease in Senegal, Charles Becker is also a generous and constructive scholar, willing to share with others in an effort to advance general knowledge. Born in the troubled Casamance region of Senegal, Angélique Becker has devoted her considerable energies toward promoting greater understanding between Christian and Muslim citizens of Senegal. I am proud to count both of them among my friends.

Many other friends and colleagues have made valuable contributions to this project. In Senegal, Mamadou Diouf, Babacar Fall, and Mohamed Mbodj shared their insights into Senegal's colonial history with me, while Saliou Mbaye, chief archivist at the Archives Nationales du Sénégal (ANS), was always ready to answer a query and solve a research problem. René Collignon kindly allowed me to consult his interview notes on aspects of health and healing among the Sereer. In France, the keen interest and support for my project from Odile Goerg, Elikia Mbokolo, and Marc Michel has been an encouragement to me. Back in North America, Jean Filipovich, Eva Neisser, and Vinh Kim Nguyen read the manuscript and offered valuable advice; so too did Jean Allman, Allen Isaacman, and the anonymous readers at Heinemann. Colleagues in the History Department and in the Department of Social Studies in Medicine at McGill tolerated my persistent questions and comments concerning bubonic plague. The list of these colleagues includes Don Bates, Pierre Boulle, Alberto Cambrosio, Gershon Hundert, Catherine LeGrand, Margaret Lock, Faith Wallis, George Weisz, Robin Yates, Alan Young, and Brian Young. My McGill students and research assistants deserve mention; they are Craig Forcese, Maureen Malowany, Ismail Rashid, Jon Roberts, Gwen Schulman, and Beth-el

Acknowledgments xiii

Tilahun. Ingrid Stockbauer helped with artwork preparation, and I received excellent copy-editing and production editing assistance from Ann O'Hear and Lynn Zelem.

Funds for overseas research in Senegal, France, and the United States of America have been generously provided by the Social Sciences and Humanities Research Council of Canada, and by the Hannah Institute for the History of Medicine. A travel grant from the Faculty of Graduate Studies and Research, McGill University, was also helpful. I consulted public archives at the ANS in Dakar, and at the U.S. National Archives in Washington, D.C., and I thank all those who assisted me at both locations.

Printed texts and journals were made available to me by the National Library of Medicine, Bethesda, Maryland, and especially by Elizabeth Dunkley and her indefatigable team at the Inter-Library Loan Department, McLennan Library, McGill University. I am grateful to the Congrégation du Saint-Esprit, Chevilly-Larue, France, for having allowed me access to missionary correspondence from Senegal, and especially to the family of the late Captain Milton H. Buehler, whose widow, Mrs. Coral Beth Buehler of McMinnville, Oregon, and son, Tim Buehler, of Brookings, Oregon, showed my wife and me wonderful hospitality, shared their recollections of Milton Buehler's stay in Dakar during the 1944 bubonic plague outbreak, and gave me permission to use family photographs pertaining to those events.

Last but not least, I thank my family for their unflagging support. They usually tolerated my sometimes graphic descriptions of the ravages of bubonic plague, and the role of rats and fleas in its transmission, although they found it necessary to prohibit the subject from being raised at the dinner table.

To all who helped me in this project, I extend the usual apology. You are not responsible for inaccuracies or my failure to heed your advice.

Abbreviations

ACSE	Archives of the Congrégation du Saint-Esprit
ADs	African Auxiliary Doctors (Médecins Auxiliaires Indigènes)
AMI	Assistance Médicale Indigène
ANS	Archives Nationales du Sénégal
BLFWA	Bacteriological Laboratory of French West Africa
CGT	Confédération Générale du Travail
DDT	Dichloro-diphenyl-trichlorothane
FEA	Federation of French Equatorial Africa
FIDES	Fonds pour l'Investissement et le Développement Économique et Social
FWA	Federation of French West Africa
ISC	International Sanitary Conference
OIHP	Office International d'Hygiène Publique
ORSTOM	Office de la Recherche Scientifique et Technique d'Outre-Mer
PI	Pasteur Institute
PID	Pasteur Institute of Dakar
SFIO	Section Française de l'Internationale Ouvrière
SICAP	Société Immobilière du Cap-Vert
WHO	World Health Organization

GLOSSARY

ceddo   Wolof and Sereer slave warriors in the service of the ruler.

chambres (kompe xoore in Soninke)   Literally great rooms, that is, boarding houses.

dara   A Qur'anic school; the house of a *marabout*, and, among the Mourids, an agricultural community of young men serving the *marabout*.

diaraf   Sereer term for chief.

escale   Emporium, a term first applied to river towns, and later, to rail centers.

gelowar   Southern Sereer aristocracy descended from Mandingo invaders from the southeast.

griot   French term for the caste of praise-singers, genealogists, and musicians found in most Sahelian ethnic groups of West Africa.

gris-gris   Charms, usually in the form of amulets.

hivernage   Rainy period from June to October in the Sahel of West Africa.

indigénat   French colonial law code of 1887 giving wide arbitrary powers to administrators.

laptot   African sailor, interpreter, or worker in the Senegal River trade.

maggal   From the verb "to celebrate or exalt," as a noun it denotes a Mourid religious celebration, especially the Grand Maggal, the major annual celebration held in the holy city of Touba to honor Shaykh Amadu Bamba Mbacké.

marabout   French term used throughout northwest Africa for a Muslim religious leader. In Senegal, a religious leader within the Sufi orders. Synonymous with *shaykh*.

Mourid Wolof Muslim religious order founded by Amadu Bamba Mbacké.

navétane Seasonal migrant worker from the interior of FWA who labored in the peanut fields of Senegal and Gambia.

niayes Coastal dunes of Senegal where fresh water in surface pools, combined with moderating sea breezes, created a humid yet moderate microclimate; in short, an oasis.

originaires Africans whose French citizenship was ultimately recognized because they or their parents had been born in one of the four communes of Senegal (Saint-Louis, Rufisque, Dakar, and Gorée).

saltigi Healer or seer.

shaykh Title for a Sufi leader.

Sufism Islamic mysticism.

taalibé A disciple of a *marabout* or a student in a Qur'anic school.

Tijaniyya A Sufi order founded in North Africa in the eighteenth century. In Senegal, the largest Muslim brotherhood.

Tirailleurs Sénégalais French West African soldiers, most of whom were conscripts.

zawiya A Sufi center usually organized around the tomb of a saintly figure.

INTRODUCTION

1

EPIDEMICS AND FRENCH COLONIAL MEDICINE

This book examines the social, political, and medical context of a recurring epidemic of bubonic plague in colonial Senegal. It is organized around four themes. The central theme examines how French colonial authorities constructed the plague epidemic, while the second contrasts French with Senegalese responses to the challenge of devastating epidemic disease. A third theme touches on urban residential policies in colonial Senegal, and how these were affected by the specter of infectious disease. The last theme addressed is the changing disease ecology of Senegal, which can be defined as the complex interaction of humans with other hosts, with the pathogen, and with their changing physical environment.

Arguing that epidemics can be constructed helps us to recognize that an epidemic cannot be understood exclusively as a medical event. As Meredeth Turshen put it over a decade ago, "bacteria and viruses may occur spontaneously in nature, but there is nothing natural or spontaneous about epidemics."[1] Concentrating exclusively on the medical dimension perpetuates the old Cartesian paradigm of clinical medicine, which stressed the individual physiology of the human body while excluding the body politic from its purview. In Senegal as elsewhere, the decision to declare a medical emergency, and to grant wide interventionist powers to health officers, was, as we will see, a political and not a medical one.

While not ignoring biological issues, this study argues that the bubonic plague epidemic in Senegal can best be understood as part of the ideological contest between conqueror and conquered. Deeply embedded in French medical assumptions was a triumphalist Enlightenment rationality which empowered Western biomedical science while contemptuously rejecting the applied knowledge of local healing specialists.[2] Also rooted in the Enlightenment was the assumption that Western sanitary measures were humanitarian acts conferring moral legitimacy on the sometimes heavy-handed European paternalist rule over "the other."³ For many Africans, on the other hand, the bubonic plague outbreak was regarded as part of the colonial conquest, biological warfare in either symbolic or concrete form. European motives for attempting disease control were questioned, and the measures often fiercely resisted, partly because they were highly intrusive yet ineffective, and partly because they were simply alien.

At the same time, this ideological dimension of colonial medicine should not be reduced to a static analysis pitting the conqueror against the conquered.⁴ French public health measures directed toward bubonic plague met tenacious resistance, but over time, as African healers were disempowered, and seasonal control measures became as regular as taxes, most Senegalese grew to accept what they could not change. A small African elite went further and came to see Western biomedicine as a measure of modernity.

Although this study is critical of the record of French colonial medicine in Senegal, it has some sympathy with a dilemma faced by the medical officials of the day. When they failed to intervene in medical emergencies they could be accused of indifference to the suffering of colonial subjects. Yet when they intervened energetically they were often charged with ignoring social and economic realities. In a similar vein, Heather Bell argues convincingly that in the epidemics which struck the Anglo-Egyptian Sudan, medical and administrative personnel faced the contradiction of public health's need for "impermeable boundaries" as opposed to the "socio-economic need for porous ones."⁵

The relationship between disease and urban residential segregation in urban Africa is our third theme. Writing about South Africa, Maynard Swanson called this relationship the "sanitary syndrome."⁶ He has shown that while the outbreaks of bubonic plague around 1900 in Cape Town and Port Elizabeth, South Africa, led many whites to insist upon urban residential segregation on medical grounds, the epidemics provided a pretext masking more deeply rooted racial prejudices.

French attitudes toward urban living in Senegal at the beginning of the twentieth century were no different from those of Europeans elsewhere on the African continent. As this study shows, precedents and policy for separating Africans from Europeans in the towns and cities of Senegal go back at least to the foundation of Dakar in 1857. Here too the "sanitary syndrome" was at work. Virtually the entire French medical community agreed that Africans should live separately from the French, and used the Dakar bubonic plague outbreak of 1914 as a paradigmatic case.

Changing disease ecology played an as yet poorly understood part in the story of bubonic plague in Senegal. Along with cholera, especially, bubonic plague benefited from transformations in the world capitalist system of the nineteenth century in its spread around the globe.[7] The epidemiological history of plague has never been amenable to simple, single-factor explanations of causation. In each of the three world pandemics of plague, often inadvertent human actions in combination with ecological shifts may have been involved. It remains impossible today to establish primary causes among such potentially relevant factors as changes in diet, work, and living patterns and the impact of these circumstances on human and animal immune systems.

Nor were the historical circumstances in which plague could expand from a limited outbreak to a raging inferno of death identical from country to country. In Senegal, no immediately obvious change in the pattern of land use within what the French came to call "the plague zone," or other impact resulting from the introduction of colonial rule and the colonial capitalist economy, can be detected.[8] Indirectly, however, the modernization of the port of Dakar and its increased international shipping activity made it more likely to attract infected rats or flea-infested goods in ships' cargoes. The so-called "Pax Gallica" of colonial rule brought with it significantly increased internal migrations of people from various regions of Senegal and from the rest of French West Africa. Voluntary or not, migration had a bearing on the susceptibility of people to disease.[9] Migration brought into the plague zone people who would not have lived there before the advent of French colonial rule.

REVIEW OF THE LITERATURE

The social history of African health and disease is a burgeoning industry. Twenty years ago, when the first modern collection of essays in what was not yet a field was published, one of the editors, David Patterson, was hard pressed to fill ten pages of text in his bibliographic essay.[10] Ten years later, two major reviews of the literature testified to a dramatic growth in the field.[11]

Several insightful works have previously addressed the themes examined in this study. In his classic investigation of a single disease over time, Randall Packard ably demonstrated how racist policies both reflected and shaped the course of tuberculosis in South Africa.[12] He shows that the curative treatments pursued by the South African medical community did not succeed against a disease of poverty like tuberculosis because they failed to address the gross inequalities endured by black

South Africans: a permanently transient labor force, overcrowded housing, inadequate sanitation, low wages, and poor health facilities. Maryinez Lyons, in her monograph on trypanosomiasis, or sleeping sickness, in the northeastern Congo during Belgian rule, has demonstrated how this quintessential "colonial disease" completely transformed local society. Not only did sleeping sickness carry a heavy death toll; intrusive health control measures such as the relocation of entire villages and the imposition of compulsory but unreliable drug therapy resulted in invasive and arbitrary social engineering.[13] Jean Comaroff has written of the dialectical linkage of the Enlightenment with nineteenth-century medicine and colonialism in South Africa. She notes how the Enlightenment's belief in the need for "rational" control over a dangerous state of nature enabled Western biomedicine to transform Africans into living laboratory specimens.[14] Most recently, in a remarkably comprehensive study of public health in the Anglo-Egyptian Sudan between 1899 and 1940, Heather Bell has examined the roles of medical researchers, practitioners, and health policy officials and their impact on sleeping sickness, yellow fever, and midwifery training. Her important contribution emphasizes the complexity of what she terms colonial medicine, and the caution which must be exercised in establishing frontiers and boundaries between the medical and the social.[15]

The theme of residential segregation has received the attention of several scholars in addition to Maynard Swanson. Studying another infectious outbreak in South Africa, the world influenza pandemic of 1918, Howard Phillips has demonstrated the important linkages of this pandemic with the furthering of discriminatory residential segregation laws.[16] Odile Goerg has discussed French and British approaches to early urban residential segregation in an essay comparing Conakry with Freetown at the beginning of the twentieth century.[17] In an essay dealing with the state of European medical knowledge and misinformation about Africa, Philip Curtin shows how colonial racism developed the myth of the diseased native, and then used it as a rationale for separating Africans from whites through residential segregation.[18] The insalubrious quarters Africans were compelled to occupy in urban areas increased their risks of contracting epidemic diseases.

In recent years, a growing number of environmental studies have testified to the importance of changing disease ecology. Although some have disagreed on whether natural or human factors have predominated during drought, famine, or the spread of disease, the arguments supporting social rather than natural factors are more persuasive.[19] James Giblin's able account of politics and environment in Northeastern Tanzania under German and then British colonialism leaves little doubt that human actions were primary in that part of East Africa.[20] Giblin demonstrates that local peasants exercised careful environmental management of their land. They were able to keep humans and tsetse flies apart to contain sleeping sickness, and to maintain elaborate patron-client relationships as a hedge against famine. With the loss of political control, local Africans also lost decision-making power over their environment; serious sleeping sickness and smallpox epidemics were the result.[21]

While these works offer a comparative perspective, they do not directly deal with bubonic plague in Africa. Despite the recurring presence of bubonic plague epidemics in the Maghreb and Egypt, and south of the Sahara in Senegal, Madagascar, Ghana, Nigeria, Kenya, Congo, Angola, and South Africa, not a single full-length monograph has yet appeared.[22] Only four articles, each of considerable merit, have been exclusively devoted to bubonic plague. The Cape Town outbreak of 1901 has been explored by Maynard Swanson and by Elizabeth van Heyningen; a study by Faranirina Esoavelomandroso covers plague in Madagascar from the 1920s to the 1940s; and Elikia Mbokolo has written on the Dakar epidemic of 1914.[23] Nancy Gallagher also includes epidemics of bubonic plague, along with cholera and typhus, as elements in her insightful study of the competition between Arab and French medicine for dominance in nineteenth-century Tunisia.[24] Very recently, Joyce Kirk has devoted a chapter to bubonic plague in her valuable monograph on African resistance to residential segregation in Port Elizabeth, South Africa.[25]

A dearth of scholarship can be also be said to apply to the history of French colonial medicine in Africa. One of the first modern critiques of French colonial medicine came from Frantz Fanon, the French-West-Indian-born psychiatrist turned revolutionary. In "Medicine and Colonialism," a short essay based on his clinical experience in Algeria, Fanon highlighted the inherent contradictions between colonial medical services and local custom and tradition.[26] He argued that local resistance to Western biomedicine was inevitable because medicine was an intrinsic part of the dominant group's values. Opposition was therefore one of the few defensive responses available to the conquered population. Yet even Fanon accepted the old notion that Western medicine and psychiatry were positive contributions, even if distorted by colonialism's inequalities.

More recently, the literature on French Africa has examined a variety of topics, but it only thinly covers the immense space of this part of the continent. William Cohen has provided a general overview of health and French colonialism and an article specifically on malaria.[27] Anne-Marie Moulin and Michael Osborne have studied the role of the Pasteur Institute as an agency of French scientific imperialism, Laurence Monnais-Rousselot has provided an overview of French medicine in Indochina, and Anne Marcovich has compared French colonial medicine in Algeria and Indochina.[28]

Three well-known scholars, Dennis Cordell, the late Joel Gregory, and Victor Piché, have offered a demographic comparison of health and disease in the Central African Republic and Burkina Faso.[29] Rita Headrick's doctoral dissertation on health and illness in French Equatorial Africa was published posthumously.[30] Two historians of the Ivory Coast, Danielle Domergue-Cloarec and Christophe Wondji, have studied health generally and a single yellow fever outbreak specifically.[31] Jean-Pierre Dozon has commented on a variety of historical issues pertaining to health.[32] Most recently, two major monographs have added significantly to our understanding of the history of disease in Francophone Africa. Jean-Paul Bado has studied French campaigns against three major endemic diseases: leprosy, trypanosomiasis, and onchocerciasis; while Eric Silla has contributed an outstanding monograph on leprosy and society in colonial and postcolonial Mali.[33]

Rather surprisingly, given Senegal's prominence in Francophone African historiography generally, no full-length studies of the history of health and disease in this country have yet been attempted. As the numerous entries in the bibliography of this book testify, Charles Becker has been an outstanding and prolific contributor to the history and sociology of health and disease in Senegal. Together with René Collignon, he has also compiled an excellent bibliography on health and demography for Senegal. We have already noted the Mbokolo article on plague. Finally, Francis Snyder has provided a historical perspective on health and the legal system in Senegal.[34]

SOURCES

The most substantial primary sources come from the National Archives of Senegal (ANS), but I have also examined primary material in France and the United States. The American sources proved particularly useful for the years 1944 and 1945, when the U.S. Army Medical Corps took the initiative against bubonic plague in the Dakar area. The private Archives des Pères du Saint-Esprit at Chevilly-Larue, near Paris, where the correspondence of French missionaries stationed within the Senegalese plague zone is located, proved of some use. Far more illuminating were some twenty interviews in Senegal which I conducted among eyewitnesses to rural plague outbreaks in the 1920s and 1930s.

Contemporary medical literature on the plague epidemics is extensive. The Collignon and Becker bibliography lists roughly one hundred entries. While I have read this material carefully, it is of limited value because most authors follow the Cartesian medical convention and avoid comment on social and political issues.

Despite their voluminous quantity, the primary sources for the history of health and disease in colonial Senegal have their limitations. Not only is there a failure to address questions of political economy, but the demographic data are scanty and unreliable until the first modern censuses after 1950. What is especially striking in the French medical record, however, is the almost total silence regarding local African healing practices. In the rare instances where local healers are mentioned, it is only to demonize them as quacks and charlatans. In his Annual Report for 1913, for example, Dr. L. Huot, head of the colony of Senegal's Health Service, railed against the "fraudulent and murderous practices of the *marabouts* and other healers who operate in inconceivable ignorance of the most elementary and banal rules of hygiene."[35] Taking into consideration what are, after all, familiar limitations of colonial record keeping, the documented source material is nevertheless a rich mine for the social historian. As the jewel in France's African crown, Senegal is particularly well served for the historian seeking to understand the role of health and disease through the prism provided by the bubonic plague epidemics. What I do not attempt in this study is to reconstruct the history of public health, a separate subject whose study is made more difficult by the limitations of the demographic and census data.

The book is organized in three parts. Part One is entitled "'Take [a Job in Dakar] if You Want to Die': The Plague Epidemic of 1914." It is dedicated to the first, and in many ways the most dramatic, plague epidemic to strike Senegal. The narrative continues through to the end of the First World War in November 1918, by which time it had become evident that plague was not going to vanish as suddenly and mysteriously as it had originally appeared. In this period, Senegalese and French perceptions of the epidemic and what to do about it were vastly at odds.

Part Two is entitled "*Kooxa Dooma Ka*: 'Acute Headaches,' 1919–38." This Sereer expression for one of the most common symptoms of bubonic plague appropriately introduces a section of the book devoted to the economic and social impact of bubonic plague between the two wars. Under investigation are the widespread ecological transformations brought about by cash-crop farming, labor migration, and other changes introduced by colonial capitalism. The periodic epidemics were highly localized, affecting a small but densely populated rectangular "plague zone" stretching from the capital of French West Africa, Dakar, to the important inland towns of Thiès, some 50 kilometers to the east, and Tivaouane, 80 kilometers to the northeast. Thiès was the railroad capital of Senegal and plague infection there represented a constant threat, unrealized as it happened, that the disease would spread deep into the hinterland of French West Africa. Tivaouane was also the Senegalese headquarters of the Tijaniyya brotherhood, and therefore a locale frequently visited by the Muslim faithful.

Part Two also examines the social impact of plague on various strata of Senegalese society. These include the emerging petty bourgeoisie of medical workers, schoolteachers, newspapermen, and politicians; the traditional healers among the Sereer and Wolof populations of the plague zone; the newly Christian Sereer Ndut communities of the district known as "Mont-Roland"; and the Tijaniyya brotherhood at Tivaouane.

Dramatic urban migration and the passage of two generations have dramatically transformed the social composition of the metropolis of Dakar and the bustling city of Thiès. In these urban locales, it was difficult to find elders who had deep roots in their neighborhoods. When they were approached and queried about past epidemics, they had no memory of plague and chose instead to speak of the polio and infuenza epidemics of the 1940s and 1950s. Fortunately, the same is not true of the Mont-Roland district, where oral interviews brought forward rich collective memories of the plague years between 1920 and 1940, as voiced by plague survivors and their kin. Chapter 8 of Part Two, entitled "Visions of the Plague: The Rural Impact," is largely based on oral evidence. In addition to revealing the emotional depths of a community under siege, this material demonstrates how bubonic plague epidemics and their accompanying control measures came to be regarded by the Senegalese population as an ongoing burden which, like death and taxes, had simply to be endured.

Part Three, entitled "'Merely a Disease of Natives': Plague, War, and Politics, 1939–45," deals with the last years of endemic plague during the Second World War, and focuses particularly on the Dakar urban epidemic of 1944. What made this epidemic markedly different from the first outbreak of 1914 was the presence in the city and on the Cape Verde peninsula of some 5,000 American military and civilian personnel, stationed in Senegal as part of the line of supply from the United States to North Africa, the Middle East, and the Soviet Union. When plague broke out, the United States Army Medical Corps requested permission to apply their new technology to combat the epidemic, and permission was reluctantly granted by the beleaguered Gaullist government. The American medics sprayed Dakar and the Cape Verde peninsula with a powerful new pesticide named DDT, and distributed sulfa drugs to plague patients. DDT successfully attacked the rat flea vector of bubonic plague and, by breaking the chain of transmission, probably became the leading factor in ending the terrible years of endo-epidemic plague in Senegal. The concluding chapter explores the retreat of plague from Senegal, and examines the disease's legacy for public health in the postcolonial era.

NOTES

1. Meredith Turshen, *The Political Ecology of Disease in Tanzania* (New Brunswick, N.J.: Rutgers University Press, 1984), 15.

2. Nancy Gallagher has argued that a similar power struggle occurred in Tunisia at the time of the French conquest, when Arab medical specialists clashed with European practitioners of Western biomedicine. See *Medicine and Power in Tunisia, 1780–1900* (Cambridge: Cambridge University Press, 1983).

3. Jean Comaroff, "The Diseased Heart of Africa: Medicine, Colonialism, and the Black Body," in *Knowledge, Power, and Practice: The Anthropology of Medicine and Everyday Life*, edited by Shirley Lindenbaum and Margaret Lock (Berkeley: University of California Press, 1993), 305–29.

4. An extensive literature has developed over tensions within these categories. See for example Frederick Cooper and Ann Stoler, eds., *Tensions of Empire: Colonial Cultures in a Bourgeois World* (Berkeley: University of California Press, 1997).

5. Heather Bell, *Frontiers of Medicine in the Anglo-Egyptian Sudan, 1899–1940* (Oxford: Clarendon Press, 1999), 10.

6. Maynard Swanson, "The Sanitation Syndrome: Bubonic Plague and Urban Native Policy in the Cape Colony, 1900–1909," *Journal of African History* 18 (1977): 387–410.

7. Whereas the cholera *vibrio* had previously been endemic mainly to Bengal, steam ships carried the pathogen along with its incubating hosts to the Near East, Africa, Europe, and the Americas. As William McNeill has pointed out, cholera's global dissemination was "the first and in many ways the most significant manifestation of the altered disease relationships created by industrialization." William H. McNeill, *Plagues and Peoples* (New York: Doubleday Anchor, 1976), 230.

8. In contrast, major plague epidemics in Manchuria in 1911 and 1921 can be attributed to political, social, and economic upheavals. See McNeill, *Plagues*, 137.

9. Randall Packard, "Maize, Cattle and Mosquitoes: The Political Economy of Malaria Epidemics in Colonial Swaziland," *Journal of African History* 25 (1984): 189–212; James Giblin, "Famine and Social Change during the Transition to Colonial Rule in Northeastern Tanzania, 1880–1896," *African Economic History* 15 (1986): 85–105.

10. K. David Patterson, "Bibliographic Essay," in *Disease in African History: An Introductory Survey and Case Studies*, edited by Gerald W. Hartwig and K. David Patterson (Durham, N.C.: Duke University Press, 1978), 238–50.

11. Steven Feierman, "Struggles for Control: The Social Roots of Health and Healing in Modern Africa," *African Studies Review* 28 (1985): 73–147; and Gwyn Prins, "But What Was the Disease? The Present State of Health and Healing in African Studies," *Past and Present*, no. 124 (1989): 158–79.

12. Randall Packard, *White Plague, Black Labor: Tuberculosis and the Political Economy of Health and Disease in South Africa* (Berkeley: University of California Press, 1989), 20.

13. Maryinez Lyons, *The Colonial Disease: A Social History of Sleeping Sickness in Northern Zaire, 1900–1940* (Cambridge: Cambridge University Press, 1992).

14. Comaroff, "The Diseased Heart of Africa," 324.

15. Bell, *Frontiers of Medicine*.

16. Howard Phillips, *"Black October": The Impact of the Spanish Influenza Epidemic of 1918 on South Africa* (Pretoria: Government Printer, 1990).

17. Odile Goerg, "From Hill Station (Freetown) to Downtown Conakry (First Ward): Comparing French and British Approaches to Segregation in Colonial Cities at the Beginning of the Twentieth Century," *Canadian Journal of African Studies* 32 (1998): 1–31.

18. Philip D. Curtin, "Medical Knowledge and Urban Planning in Tropical Africa," *American Historical Review* 90 (1985): 594–613.

19. The question of drought and famine is a case in point. Drawing on the seminal "entitlements" hypothesis of Amartya Sen, which attributes famine not to absolute shortage of food, but to relative lack of access among the less privileged, research in southern Africa has demonstrated the primacy of socioeconomic and political factors. See Elizabeth Eldredge, "Famine and Disease in Nineteenth-Century Lesotho," *African Economic History* 16 (1987): 61–93; Diana Wylie, "The Changing Face of Hunger in Southern African History, 1880–1980," *Past and Present*, no. 122 (1989): 159–99; and Henrietta Moore and Megan Vaughan, *Cutting down Trees: Gender, Nutrition, and Agricultural Change in the Northern Province of Zambia, 1890–1990* (London: James Currey, 1994). For an argument stressing the primacy of natural phenomena, see Charles Ballard, "Drought and Economic Distress: South Africa in the 1800s," *Journal of Interdisciplinary History* 17 (1986): 359–78.

20. James L. Giblin, *The Politics of Environmental Control in Northeastern Tanzania, 1840–1940* (Philadelphia: University of Pennsylvania Press, 1992).

21. Giblin, *Environmental Control*, 121 and 128–29. On sleeping sickness, for an essay in which the pioneering work of John Ford on the ecology of sleeping sickness is clearly explained, see James L. Giblin, "Trypanosomiasis Control in African History: An Evaded Issue?" *Journal of African History* 31 (1990): 59–80.

22. The statement applies only to published material. The bibliography lists roughly a dozen master's and doctoral theses on Senegalese health issues generally, which have proved helpful to this study.

23. Faranirina Esoavelomandroso, "Maladie et politique en situation coloniale: La peste à Madagascar," *Annales ESC* 36, no. 2 (1981): 168–90; Elikia Mbokolo, "Peste et société urbaine à Dakar: L'épidèmie de 1914," *Cahiers d'Etudes Africaines* 22 (1982):

13–46; Swanson, "The Sanitation Syndrome," 387–410; and Elizabeth van Heyningen, "Cape Town and the Plague of 1901," in *Studies in the History of Cape Town*, vol. 4, edited by Christopher Saunders, Howard Philips, and Elizabeth van Heyningen (Cape Town: University of Cape Town, 1981).

24. Gallagher, *Medicine and Power in Tunisia*.

25. Joyce F. Kirk, *Making a Voice: African Resistance to Segregation in South Africa* (Boulder, Colo.: Westview Press, 1998).

26. Frantz Fanon, "Medicine and Colonialism," in *A Dying Colonialism* (New York: Grove Press, 1965), 121–45.

27. William Cohen, "Malaria and French Imperialism," *Journal of African History* 24 (1983): 23–36; William Cohen, "Health and Colonialism in French Africa," in *Etudes africaines offertes à Henri Brunschwig*, edited by Jan Vansina et al. (Paris: Editions de l'Ecole des Hautes Études en Sciences Sociales, 1982).

28. Anne-Marie Moulin, "Patriarchal Science: The Network of the Overseas Pasteur Institutes," in *Science and Empires: Historical Studies about Scientific Development and European Expansion*, edited by Patrick Petitjean, Catherine Jami, and Anne-Marie Moulin (Dordrecht, Holland: Kluwer, 1992), 307–21; and Moulin, "Tropical without the Tropics: The Turning-Point of Pastorian Medicine in North Africa," in *Warm Climates and Western Medicine: The Emergence of Tropical Medicine, 1500–1900*, edited by David Arnold (Atlanta: Rodopi B.V., 1996), 160–80; Michael A. Osborne, "Resurrecting Hippocrates: Hygienic Sciences and the French Scientific Expeditions to Egypt, Morea and Algeria," in *Warm Climates and Western Medicine: The Emergence of Tropical Medicine, 1500–1900*, edited by David Arnold (Atlanta: Rodopi B.V., 1996), 80–98; Laurence Monnais-Rousselot, *Médecine et colonisation: L'aventure indochinoise, 1860–1939* (Paris: Éditions CNRS, 1999); Anne Marcovich, "French Colonial Medicine and Colonial Rule: Algeria and Indochina," in *Disease, Medicine and Empire: Perspectives on Western Medicine and the Experience of European Expansion*, edited by Roy MacLeod and Milton Lewis (London: Routledge, 1988), 103–17.

29. Dennis D. Cordell, Joel W. Gregory, and Victor Piché, "The Demographic Reproduction of Health and Disease: Colonial Central African Republic and Contemporary Burkina Faso," in *The Social Basis of Health and Healing in Africa*, edited by Steven Feierman and John M. Janzen (Berkeley: University of California Press, 1992), 39–70.

30. Rita Headrick, *Colonialism, Health and Illness in French Equatorial Africa, 1885–1935* (Atlanta: African Studies Association Press, 1994).

31. Danielle Domergue-Cloarec, *La santé en Côte d'Ivoire, 1905–1958* (Toulouse-Le Mirail: Association des Publications Universitaires, 1986); Christophe Wondji, "La fièvre jaune à Grand-Bassam, 1899–1903," *Revue Française d'Histoire d'Outre-Mer* 59 (1972): 204–39.

32. Jean-Pierre Dozon, "D'un tombeau à l'autre," *Cahiers d'Etudes Africaines*, 121–22, vol. 31 (1991): 135–57; Dozon, "A propos de l'ouvrage de Danielle Domergue-Cloarec: La santé en Côte d'Ivoire 1905–1958," *Psychopathologie Africaine* 31 (1986–87): 211–17; and Dozon, "Quand les Pastoriens traquaient la maladie du sommeil," *Sciences Sociales et Santé* 3 (1985): 27–56.

33. Jean-Paul Bado, *Médecine coloniale et grandes endémies en Afrique, 1900–1960: Lèpre, trypanosomiase humaine et onchocercose* (Paris: Karthala, 1996); Eric

Silla, *"People Are Not the Same": Leprosy and Identity in Twentieth Century Mali* (Portsmouth, N.H.: Heinemann, 1998).

34. René Collignon and Charles Becker (with the collaboration of Ellen Brickwedde, Didier Fassin, and Christine Henry), *Santé et population en Sénégambie des origines à 1960: Bibliographie annotée* (Paris: Institut National d'Etudes Démographiques, 1989); Francis Snyder, "Health Policy and the Law in Senegal," *Social Science and Medicine*, 8 (1979): 11–28.

35. Archives Nationales du Sénégal (ANS), Dakar, Senegal, ANS\2G13\26, Saint-Louis, Dr. L. Huot, Annual Medical Report for 1913, 20 September 1914, 253 pp. (hereafter cited as Huot Report for 1913). All translations of material from the French Archives are by the author.

2

BACKGROUND TO THE SENEGALESE BUBONIC PLAGUE EPIDEMICS, 1880–1914

> [The migrant laborers] sleep anywhere, eat anything, crowd inside tiny houses, supplying daily labor that is often poorly done, and they end their evenings by singing and dancing to their tam-tams.[1]

This chapter provides the historical context for the bubonic plague epidemics which were to strike Senegal with such devastating force beginning in 1914. It is organized in three sections. First, while this is a social rather than a natural history of plague, it is worthwhile examining briefly the pathogen, its rodent hosts, its insect vector, and its occasional human victim. Such a technical discussion should not blind us, however, to new risks to public health resulting from such human activities as the military conquest of the region, the building of railways and steamships, and the establishment of large, overcrowded urban centers. Indeed, Senegal, like the rest of Africa, experienced a medical crisis in the years from 1880 to 1920 and the second section of the chapter examines this subject. Third, the chapter studies the unique role played by Senegal's limited system of electoral politics. In May 1914, an obscure African civil servant named Blaise Diagne shocked the French African empire when he was elected to the French National Assembly as Deputy for Senegal. His stunning electoral victory coincided with official recognition that a bubonic plague epidemic was under way in

Dakar. This remarkable conjunction of political and biological events was to prove a major watershed in the history of the country.

ETIOLOGY OF BUBONIC PLAGUE

Few if any infectious diseases have struck greater fear in the European collective memory than bubonic plague. Over the centuries, Western intellectuals from Boccaccio through Defoe and Camus to the present-day South African novelist André Brink have used bubonic plague as a metaphor for both political and social disaster and as an epidemiological catastrophe in its own right.[2] Most of the Western literature on plague refers to what epidemiological historians have labeled the second pandemic of bubonic plague, the so-called "Black Death," which carried off between one-quarter and one-half of the total population of Europe, North Africa, and the Middle East in the middle of the fourteenth century.[3] The world's first bubonic plague pandemic, often called Justinian's plague because the Emperor himself was stricken but recovered, broke out in Egypt, then part of the eastern Roman Empire, in 542 C.E.[4] Plague in twentieth-century Senegal was part of the third plague pandemic, which first exploded onto the world stage in Hong Kong in 1894.

Although the third pandemic is less well known today to the general public in the West, it struck with great intensity. Plague killed roughly 13 million people on every continent before slowing down in the second quarter of the twentieth century.[5] Two factors help explain this relative silence. First, extensive though it was, the third pandemic's time line was extremely lopsided. For the world as a whole, the third pandemic case rate peaked around 1910, fell off dramatically during the First World War, rose sharply again in the early 1920s, and then dropped off sharply again until, by 1950, plague seemed to have virtually disappeared as a major human disease. The second factor has to do with place. Stated bluntly, plague was simply not a white man's disease in the twentieth century. Of the 9.6 million officially recorded deaths from plague in the twentieth century, over 90 percent, or close to 9 million, occurred on the Indian subcontinent. Indonesia and China each suffered roughly 150,000 deaths, the same number as occurred on the African continent as a whole.[6] In comparison, Europe's death toll was slightly more than 7,000, while the total in the Americas was roughly 38,000, mostly in South America. In the neo-Europes overseas, mortality figures were similarly low. Ann Carmichael has every reason therefore to describe plague outbreaks in the West as "relatively minor, but nonetheless panic-inspiring, epidemics."[7]

Bubonic plague was the most persistent and dramatic infectious disease to strike Senegal in the twentieth century, even if chronic diseases such as malaria and dysentery killed more people. From the time plague first appeared in 1914 until its final departure in 1945, scarcely a year went by without a recorded outbreak in either rural or urban areas. Yellow fever, it is true, was also a great threat to public health, but its outbreaks remained hidden except for the major Dakar epidemic of 1927–28.[8] The human and financial costs of the terrible scourge of plague cannot be measured. Recorded Senegalese deaths from plague exceeded 35,000 over thirty-two years, but this figure represents an unknown fraction of the real toll. Senegal may have suffered the highest case rates per 10,000 people in Africa, and rates second only to India worldwide.[9]

The microbial agent responsible for bubonic plague is *Yersinia pestis*.[10] Although it is a "simple" bacterial organism, its history and epidemiology are exceedingly complex, which accounts in part for the numerous misconceptions surrounding this disease over the past fifteen centuries. While a vantage point at the beginning of this new millennium offers definitive explanations concerning many of plague's aspects, other features remain as mysterious and perplexing as they were to our predecessors.

Bubonic plague is a zoonosis, a shared infection of wild rodents and other small ruminants, on the one hand, and humans on the other. Zoonoses, or "cross-over" diseases, include many of the most important human diseases globally. The agents of roughly 80 percent of all described infections of humans are shared in nature by other vertebrate animals.[11] Like other zoonoses, such as yellow fever, which have permanent animal hosts, bubonic plague can cross over to humans as a result of a series of particular ecological changes which can affect the ecosystem of one or more of four categories of living species: the bacillus itself; its wild rodent hosts; the fleas which these rodents harbor in their fur; and humans as prospective alternative recipients of flea bites.

Small sylvatic mammals, which include at least 230 species of wild rodents worldwide, serve as the enzootic reservoir species: a population in which *Y. pestis* is permanently present because these species can survive and reproduce while infected.[12] A large die-off, or epizootic, occurs when the organism is transmitted to a new, less resistant rodent population, either by the bite of an infected flea, or because the bacteria have been able to survive within the sheltered microclimate of warm rodent burrows.[13] It is not necessary that the enzootic and epizootic animals be of different species, but merely of different population groups.[14]

Among those rodents which have been historically subject to bubonic plague epizootics are the common "black" or "brown" house rats (respectively, *Rattus rattus* and *Rattus norvegicus*), sometimes called "commensal" rodents because they have found food sources by living in proximity to humans. Both species are highly susceptible to *Y. pestis* and have been transported by modern navigation throughout the world.[15] Both were present in Senegal during the plague years, as were a wide variety of field rodents which could serve as potential reservoirs of infection. These include the giant rat, *Cricetomys gambianus*; the shrew mouse, *Crocidura stamfii*; and the palm rat, *Xerus erythropus*.[16]

Several species of flea have been found to infest the fur of both wild and commensal rodents, and to be capable of transmitting *Y. pestis* to their hosts with varying degrees of effectiveness. Some observers maintain that the introduction of the more efficient vector subspecies, *Xenopsylla cheopis*, which replaced its competitor, *Xenopsylla astia*, was responsible for the plague conflagration which swept over western India and left 6 million dead within one decade after 1896.[17] Widely distributed in Senegal, *X. cheopis* is the most dangerous of the flea vectors of plague, and, among the various complex factors which accounted for the years of endo-epidemic plague in Senegal, its role may have been decisive.[18] *X. cheopis* does not flourish when the weather is hot, or when humidity drops below 70 percent. Plague, as a result, is most definitely a seasonal illness, with risk rising in slightly cooler, more humid months of the year, diminishing in hot, dry periods, and disappearing completely in cold seasons when the mercury drops below 15 degrees Celsius.[19]

For all their historical severity, plague infections in humans are largely accidental events. Humans are not a critical link in the life cycle of the *Y. pestis* organism, as they are for bilharzia or malaria, for example. In order for bubonic plague to spread among humans, three essential conditions must be present. The first is the presence of a reservoir, a *Y. pestis*-infected flea population cohabiting with a nonsusceptible rodent population. Second, a vulnerable, highly susceptible population of commensal rodents must become infected through accidental contact with the first population. Third, these vulnerable new hosts must be close enough to humans that, when they die in large numbers, their fleas, having ingested large numbers of *Y. pestis*, will migrate to humans in search of a blood meal. The critical secondary variable of climate helps determine the degree to which these primary conditions can be fulfilled. The fleas are at their most active biting stage in warm, dry weather, suggesting a specific season in which rodent epizootics and human epidemics might be anticipated. Some regions are simply too hot, too cold, or too moist ever to provide optimal conditions for flea activity.

Human outbreaks of bubonic plague are sporadic in incidence and confined to household units whose shelters contain infected fleas. Once removed from such locations and separated from the critical vectors, persons carrying bubonic plague are unlikely to contaminate others. It was once believed that inter-human transmission of plague, which is possible in the highly contagious pulmonary form, could also sustain a human epidemic. What happens, however, is that the very virulence of such cases produces a burn-out effect. In short, to sustain an epidemic, a large infected rodent population must be present.

Without antibiotic therapy, bubonic plague infection in humans is fatal within seven days in at least 60 percent of all cases. The most characteristic first symptom, which gives the disease its name, is the early appearance of buboes, usually distributed in the groin, the armpit (axilla), or even the cervical lymph nodes. Occasionally, the *Y. pestis* organisms will invade the lungs and produce pulmonary or pneumonic plague. More rarely, *Y. pestis* organisms may infest the bloodstream to such an extent that the lymph nodes are overwhelmed before they swell, producing a particularly lethal variety known as septicemic plague. If either pulmonary or septicemic plague is not treated with antibiotics within twenty-four hours of its appearance, death is almost inevitable.[20] Cases of bubonic plague may vary in intensity from a sub-clinically mild indisposition to violent death. Variables include the type of flea vector, the location and effectiveness of the vector's bite, the number of bacilli present, and, more controversially, the condition of the patient's immune system.

Immediate diagnosis of bubonic plague through observation is not easy, despite the characteristic appearance of large buboes within roughly four days of infection. The buboes can be the size of an egg, an orange, or even a grapefruit, and are excruciatingly painful. Sometimes, hemorrhagic sepsis can occur, blackening large areas of the surface of the body and producing the repulsive appearance that gave the second pandemic the label, "Black Death."[21] Laboratory diagnosis based on standardized Gramm staining procedures became the accepted and eventually the only method of officially determining the presence of *Y. pestis* infection after the beginning of the twentieth century.[22]

Human vulnerability to *Y. pestis* is variable. People living in conditions of poverty, overcrowding, and malnutrition are at greater risk than others, both because their immune systems are undermined by their circumstances and because their adverse living conditions promote the presence of rodents and fleas.[23] Most humans at most times, like commensal rodents, constitute a population highly susceptible to *Y. pestis*. On the other hand, in a few specialized circumstances, humans may either acquire or inherit immunity.[24]

Occupations are also a factor. Dock workers, grain handlers, and bakers are more exposed to commensal rodents that feed on grain supplies. A gendered factor places women at more risk than men since they spend more time in dwellings in which infected rodents and fleas may be present.[25] In rural areas, farmers, hunters, and trappers may all be at risk from sylvatic plague.

Attempts to prevent, control, and treat bubonic plague are no doubt as old as the the disease itself. During the second pandemic, the empirical response of medieval authorities was either to evacuate or to isolate victims. Flight was, in fact, an effective response so long as it distanced humans from infected fleas. Isolation, however, was not helpful, and it was downright harmful when patients were confined to homes together with infected fleas and as yet uninfected relatives. In time, isolation hostels, called lazarettos, emerged in Italy as part of the general quarantine regulations which developed there.[26] Public officials did not learn from others' experiences. In 1666, at Eyam in Derbyshire, England, the parish rector persuaded his congregation to remain in the village in the middle of a severe plague outbreak, with the result that four out of every ten inhabitants died.[27] Before 1894, neither public health control nor direct medical measures proved effective against plague.[28]

At the turn of the twentieth century, however, public expectations of a breakthrough in the control of plague were high. The new scientific advances were immediately applied to plague after its reappearance in Hong Kong, where Alexandre Yersin, a Franco-Swiss microbiologist and student of Pasteur, won a race against Shibasaburo Kitasato, the Japanese microbiologist who had studied with Robert Koch, to isolate the plague bacillus. Yersin also suggested that rats were a major factor in the transmission of the disease.[29] In Bombay in 1897, the Frenchman Paul-Louis Simond and a Ukrainian Jew in British employment, Waldemar Haffkine, confirmed that rats were a key vector. A year later, Simond put forward the theory that fleas were the vector of *Y. pestis*, although it took a decade or more before a scientific consensus emerged.[30]

If the research response to the resurgence of plague was swift, so too was the action of the scientific community at the formal international level. In 1897 an International Sanitary Conference was held at Venice to deal with the new threat to the world's well-being, and a second meeting took place in Paris in 1903.[31] The plague control measures which emerged proved disappointing; they harkened back to the past, rather than looking to the future.[32] In addition to quarantine, the other standard control measures continued to be fumigation and burning of potentially infectious goods and property. As in the past, these measures continued to be ineffective against such a tenacious adversary as *Y. pestis.*

In the early years of the new century, two new procedures, growing out of the biomedical revolution, seemed to be much more promising. Rat control by means of trapping and poisoning was the logical result of the discovery of the plague vector. Yet it seemed pedestrian when set alongside the second measure, mass inoculation with an anti-plague vaccine. As it happened, however, these control techniques produced mixed results. Rodent kills reached millions annually but had little impact on the fecundity of rodents.[33] Rat control through better construction did succeed in port cities, especially in Western cities which might otherwise have been vulnerable to plague importation.[34] Meanwhile, in India during 1897, Waldemar Haffkine produced a practical and inexpensive anti-plague vaccine from a broth colony killed by heat. Compared with tetanus or diphtheria, for example, which were quickly neutralized by effective vaccines by the turn of the century, the immunological aspects of bubonic plague proved to be much more daunting. Like other early vaccines, the Haffkine formulation had unpleasant side effects, and did not provide complete protection, though it was said to have reduced risk by up to 50 percent.[35] The alternative, a live strain of nonvirulent *Y. pestis*, was not developed until the 1930s, but this type was found to provoke even more severe reactions than other vaccines. The E.V. 76 strain in Madagascar, for example, resulted in the hospitalization of several recipients.[36] Thus, despite the heightened efforts against bubonic plague internationally, half-way through the twentieth century Western biomedicine had no effective treatment to combat the devastatingly high mortality rates of infected patients. This situation was to change dramatically and abruptly, beginning in 1945.

Although the third pandemic was everywhere in retreat by the end of the Second World War, probably as a result of natural burn-out as much as because of heightened international public health measures, two new elements dealt it a final blow. One was the development of antibiotics to treat infected patients. The broad-based antibiotic streptomycin has proven to be dramatically successful even against the most virulent *Y. pestis* infections since it was first administered in 1945, and indeed remains the recommended therapy today, almost half a century later.[37] The other breakthrough was the arrival of a sensational new insecticide, DDT, which destroyed the plague transmission cycle by attacking the flea vector.[38] By the 1950s, DDT had become the standard insecticide employed against sporadic outbreaks of bubonic plague and other insect-borne diseases the world over.[39] Excessive use of this miracle insecticide has, however, had two sobering consequences. First, some vector resistance has developed; second, DDT and related chlorinated pesticides have carried dangers to wildlife, and potentially to humans.[40]

FRENCH CONQUEST AND THE MEDICAL CRISIS IN SENEGAL

While they did not produce anything like the demographic disaster that the European conquest of the Americas unleashed, the conquest of Africa and the imposition of the new capitalist economic system did trigger a serious medical crisis throughout the continent between 1880 and 1920.[41] East and Central Africa appear to have been hardest hit by epidemics which can be directly or indirectly attributed to the structural changes which occurred during this traumatic period.[42] In Senegal, the conquest period brought profound changes. The host population was subjected to conquest and occupation armies, the introduction of the railway, new demands for labor, and hence for labor migration, and shifts in agriculture away from staples and toward cash crops, especially peanuts. Women felt these changes most, having to subsist on smaller, deteriorating plots of land as men were drained away into migration by often coercive colonial labor policies. From a health perspective, the Senegalese no longer controlled their natural environment.[43] The French now implicitly and sometimes explicitly dictated how the land should be apportioned and exploited. The French colonial government not only denied the validity of African healers and therapies, it delegitimized them, and made it more difficult for them to meet the medical needs of a population moving to towns and being struck down by new and by old but modified epidemic diseases.

While structural changes were fundamental, at the same time, natural forces also contributed to immiseration. The sahelian and savanna regions of Senegal passed through a climatic cycle extremely unfavorable to the practice of agriculture and even pastoralism. The first decades of colonial rule coincided with complaints by Africans of unusually low rainfall, together with visual evidence of aridity.[44] Military conquest, coupled with diminishing rainfall and locust plagues, led to widespread famine throughout the Sahel in 1900–1903.[45] Drought struck again from 1910 to 1915, with a terrible famine after poor harvests in 1913 and 1914, exacerbated by epizootics and epidemics. Administrators noted the high death rates and the massive migrations as people traveled in search of food and work.[46]

The medical impact of the European intrusion in Senegal cannot be isolated from the overall epidemiological history of the region, which experienced the arrival of new pathogens and the resurgence of old ones. Among the diseases familiar to the Senegalese, malaria was by far the biggest scourge, with smallpox and yellow fever also prominent on the list of killers, as were infantile diseases like measles and whooping cough. Endemic rather than epidemic, malaria took its highest toll among infants and young children. Those who survived their first attacks developed sufficient antigens to enjoy some protection later in life. Because few such adults died, malaria was often overlooked in European statistical assessments of the health of the Senegalese population, although it remained, along with yellow fever, the biggest killer of unseasoned foreigners in the country. For the host adult population, then, malaria was an endemic rather than an epidemic disease.

Smallpox represented an epidemiological puzzle for Senegal. The disease was certainly present there for centuries, but the strain cannot be determined. It is entirely possible that, as in Kenya and other parts of East Africa, West African smallpox was the more moderate *Variola minor*, with mild symptoms and a death rate of 1 percent or less, rather than the more virulent *Variola major*, a killer with mortality rates commonly approaching 30 percent.[47] The arrival of Europeans in greater numbers, and especially the heightened commercial activity resulting from steamship navigation and trade expansion, may have introduced a more virulent smallpox strain to the country. In 1835–36, a smallpox outbreak was reported for the middle Senegal valley.[48] The Saint-Louis region was struck by serious if localized smallpox outbreaks eight times between 1858 and 1898.[49] The most serious of these occurred in 1888–89, when thirty deaths among 120 reported cases were registered in Saint-Louis itself.[50]

The history of yellow fever in Senegal is another mystery. This viral disease was probably imported to Senegal and the rest of West Africa, perhaps as early as the sixteenth century, as a by-product of the increased contact between the Americas and Africa resulting from the slave trade. By the nineteenth century, it too had become endemic, but effects on Africans were much less severe than for malaria.[51] For the unseasoned French adults in Senegal, on the other hand, yellow fever was the most feared disease, and for good reason. The small French colony was racked by yellow fever epidemics on over twenty occasions from the mid eighteenth century to the beginning of the twentieth century.[52] Because it threatened France's very ability to occupy and govern the colony, and because the health of Europeans was the primary objective of public health policy as it emerged in the colony, yellow fever established important precedents for the control of infectious diseases well into the twentieth century.

Two virulent diseases new to Senegal and the rest of tropical Africa in the nineteenth century were bubonic plague and cholera.[53] In fact, the first confirmed cases of bubonic plague in Senegal did not occur until the 1914 epidemic broke out, even if French health officials were on their guard against plague after a mild outbreak took place in Grand Bassam, Ivory Coast, in 1899.

Cholera made two major epidemic appearances in Saint-Louis and the Senegal River Valley, first appearing in 1868–69, and again in 1893.[54] Each time the disease broke out in Saint-Louis, and then spread rapidly upriver as far as Dagana, Matam, and Podor, and south to Dakar, Gorée, and Rufisque. In the first cholera epidemic, death was not confined to the poor and downtrodden. Two of the ninety-two Europeans who lost their life were the governor, Pinet-Laprade, and a physician, Dr. Maurel.[55] Such was not the case during the 1893 cholera outbreak, which struck Africans much more severely than Europeans.[56] The wide discrepancy between African and European deaths in Saint-Louis drew a dramatic explanation from Roman Catholic missionaries. The Sisters of the Congregation of Saint-Joseph de Cluny had erected a statue of St. Roch, patron saint of epidemic victims, and wrote triumphally that "the Virgin Mary rewarded our confidence, and we escaped the disaster. The *marabouts*, taken by surprise, expressed their amazement for the fact that the Christians did not die, while their own devotees died at the rate of 50 to 60 a day."[57] No response from the Muslim community of Saint-Louis has been recorded, but the traditional Muslim view held that both the bringing of affliction and the protection of the faithful were manifestations of God's Will. Second, some might have noted that the better-off Europeans and Creoles of Saint-Louis, most of whom were Christian, escaped cholera in 1893, while the urban poor were victimized. Class and ethnicity, not religion, were the operative variables in the 1893 cholera outbreak.

Like people with premodern medical systems the world over, Africans had few effective weapons against these devastating epidemics. Instead, their practices fell within what some have called a precolonial African public health system geared more toward prevention or containment of infectious disease than toward cure.[58] One preventive measure against smallpox was variolation, first developed in China, from where it spread to the Middle East and then to parts of Africa. By the nineteenth century it was being practiced in Senegal, and at the end of the century it remained widespread despite French efforts to stop it and replace it with vaccination.[59]

Senegalese patients in "quest of therapy," to use John Janzen's apt phrase, did have a series of choices.[60] In virtually every household there existed a broad empirical understanding of herbal remedies. One French physician counted no less than forty-seven plants and medicines used to deal with various medical problems ranging from fevers to eye infections to venereal diseases when he visited the herbalists' stalls in the Saint-Louis market in 1876.[61] Consultations with specialist healers, on the other hand, while varying from group to group, usually meant a visit at one stage to a Muslim therapist. A minority of learned scholars were probably familiar with the Galenic system as filtered through Islamic medicine, although there is no evidence for this. Most Muslim healers would have been located within the prophetic tradition of healing through special prayers, and the distribution of amulets and talismans carefully inscribed with the names of God, Muslim saints, and the patient's parents, together with the name and age of the patient. Others would be skilled in the interpretation of nightly dreams and in predictive specialties such as astrology, geomancy, and palmistry.[62]

Although Senegalese living in the towns could choose French medical therapies, fragmentary evidence suggests that they usually avoided this option. In an effort to thwart African healers, the French promulgated a decree on 17 August 1897 which made biomedicine the official medical system. Yet, as late as 1913, Senegalese patients were going to the French hospitals in Saint-Louis, Dakar, and Rufisque only as a last resort, if at all.[63] The same was true for births. French authorities held African midwives responsible for the low numbers of women seeking delivery in the colonial hospitals.[64] French missionaries also complained about the popularity of their Muslim competitors as healers, even though missionary medicine was not extensively offered in Senegal, unlike British East Africa, for example.[65] Around the mid nineteenth century, the Abbé Boilat, at least, was able to concede that some Muslim *marabouts* were knowledgeable about healing, unlike the charlatan *marabouts* who sold "fetishes" for profit, and misled people.[66] As late as 1909, Christian missionaries in Saint-Louis complained that even their own parishioners were known to consult Muslim and pagan healers, and they bemoaned this superstitious faith in "sorcery" as the "remnants of savagery."[67] The colonial administration joined in the chorus of disapproval, describing *marabout* healers as "dangerous troublemakers" in 1913, and recommended tight surveillance to reduce their "disastrous and deadly" influence.[68] While some charlatans no doubt sprang up with the commoditization of healing after the creation of the French West African Federation in 1895, Kalala J. Ngalamulume argues persuasively that the spirited attacks by missionaries and the colonial administration were inspired by the strong following the Muslim healers enjoyed in the Saint-Louis region.[69] The same situation no doubt applied in the port towns of Rufisque and Dakar to the south.

Despite these religious tensions, it should not be assumed that African and French approaches to healing at the turn of the century were in philosophical contradiction to each other. Ironically, African and French healers had more in common with each other than either did with the new microscope-based laboratory medicine which was just then emerging in the avant-garde research centers of Paris or Berlin. Many French clinicians held, for example, that invisible "miasmata" caused disease, while African healers attributed numerous illnesses to invisible spirits.[70] Such external parallels were no doubt irrelevant to both the French and the African communities. For non-Muslim Senegalese, and probably for a good percentage of Muslims as well, what was more significant was the way in which good health was seen as part of a much larger social reality. Good health was a measure of the equilibrium which should extend beyond the individual within the extended family to the larger society, the natural environment, and the supernatural world. Ill-health represented disequilibrium in one element or a series of elements in this universe, so that diagnosis and therapy was a complex process involving more than just the individual patient.[71]

In fact, the conflict between the two systems was political rather than medical, as Meredeth Turshen has argued.[72] Colonial administrations were not prepared to see the authority of the African healer enhanced at the expense of their own appointed African officials. On the contrary, the object was to demonize healers, herbalists, and spirit mediums as evil embodiments of African superstition.

A gendered dimension was also prevalent in colonial policies. African women were disadvantaged not only because the colonial impact placed increased burdens on them, but also because women were often adept as healers. While their position of subordination in precolonial social formations should not be disregarded, African women therapists found their social status challenged and often eroded under colonialism.

Thus, the two communities, French and African, stood completely apart on medical issues. The Africans saw nothing in French medicine that moved them to abandon their own therapies. The French attitude, shared by Europeans all over Africa in the late nineteenth century, was to reject African empirical knowledge about herbal medicine and the natural environment, and social healing methods which were sensitive to local beliefs. African healers were to be cast aside and replaced by Western practitioners, rather than being understood, let alone appreciated.

EARLY FRENCH PUBLIC HEALTH MEASURES

As the twentieth century dawned, little resembling a modern public health policy existed in Senegal. Its beginnings coincided with the arrival of the new governor-general, Émile Roume, whose enthusiasm for public health works matched his commitment to a new port for Dakar and the extension of the railway.[73] A few of the health reforms had implications for rural French West Africa (FWA), but far greater emphasis was placed on urban centers, where the French lived together with, or preferably apart from, their "unsanitary" African neighbors. For example, the creation of the Assistance Médicale Indigène (AMI), was supposed to bring health care to the rural areas. While consultations increased dramatically, they were essentially confined to key towns like Thiès. On the other hand, the AMI was almost invisible in the Upper Senegal Valley, and Diourbel did not get its AMI post clinic until 1910.[74] For the entire FWA territory, only twenty military and civilian doctors were recruited in 1905. The difficulty in recruiting medical staff led the following year to the creation of a corps of African medical assistants, trained locally to work alongside French doctors as interpreters, and to run smaller medical posts when necessary.[75]

Roume's rhetorical commitment to medical reform was part of what he saw as France's "civilizing mission." Alice Conklin is convinced that Roume was sincere, and points out that he allocated significant sums to health in the 1903 and 1906 colonial loans he negotiated on behalf of FWA.[76] On the other hand, rhetorical flourishes regarding Africa's "moral and material regeneration" were also code words used by outright scoundrels like the Belgian King Leopold II and his cronies to justify their massive exploitation of the Congolese population in Central Africa.[77] Conklin concedes, in fact, that Roume was by no means free of bias against West Africans. In rejecting the possibility of establishing a medical school in Dakar similar to those in Madagascar or Indochina, Roume justified the decision not on financial grounds but because of the "insufficient development of our African population."[78]

Nor was it the case that French officials were prepared to live side-by-side with their African "children." Indeed, medical and lay observers were virtually unanimous regarding the need to separate African from European residences. In his manual, *Colonial Hygiene*, Dr. Alexandre Kermorgant had been emphatic: "The native villages constitute a permanent danger for Europeans because of the numerous transmissible illnesses which their inhabitants frequently suffer from, so that we can only counsel building European dwellings at a certain distance from native groupings."[79] Georges Ribot and Robert Lafon were equally explicit, stating that "segregation should include the absolute separation of Dakar into two quarters, a European city and a native city."[80] Still others drew unflattering attention to Dakar's "smell of rotten fish and odours not yet ever encountered," or to the beaches soiled by garbage in Saint-Louis.[81] Rufisque lacked an abattoir and animals were butchered on the open sands, a paradise for insects and vermin but not for humans.[82] Even Gorée, once regarded as a relatively healthy place for convalescent Europeans, had become dilapidated, and garbage had been allowed to accumulate at the end of the streets leading to the sea.[83] Why Africans were singled out as the sole polluters was never made clear in the French sanitary rhetoric. The easiest solution was to move the indigenous population out.

Precedents for the relocation of Africans away from European sections of town had occurred steadily from the time of Dakar's foundation in 1857. The very next year, the Lebu villages closest to the water's edge, notably Ngaraf, Thiérigne, and Hock, were moved inland. The yellow fever outbreak of 1900–1901 drove the French authorities to move large portions of Kaye and Hock once again, and in 1905 and 1908, on the grounds of health and space, officials forced the Lebu communities at Bakonda (near Santiaba) and Thiérigne (now located near Yakhadieuf) to relocate further away from the center of Dakar.[84] Alain Sinou, a historian of urban planning, maintains that by 1904, colonial officials in Dakar were planning buffer zones of "non-edificandi" to protect the European community on both hygienic and social grounds.[85] Indeed, Governor-General Ponty lent his voice to what had become a chorus of support for residential segregation when he observed in 1909: "We must continue to repeat the same advice until it finally penetrates the consciousness of all of the necessity for Europeans to live apart from natives, and to protect their sleep with good quality mosquito netting."[86]

The principle of residential segregation went from planning to practice when French legislation passed on 21 May 1905 provided a new building code for each city and town in Senegal. The code prohibited construction in straw and wood in European zones, but not in "native" zones, in the urban areas of Dakar, Saint-Louis, and Rufisque. In the trading centers of Thiès, Tivaouane, and Louga, the new building code applied to the town centers where the European homes were built.[87]

The toponymy of Thiès and its segregated districts speaks volumes about African bitterness over their compulsory relocation. The original village of Thiès-None, located right beside the French trade center, was removed and transferred south of the rail line to provide room for merchants to expand their construction around the *escale* (emporium) itself. Africans in Thiès gave their transplanted quarter the Wolof name of Randoulène, a label which would forever reflect their resentment: it means "go away and stay away!"[88] Randoulène and other African quarters, in these early years, were unsanitary and overcrowded. Garbage accumulated everywhere, and hastily erected straw and wooden constructions had to suffice for a generation or more before more solid adobe structures were built.[89]

Demographic indicators of early urban life in Senegal are fragmentary and difficult to use, since the French took no formal censuses and instead produced a series of estimates. Several writers have attempted to use these data, some even going so far as to calculate birth and death rates, but the exercise is flawed.[90] What can be extrapolated is that rapid urban population growth, coupled with acute housing shortages, was producing overcrowding and unsanitary conditions of life in general. Contrary to colonialist prejudices, the new African arrivals did not choose to live in such conditions on cultural grounds. Their unsanitary situation was imposed on them by the colonial economy.

Dakar, a new port, was the fastest rising town, or commune, as French law put it. Its selection in 1902 as the site of the capital of the entire territory of French West Africa was the final recognition of its growing economic and military importance. The large federal bureaucracy headed by the governor-general of FWA and the growing number of French commercial firms associated with the peanut trade made Dakar the town with the highest proportion of Europeans, roughly 10 percent of the total population of 20,000 by 1905. By that time, the four communes included a population of roughly 68,000, about 6 percent of the population of the entire colony.[91]

A great many of the new immigrants to the towns, probably a majority, were former slaves.[92] These new arrivals were regarded with trepidation both by the autochthonous Lebu population and by the French. The Lebu called the urban migrants *dokhendem* (from *dokh*, to walk, and *endem*, to go away), and feared they would be displaced by the newcomers.[93] The migrants' numbers cannot be determined, but it is worth noting that, for 1910, while official statistics estimated that Dakar had a population of 17,000, when the "transients" were counted the estimated figure jumped to 30,000.[94] For the French writer C. Jojot, these new arrivals were seen as a transient "floating population," "an invasion of stranger elements of doubtful value," who lived a wretched existence. "Their misery is only too frequent. Many blacks don't eat enough to curb their hunger, biscuits soaked in water, a little rice and sugar. Most are poorly dressed and if they pay a high price in the winter season with respiratory infections, this is because they are cold. Many live in insalubrious houses where the rains penetrate."[95]

Providing housing for the urban influx from the countryside and from France itself proved to be a difficult task after 1901. Between 1903 and 1908, some 440 new buildings were erected by the private sector, both European and African. While Europeans were responsible for 150 new houses and 800 rooms, African entrepreneurs almost doubled this capacity, putting up 285 houses with 1400 rooms.[96] Rents were high, given the laws of supply and demand, with an unfurnished dwelling of three to five rooms going for anywhere from 150 to even 300 francs monthly. European workers and minor bureaucrats who could not afford these rates were obliged to live in "native" housing.[97] The General Council complained in 1908 that rents had become a heavy burden for Dakar residents.[98] Contributing to the housing shortage was a rigorous application of health legislation in 1905 when a new outbreak of yellow fever was feared. The medical head of the Municipal Hygiene Service in Dakar ordered the destruction of some 1,060 dwellings, of which 43 were of brick construction and the rest were of straw or wood.[99]

The year 1905 also saw new developments in the continuing saga of Lebu land ownership within the city of Dakar. Despite periodic French assertions that they had taken ownership of the Cape Verde peninsula by right of conquest from the Wolof *damel* or ruler of Kajoor, the change of sovereignty did not alter the fact that Lebu families held possession of land on which their private properties stood.[100] In 1891, a French commission declared that since most inhabitants of Dakar had neither deeds nor other proof of ownership, most land could rightly be claimed by the French state.[101] A convention of 23 June 1905 took the further step of transferring a considerable block of land known as the Tound to French control in return for the creation of a village on the land and the provision of an annual amount of 1,800 francs to be paid into a collective fund.[102]

This 1905 agreement between the French and a portion of the Lebu community created division. Those who had benefited from the French presence accepted the commission's views and the 1905 settlement. More traditional elements saw the agreement as a betrayal, and sought to have it annulled. From its first appearance in 1913 onward, the opposition journal, *La Démocratie*, led the fight for the restoration of Lebu rights to the Tound. This was also a principal theme of Blaise Diagne's election campaign in 1914.[103] Traditionally minded Lebu would link the destruction of their homes by health officials, the declaration of the plague emergency in 1914, and the contesting of Blaise Diagne's electoral victory as elements in a conspiracy to cheat them out of their property.[104]

The restrictive building codes were part of the new health legislation after 1904 which stressed urban sanitary reform. Municipal clean-up efforts in the four Senegalese communes were organized on the basis of two campaigns: from 1904 to 1908; and from 1909 to 1920. In the first period, efforts were concentrated on the drainage of marshes, the building of a network of sewers, the widening of existing streets, and the building of new ones. In Dakar, an effort to expand the fresh water supply was also included, and a modern abattoir and a new Muslim cemetery were opened.[105] The second campaign involved hospital and clinic maintenance and expansion, as well as the establishment in Dakar of the new Bacteriological Laboratory. But the coming of plague and war in 1914 ate up the funding and few improvements were actually made.[106] As a result, Dakar in 1914 still lacked a regularized garbage removal service using metal containers, and a periodic flushing system for its sewers. The first public toilets, begun in 1909, had reached the minuscule number of fourteen for a city of over 30,000, and fecal matter was collected in unsanitary "honey-pot" wagons and dumped directly into the sea. For the most part, Dakar and the other three communes relied on *marseillaises*, vases containing human waste which were dumped directly into the sea. The water supply at Hann was also insufficient for the large town Dakar had become.[107]

Saint-Louis had not been transformed into a colonial "garden city." In 1911, Maliseye Niang, a representative of the mayor's office, and a contractor named Raumégana were asked to report on residents' compliance with the new sanitary measures. They found that the streets leading to the river in the northern part of Saint-Louis had become dead ends, clogged by the accumulation of garbage to a height of one meter.[108]

The only change was the enforcement of what appeared to the African population to be new and draconian health ordinances. The most serious of these new laws appeared in 1912, inspired no doubt by successful efforts in the Americas to rid cities of stagnant water sites in which the yellow fever vector, *Aedes aegypti*, could breed. Known in Senegalese oral tradition as the "law of the three interdictions," the 1912 legislation prohibited the collection of rainfall on house roofs, in bottles on walls, or in ground-level containers.[109]

Particularly galling was the enforcement of health regulations in a manner prejudicial to Africans. That same year, in Thiès, when a European was fatally struck down with yellow fever, health agents burnt and disinfected all the African homes surrounding his lodgings, but avoided burning or tearing down property of the Europeans.[110] In Dakar, the Health Service was actively imposing municipal fines for offenses ranging from failure to cover wells and allowing stagnant water on property to failure to remove waste and rotting matter. Between 1907 and 1920, an annual average of roughly 770 fines were handed down; in 1911, the number soared to a record 1,666 fines.[111]

African responses to these new health measures were generally unenthusiastic to say the least. Drinking water was always in short supply, especially in a desert-side town like Saint-Louis, so the prohibition on collecting rainwater represented not only a serious imposition but also a callous insensitivity to popular needs.[112] The attempt to impose smallpox vaccinations, and to ban local practices of variolation, also met with resistance. In Dakar in 1907, when only 437 vaccinations were carried out, the mayor complained that the law did not permit him to force Muslim citizens to vaccinate their children.[113] That same year, the Health Service reported that many people who had been forced in one way or another to take the smallpox vaccine were attempting to wash out the vaccine with soap or with acidic vegetal liquids.[114]

What must have particularly rankled was the use of health procedures as a form of social control by linking something Africans desired, like educational advancement, to something they did not, like smallpox vaccination.[115] In 1904, the governor of Senegal issued a decree reiterating that the smallpox vaccination was compulsory for all children attending school, and obliging school principals to report on the incidence and types of infectious diseases encountered among their pupils.[116] The majority of Africans did not have access to schools, but the compulsory vaccination program may have dissuaded some from sending their children to school. What was clear was that as late as 1914, French medical authorities were complaining that the majority of Africans continued to resist vaccination.[117]

One of the most poignant pieces of evidence surviving from this period is a letter addressed to the governor-general of FWA by a group of Dakar women on 8 January 1909. The self-effacing tone aside, what becomes clear is that French medical personnel were totally insensitive to the African public on the receiving end of French medical and social engineering:

> We have heard talk about your noble heart. That is why we are asking for your protection as our dear father. We have nothing left to eat, but despite our great misery, they are forcing us to repair our houses; we cannot do this. They also want us to build foundations of masonry on which to place our lean-tos; this we cannot do.
>
> The doctor from the health service comes to visit our homes three times a day. He empties our water or places petroleum inside the containers, disturbs our utensils and commits many other excesses of power but we beg you, Monsieur le Gouvereur-Général, please ask this doctor to use a little more tact in the carrying out of his delicate duties.[118]

THE POLITICAL SETTING IN 1914

What made Senegal unique among French colonies in Africa was its historical claim to political representation. With the birth of the Third

Republic in France and the introduction of political democracy (for males only) after 1871, Senegal, along with the other "old" colonies such as Martinique, Guadeloupe, and Réunion, was given the right to elect a deputy to the French National Assembly. Electors living in the four communes of Saint-Louis, Dakar, Rufisque, and Gorée could vote in elections for mayor, for representatives to the municipal councils and the General Council, and, most importantly, for Deputy to the French National Assembly in Paris.[119] The male African electors were dubbed *originaires*, a term which alluded to their descent from those living in the two original port towns of the old colony. Early Senegalese elections were patronage contests among competing political clans composed of French and Creole business interests, with the colonial administration as a frequent participant.[120]

Electoral politics became an important battleground in Senegal after the turn of the century, and especially after William Ponty replaced Roume as governor-general of FWA in 1908. Hand-picked by Roume on the basis of his success as governor of Soudan, the young, dynamic Ponty would serve in the top post in FWA from 1908 until his death in office in 1915. Highly intelligent if strongly paternalist, Ponty proved more flexible and politically astute than most French proconsuls in Africa before or after his time.[121]

One of Ponty's prime objectives was to undermine what he perceived as a growing threat from the *originaires*. In 1907, the governor of Senegal had managed to reduce the number of African voters on the municipal electoral rolls by one half. From then until 1914 a series of anti-*originaire* measures were introduced. These included the loss of voting rights; the application of a head tax for all Africans without exception living in the communes; the subjection of *originaires* to "native" courts when living or traveling outside the four communes; and their systematic exclusion from French schools. Also, in a decision which would soon become a major subject of confrontation, in 1911 all *originaires* were summarily dismissed from the French metropolitan army and obliged to serve with the Tirailleurs Sénégalais, units formerly restricted to the African non-*originaire* population.[122] Finally, and most seriously, Ponty in 1913 launched a legal challenge in French courts to settle the vexed question of *originaire* rights once and for all. Ponty wished to confine citizenship to the tiny number of Africans who had moved away from Islam and were willing to accept French civil statutes exclusively. This had been the manner in which the overwhelmingly Muslim population of Algeria had been kept from acquiring French citizenship. These issues had not been resolved before the First World War, and the prospects for the *originaires* did not look bright, at least not until Blaise Diagne made his dramatic entry onto the political scene in 1914.

The context for Diagne's rise was provided by the stepped-up anti-*originaire* campaign. In 1912, a group of newly militant Africans, calling themselves the "Young Senegalese" in conscious imitation of Kamal Ataturk's "Young Turks," rose to prominence in Saint-Louis as the colony's first African political group.[123] Deeply troubled by the colonial administration's efforts to remove their voting rights and citizenship, these clerks, teachers, interpreters, and letter-writers were reformers rather than nationalists. They resented the lower pay they received for doing the same work as Frenchmen and Creoles, and railed against the racial discrimination which blocked their advancement in the colonial bureaucracy and the private sector. In addition to Lamine Guèye, the first African lawyer in French West Africa, who would have a significant political career spanning the next forty years, the group included Amadou Duguay-Clédor, Amadou Assane Ndoye, and Papa Mar Diop. As their president, they chose the elderly Thiécouta Diop, a Wolof notable whose halting French obliged him to use an interpreter in his dealings with the administration.

The most influential and inspirational of the new breed of Senegalese politicians was Galandou Diouf. In 1909, he had surprised every one by getting elected to the General Council.[124] His willingness to bring African grievances forward at the General Council inspired the Young Senegalese. In late 1913, they became active contributors to a new opposition newspaper which had just emerged, *La Démocratie*, whose editor was a French adventurer named Daramy Jean D'Oxoby, and whose principal financial backer was a French tavern keeper in Dakar, Jules Sergent.[125] The pages of *La Démocratie* were devoted to issues dear to small businessmen who resented the powerful Bordeaux trading houses. Increasingly, however, the newspaper began to champion the cause of underdogs in general, including the Lebu of the Cape Verde peninsula, whose property rights were being steadily encroached upon. The paper reported, for example, that the French Colonial Army had evicted many Lebu from their fields near Ouakam so that the army could perform maneuvers, and had not paid any compensation.[126]

Even more important than their willingness to risk censure and possible retribution for openly opposing the French administration, the Young Senegalese in 1913 began to consider the prospect of breaking the Creoles' hold on the deputyship. The challenger to Creole hegemony was a young Gorée-born African named Blaise Diagne.

Blaise Diagne was born in 1872 to humble parents, Niokhar Diagne, a Sereer cook, and Gnagna Preira, a housemaid whose paternal ancestors may have been of mixed Portuguese descent, but whose maternal line was Lebu.[127] Young Blaise did very well at the local Catholic school on Gorée, and at the short-lived secondary school in Saint-Louis. He then joined the French colonial customs service, and for the next twenty years received postings to a wide range of locales which included Dahomey, French Congo, Gabon, Réunion, Madagascar, and finally French Guyana. Wherever he went, he caused trouble for his superiors and came close to being fired. Each time, it was his acute sensitivity to issues of race and discrimination which lay at the core of his conflicts.[128] What probably saved Diagne from dismissal from colonial service was his total devotion to the French assimilationist principle, together with an awareness of his legal rights, and his wise political instincts in cultivating people who had influence.[129]

Throughout his long service, Diagne had never returned to Senegal, but he had kept in touch with several old schoolmates who kept him abreast of political happenings. In April 1913, *L'AOF* ran a story listing Diagne as an outside candidate among several others preparing to challenge the Creole Deputy François Carpot for the Senegalese seat in the 1914 elections. After testing the waters carefully, on 30 January 1914, Diagne sailed from Marseille for Dakar and his rendezvous with destiny.

Diagne had only three months to campaign, but he owed his success both to his fiery oratory and to the serious mistake his opponents made in underestimating him.[130] Carpot contemptuously dismissed Diagne and alluded to his humble origins by referring to him as the "Sereer candidate."[131] But although Carpot had the informal backing of both the governor of Senegal, Henri Cor, and Governor-General Ponty, his main Creole rival, Justin Devès, not only opposed Carpot but persuaded the Devès family's Alsatian-born lawyer in Paris, Henri Heimburger, to enter the race. The Creole vote was to be split still further when Georges Crespin, a young Saint-Louis lawyer, son of a former mayor of Saint-Louis, threw his hat into the ring. A third Creole candidate was Louis Pellegrin, a merchant and member of an old Creole trading family.

Blaise Diagne's candidacy had mixed support. Aside from a tiny handful of Young Senegalese, he was without backing in Creole-dominated Saint-Louis. Galandou Diouf's support gave him some following in Rufisque, but Gorée and Dakar proved to be his strongholds. The important Lebu leader, Imam Assane Ndoye, and his uncle, Shaykh Youssou Bamar Guèye, decided to abandon the Marsat-Masson machine and back Diagne as a fellow African.[132] They brought with them the entire Dakar Lebu assembly, with the notable exception of the highest-ranking Lebu Muslim in Dakar, Serigne Alpha Dial, who remained loyal to Marsat.

Diagne could also rely on the support of fellow Africans in the colonial bureaucracy such as Papa Konaré Jouga, a customs officer like himself.[133] Also in his camp was the outspoken French journalist Jean D'Oxoby, who had named Diagne "political director" of *La Démocratie*.[134] Helping fund Diagne's campaign were monies originating with the Mourid brotherhood of Ahmadu Bamba Mbacké.[135] Although the brotherhood was largely rural at this time, and few of its members were qualified to vote, the Mourid alliance with Diagne was to prove extremely useful to him in obtaining the respect of the great majority of Senegalese subjects, and in helping him to hold on to his deputyship until his death in 1934.

It was not difficult for Diagne to find campaign issues. For the Lebu, he promised to see their land claims in Dakar made good. He told the Sereer that he would see to it that their informal occupation of vacant land nominally belonging to the old Wolof state of Kajoor in the Lake Tamma and Thiès regions would be officially recognized.[136] For the aspiring African elite, nervous about the erosion, threatened and real, of their rights, Diagne promised to repeal discriminatory legislation and to get the French National Assembly to recognize the *originaires* as citizens once and for all. He scored telling points against Carpot during the campaign by suggesting that the incumbent had supported the infamous decree of 12 August 1912, which had threatened to remove African voting rights for the deputyship. In fact, the initiative had come from the Ministry of Colonies in Paris, but Carpot never succeeded in disassociating himself from the notion that he opposed the African franchise.[137] Aware that he would not have their support, Diagne loudly attacked the Bordeaux trading houses for having exploited Senegal. Few could have realized in 1914 that in the interwar period Diagne would become their spokesman.[138]

The election campaign leading up to the first ballot on Sunday, 26 April, generated the most interest ever in Senegalese electoral politics. When the votes were tallied, the results shocked complacent French observers. Governor Cor had written in an undated memo that Diagne "has no chance of success."[139] Yet Diagne led all the candidates with 1,910 votes, just under 40 percent of the total. Carpot, Heimburger, and Marsat, with 671, 668, and 516 votes respectively, all under 14 percent, had been soundly beaten.[140] Only the concentrated support of all anti-African voters behind a united candidate in the second round of voting would avert what many believed to be a disaster. When the obstinate Carpot refused to withdraw his candidacy in favour of the Devès man Heimburger, he sealed the fate of the opposition to Diagne.[141]

The short run-off campaign, culminating on Sunday, 10 May 1914, was vicious. French merchants withheld credit from African customers who would not agree to support Heimburger. In Dakar, Mayor Masson threatened to cut off the water and electricity of Africans unless they stopped campaigning for Diagne. Rumors flew that all appointed African chiefs and civil servants would be sacked if Diagne won.[142] To the African electors, Diagne was depicted as a man who preferred the vest to the *boubou*, wine to lemonade, and cognac to milk in his coffee.[143]

Diagne responded with threats of his own. If the water were cut off and the Bordeaux houses stopped giving credit to Africans, then he would persuade African food merchants not to open their stalls in the market, and he would even call for a general strike unless the French desisted.[144] In mellower moments, he declared himself the candidate of all parties and groups. Noting that his French wife was white, and therefore his children were Creole, he proclaimed himself in favor of reconciliation among all three communities in Senegal.[145]

When the votes of the run-off election were counted, Diagne defeated Heimburger by only 175 votes, a margin of less than 3 percent of the total votes cast. Carpot finished a distant third; except for his obstinacy, most of his support (472 votes) would have probably gone to Heimburger and prevented Diagne's victory.[146] Few realized at the time that the election of 10 May 1914 marked the end of Creole political dominance in Senegal and the ascendency of African electoral control. Fewer still, whether rich or poor, powerful or weak, realized that at precisely that time, a second major surprise was about to occur: the outbreak of bubonic plague.

NOTES

1. Georges Ribot and Robert Lafon, *Dakar. Ses origines, son avenir* (Bordeaux: G. Delmas, 1908), 43–44.

2. Giovanni Boccaccio, *The Decameron*, translated by G. H. McWilliam (Harmondsworth, England: Penguin, 1972); Daniel Defoe, *A Journal of the Plague Year* (Harmondsworth, England: Penguin, 1966; original edition, 1722); Albert Camus, *The Plague*, translated by Hamish Hamilton, 1948 (Harmondsworth, England: Penguin, 1960); André Brink, *The Wall of the Plague* (London: Fontana, 1985). See also Raymond Crawfurd, *Plague and Pestilence in Literature and Art* (London: Oxford University Press, 1914); and A. M. Campbell, *The Black Death and Men of Learning* (New York: AMS Press, 1931).

3. The second is by far the best documented of the three plague pandemics. The best recent overview is Robert S. Gottfried, *The Black Death: Natural and Human Disaster in Medieval Europe* (New York: The Free Press, 1983), which stresses the

newer environmental approach more than does Philip Ziegler, *The Black Death* (Harmondsworth, England: Penguin, 1970). For estimates of its overall mortality, see Katharine Park, "Black Death," in *The Cambridge World History of Human Disease*, edited by Kenneth Kiple (New York: Cambridge University Press, 1992), 613.

4. Pauline Allen, "The 'Justinianic' Plague," *Byzantion* 49 (1979): 5–20; Jerry H. Bentley, "Hemispheric Integration, 500–1500 C.E.," *Journal of World History* 9 (1998): 237–54.

5. With the exception of India, relatively few specific historical studies of the third pandemic exist. One of the rare available monographs is Peter Curson and Kevin McCracken, *Plague in Sydney: Anatomy of an Epidemic* (Kensington, N.S.W.: New South Wales University Press, 1989). For the pandemic's beginnings in China, see Carol Benedict, *Bubonic Plague in Nineteenth-Century China* (Stanford, Calif.: Stanford University Press, 1996). A chapter of Elizabeth Sinn's, *Power and Charity: The Early History of the Tung Wah Hospital* (Hong Kong: Oxford University Press, 1989), is devoted to the 1894 Hong Kong outbreak. A chapter on San Francisco's 1900 plague outbreak is included in Charles J. McClain, *In Search of Equality: The Chinese Struggle against Discrimination in Nineteenth Century America* (Berkeley: University of California Press, 1994). The plague in Cape Town is ably treated in Elizabeth van Heyningen, "Cape Town and the Plague of 1901," in *Studies in the History of Cape Town*, vol.4, edited by Christopher Saunders, Howard Philips, and Elizabeth van Heyningen (Cape Town: University of Cape Town, 1981), 66–107. Surprisingly little comparative work has yet been done, although the research of Mary Sutphen offers a promising beginning. See her "Rumoured Power: Hong Kong, 1894 and Cape Town, 1901," in *Western Medicine as Contested Knowledge*, edited by Andrew Cunningham and Bridie Andrews (Manchester: Manchester University Press, 1997), 241–61; and by the same author, "Not What, but Where: Bubonic Plague and the Reception of Germ Theories in Hong Kong and Calcutta," *Journal of the History of Medicine and Allied Sciences* 52 (1997): 81–113. As a follow-up to the current study, I am planning a monograph comparing the impact of the third pandemic between 1894 and 1900 on selected international ports.

6. Unless otherwise stated, all data are from Ernst Rodenwaldt and Helmut J. Jusatz, eds., *Welt-Seuchen Atlas (World Atlas of Epidemic Disease)* (Hamburg: Falk-Verlag, 1961, vol. 2, 47–48; and vol. 3, 86–87). For India alone, more recent estimates run over 12 million, which is about 25 percent higher than earlier figures. See David Arnold, *Colonizing the Body: State Medicine and Epidemic Disease in Nineteenth Century India* (Berkeley: University of California Press, 1993), 201–03.

7. Ann G. Carmichael, "Bubonic Plague," in *The Cambridge World History of Human Disease*, edited by Kenneth Kiple (New York: Cambridge University Press, 1992), 631.

8. For accounts of this outbreak, see F.P.J. Sorel, "L'épidémie de fièvre jaune à Dakar," *Compte-Rendu de l'Académie des Sciences* 12 (1932): 545–55; F.P.J. Sorel, "La fièvre jaune chez les indigènes à Dakar en 1927," *Bulletin de la Société de Pathologie Exotique* 21 (1928): 509–11; and George H. Ramsey, "Yellow Fever in Senegal, with Special Reference to 1926 and 1927 Epidemics," *American Journal of Hygiene* 13, no. 1 (1931): 129–63.

9. Comparisons are difficult, both because general population censuses were not scientific and because people hid their sick and dying from authorities everywhere.

Two German epidemiologists have suggested the following case rates per 10,000 during the third plague pandemic: India, 427; Senegal, 269; Hong Kong, 244; Mauritius, 227; Burma, 122; Madagascar, 116; Madeira, 108; Uganda, 88; Ecuador, 50; and Indonesia, 42. Rodenwaldt and Jusatz, *World Atlas of Epidemic Disease*, vol. 2, 47–48; and vol. 3, 86–87.

10. The scientific literature on bubonic plague is voluminous and is drawn from such disparate fields as the history of medicine, human and veterinary medicine, biology, and entomology. This section is based on the following: James R. Busvine, *Disease Transmission by Insects: Its Discovery and 90 Years of Effort to Prevent It* (Berlin: Springer-Verlag, 1993); Thomas C. Butler, *Plague and other Yersinia Infections* (New York: Plenum Medical Book Co., 1983); Carmichael, "Bubonic Plague"; Fabian L. Hirst, *The Conquest of Plague: A Study of the Evolution of Epidemiology* (Oxford: Clarendon Press, 1953); R. Pollitzer, *Plague* (Geneva: WHO, 1954); and Calvin W. Schwabe, *Veterinary Medicine and Human Health*, third edition (Baltimore: Williams and Wilkins, 1984).

11. Schwabe, *Veterinary Medicine*, 94.

12. Butler, *Plague*, 48.

13. Carmichael, "Bubonic Plague," 628.

14. The levels of tolerance toward *Yersinia pestis* among rodents varies enormously, influenced by variables such as group behavior, changing seasons, and food supply. See J. B. Calhoun, *The Ecology and Sociology of the Norway Rat* (Baltimore: U.S. Public Health Service, 1963).

15. The dominant species could vary. In Angola, *R. rattus* prevailed, while in São Tomé *R. norvegicus* dominated. Ricardo Jorge, *Les faunes régionales des rongeurs et des puces dans leurs rapports avec la peste. Résultats de l'enquête du comité permanent de l'Office International d'Hygiène Publique, 1924–27* (Paris: Masson, 1928), 53–54.

16. Jean-Marc Duplantier and Laurent Granjon, *Les rongeurs du Sénégal* (Dakar: ORSTOM, 1993).

17. Although it is only one of several hypotheses, an ecological argument associated with the introduction of a new species of flea vector is intriguing. See H. King and C. Pandit, "Summary of Rat-Flea Survey of Madras Presidency," *Indian Journal of Medical Research* 19 (1931): 357–92.

18. No scientific research on fleas took place in Senegal before the 1920s, and the timing of *Xenopsylla cheopis*'s arrival remains a mystery. This question is taken up again in chapter 7. For differing hypotheses, see Marcel Advier, "Étude expérimentale du rôle du *Synosternus pallidus* dans la transmission de la peste," *Bulletin de la Société de Pathologie Exotique* 30 (1937): 643; Leo Kartman, "A Note on the Problem of Plague in Dakar, Sénégal, French West Africa," *Journal of Parasitology* 32 (1946): 30–35; and Alexandre Wassilieff, "Observations sur les puces de la région de Cayor," *Bulletin de la Société de Pathologie Exotique* 23 (1930): 474–78.

19. For a full description of how fleas transmit *Y. pestis*, see Busvine, *Disease Transmission*, 65; and Pollitzer, *Plague*, 322–24, 330, 334.

20. Butler, *Plague*, 112; and Carmichael, "Bubonic Plague," 628.

21. Carmichael, "Bubonic Plague," 630.

22. Andrew Cunningham, "Transforming Plague: The Laboratory and the Identity of Infectious Disease," in *The Laboratory Revolution in Medicine*, edited by Andrew

Cunningham and Perry Williams (Cambridge: Cambridge University Press, 1992), 209–44.

23. Malnutrition depresses immune reactions, while other infections, such as malaria and tuberculosis, may also suppress immune responses to plague, according to Butler, *Plague*, 53–54.

24. Some geneticists argue for immunity basing their arguments not on empirical research among plague survivors but on experimental laboratory work. See G.V.J. Nossal, *Antibodies and Immunities*, second edition (New York: Basic Books, 1978); Carmichael, "Bubonic Plague," 629; and Ira Klein, "Plague, Policy and Popular Unrest in British India," *Modern Asian Studies* 22 (1988): 755.

25. For the impact of the second pandemic on women, see J. Bean, "Plague, Population and Economic Decline in England in the Later Middle Ages," *Economic History Review*, 2nd series, 15 (1962–63): 423–37. The consensus among modern researchers is that exposure rather than gender is the key variable. Butler, *Plague*, 43.

26. The term "lazaretto" derives from the island of San Lazaretto, where the first quarantine buildings were located at the entrance to Venice. For more on Italian defense against plague, see Carlo Cipolla, *Fighting the Plague in Seventeenth-Century Italy* (Madison: University of Wisconsin Press, 1981); and Ann G. Carmichael, *Plague and the Poor in Renaissance Florence* (New York: Cambridge University Press, 1986).

27. Paul Slack, *The Impact of Plague in Tudor and Stuart England* (Oxford: Clarendon Press, 1985), 268.

28. In the early nineteenth century, once the success of Jenner's vaccination procedure for smallpox had become established, experiments with plague vaccines were tried without success, notably in Egypt during the 1834–35 plague outbreak there, with condemned prisoners inoculated with blood from victims, or made to sleep in victims' bedding. Busvine, *Disease Transmission*, 63. We are left to ponder the wry wisdom of the sixteenth-century Sicilian physician, Giovanni Ingrassia, who remarked that the only remedies against plague were "pills made of three ingredients called *cito, longe, and tarde* (swiftly, far, and tardy), namely, run swiftly, go far and return tardily." Quoted in Carlo Cipolla, *Cristofaro and the Plague: A Study in the History of Public Health in the Age of Galileo* (Berkeley: University of California Press, 1973).

Jean-Noël Biraben suggests that quarantine regulations played a significant part in ending epidemic plague both in Europe and in North Africa; somewhat more cautiously, Carlo Cipolla makes the same point. But Ann Carmichael has the weight of scientific evidence on her side when she disputes such claims. See Jean-Noël Biraben, *Les hommes et la peste en France et dans les pays européens et méditerranéens*, vol. 1, *La peste dans l'histoire* (Paris: Mouton, 1975); Carlo Cipolla, *Public Health and the Medical Profession in the Renaissance* (Cambridge: Cambridge University Press, 1976); and Carmichael, "Bubonic Plague," 630.

29. For differing analyses of the Yersin-Kitasato controversies, see Henri Mollaret and Jacqueline Brossolet, *Alexandre Yersin, le vainqueur de la peste* (Paris: Fayard, 1985); Norman Howard-Jones, "Kitasato, Yersin and the Plague Bacillus," *Clio Medica* 10 (1975): 23–27; Noël Bernard, *Yersin: Pionnier-Savant-Explorateur (1863–1943)* (Paris: Albin Michel, 1961); David J. Bibel and T. H. Chen, "Diagnosis of Plague: An Analysis of the Yersin-Kitasato Controversy," *Bacteriological Review*

40 (1976): 633–51; and Alexandre Yersin, "La Peste bubonique à Hong Kong," *Annales de l'Institut Pasteur* 8 (1894): 662–67.

30. That same year, Yersin, along with Pasteur's successor, Émile Roux, went public with the conclusion that bubonic plague was a disease of rats which could also infect humans, and that the best public health response was to destroy rats. Within a very short time, Robert Koch expressed the same opinion following a short visit to India, and Patrick Manson added his influential views soon after. Hirst, *The Conquest of Plague*, 161.

31. Cholera had been the target of earlier conferences, beginning with Paris in 1851, which was attended by delegates from eleven European nations and the Ottoman Empire. Roy Porter, *The Greatest Benefit to Mankind: A Medical History of Humanity from Antiquity to the Present* (London: Harper Collins, 1997), 485–86. See also Norman Howard-Jones, *The Scientific Background of the International Sanitary Conferences, 1851–1938* (Geneva: WHO, 1975).

32. Mary Sutphen has shown that, despite the bacteriological revolution, health officials in the colonies commonly continued using disease control routines based on an older environmentalist framework. Sutphen, "Rumoured Power," 241–61; and Sutphen, "Not What, but Where," 81–113.

33. Hirst, *The Conquest of Plague*; Busvine, *Disease Transmission*, 195–96.

34. Busvine, *Disease Transmission*, 198.

35. Haffkine's vaccine, injected subcutaneously, produced fever, localized swelling, and abnormal flushing of the skin (erythema). Despite improvements in the interwar years, this vaccine left most vaccinated persons incapacitated for a day or two, while an unfortunate few developed plague infections. Busvine, *Disease Transmission*, 194; and Butler, *Plague*, 199.

36. K. F. Meyer, D. Cavanaugh, O. Bartelloni, and J. Marshall, "Plague Immunization I. Past and Present Trends," *Journal of Infectious Diseases* 129 (Supplement) (1974): 513–18.

37. *The 1991 Red Book: Report of the Committee on Infectious Diseases*, 22nd edition (Elk Grove, Ill.: American Academy of Pediatrics, 1991), 371.

38. DDT was first synthesized in 1874, but its insecticidal powers were only discovered in the mid 1930s by Paul Müller, working for the Geigy Company in Switzerland. It was first administered on a large scale by United States Army medical units to combat an outbreak of typhus in Naples in 1943. Its employment during the bubonic plague epidemic of Dakar in 1944 was, therefore, one of its earliest uses anywhere. Simultaneously with its application in Dakar, DDT was used against malaria-bearing anopheles mosquitoes in Italy. Busvine, *Disease Transmission*, 216–18.

39. For Senegal, see chapter 10. For DDT use around the world, see Busvine, *Disease Transmission*, 291–92.

40. For vector resistance, see Busvine, *Disease Transmission*, 293. For possible dangers, see Rachel Carson, *Silent Spring* (Boston: Houghton Mifflin, 1962); and Barry Commoner, *Making Peace with the Planet* (New York: Pantheon, 1990), 50.

41. Alfred W. Crosby, *The Columbian Exchange: Biological and Cultural Consequences of 1492* (Westport, Conn.: Greenwood Press, 1972); and John Iliffe, *Africans: The History of a Continent* (Cambridge: Cambridge University Press, 1995), 208–11. See also Joseph Miller, "Demographic History Revisited: Review Article," *Journal of*

African History 25 (1984): 93, for what he calls "the epidemiological, epizootic, and subsistence crises of 1880–1920."

42. See two articles by Marc H. Dawson: "Disease and Population Decline of the Kikuyu of Kenya, 1890-1925," in *African Historical Demography*, vol. 2, edited by Christopher Fyfe and David McMaster (Edinburgh: Centre for African Studies, University of Edinburgh, 1981), 121–38; and "Health, Nutrition, and Population in Central Kenya, 1890–1945," in *African Population and Capitalism*, edited by Dennis D. Cordell and Joel W. Gregory (Boulder, Col.: Westview Press, 1987), 201–17.

43. One of the best case studies of this process elsewhere in Africa is James L. Giblin, *The Politics of Environmental Control in Northeastern Tanzania, 1840–1940* (Philadelphia: University of Pennsylvania Press, 1992). A similar study of Senegambia is overdue.

44. Andrew Clark, "Environmental Decline and Ecological Response in the Upper Senegal Valley, West Africa, from the Late Nineteenth Century to World War I," *Journal of African History* 36 (1995): 197–218.

45. Boureima Alpha Gado, *Une histoire des famines au Sahel* (Paris: Harmattan, 1993), chapter 5.

46. Gado, *Une histoire des famines*, chapter 5; Marc Michel, *L'appel à l'Afrique: Contributions et réaction à l'effort de guerre en A.O.F., 1914–1919* (Paris: Publications de la Sorbonne, 1982), 154–55.

47. Marc H. Dawson, "Disease and Social Change: Smallpox in Kenya, 1880–1920," *Social Science and Medicine* 13B (1979): 245–51.

48. Charles Becker, "Notes sur les conditions écologiques en Sénégambie aux 17e et 18e siècles," *African Economic History* 14 (1985): tables, 168–69.

49. The years were 1858, 1859, 1883, 1889, 1891, 1895, 1897, and 1898; the outbreak in 1895 was the most severe. The smallpox season usually ran from mid November to the end of May. Mamadou Moustapha Dieng, "Les épidémies au Sénégal au XIXe siècle: Méthodologies et perspectives de recherches" (rapport de D.E.A. en Histoire, Université de Dakar, October 1984), 36.

50. Kalala J. Ngalamulume, "City Growth, Health Problems, and Colonial Government Response: Saint-Louis (Senegal) from Mid-Nineteenth Century to the First World War" (Ph.D. dissertation, Michigan State University, East Lansing, 1996), 289–90.

51. Philip D. Curtin, *Disease and Empire: The Health of European Troops in the Conquest of Africa* (Cambridge: Cambridge University Press, 1998), 10.

52. Charles Becker, "L'apparition du SIDA et la gestion des épidémies du passé au Sénégal," in *Les sciences sociales face au Sida en Afrique. Cas africains autour de l'exemple ivoirien*, edited by Jean-Pierre Dozon and Laurent Vidal (Abidjan: GIDIS-CI-ORSTOM, 1993), p. 74; Curtin, *Disease and Empire*, 78–82.

53. Before 1800, cholera was confined to the Indian subcontinent. The question as to whether bubonic plague was present in precolonial Senegal cannot be definitively answered, but a good case can be made that it was not. See John Iliffe, *Africans*, 67; and Myron Echenberg, " 'Scientific Gold': Robert Koch and Africa, 1883–1906," in *Agency and Action in Colonial Africa: Essays for John E. Flint*, edited by Chris Youé and Tim Stapleton (London: Palgrave, 2001), 34–49.

54. Angélique Diop, "Santé et colonisation au Sénégal, 1895–1914" (Thèse de troisième cycle, Université de Paris I, Paris, 1982), 100; Dieng, "Les épidémies," 37–39; Becker, "L'apparition du SIDA," table.

55. Ngalamulume, "City Growth," 228.

56. For more details see Ngalamulume, "City Growth," 231–34; and the views of Dr. Charles Carpot, a member of a noted Creole clan of businessmen, published in the *Journal Officiel du Sénégal*, 8 July 1893, 30–32.

57. Quoted in Ngalamulume, "City Growth," 235.

58. Gloria Waite, for instance, notes how some states privileged healers and gave them control over the location of villages in relation to water supply. John Iliffe observes that in Asante and in the empire of Mwanamutapa, healers and herbalists, respectively, sat on the highest councils of state. Gloria Waite, "Public Health in Precolonial East-Central Africa," in *The Social Basis of Health and Healing in Africa*, edited by Steven Feierman and John M. Janzen (Berkeley: University of California Press, 1992), 212–31; John Iliffe, *Africans*, 114.

59. Variolation involved the injection of the live smallpox virus, taken from the pustules of an active case, into a healthy individual so that the transfer would attenuate the agent and produce only a mild case of the disease in exchange for permanent immunity. See Guenter B. Risse, "History of Western Medicine from Hippocrates to Germ Theory," in *The Cambridge World History of Human Disease*, edited by Kenneth Kiple (Cambridge: Cambridge University Press, 1993), 17. For Senegal, see Ngalamulume, "City Growth," 116–17.

60. John Janzen, *The Quest for Therapy: Medical Pluralism in Lower Zaire* (Berkeley: University of California Press, 1978).

61. Ngalamulume, "City Growth," 153–55.

62. Ismail H. Abdalla, *Islam, Medicine, and Practitioners in Northern Nigeria* (Lewiston, N.Y.: Edwin Mellen Press, 1997), 69–88.

63. ANS\2G13\26, Dr. L. Huot, Annual Medical Report for 1913. A decade previously, Huot's predecessor noted that Africans alternated among "fetishists," Muslim healers, and French physicians, choosing the last-mentioned for accidents requiring surgery. ANS\2G7\18, Dr. Merveilleux, Annual Medical Report for 1904.

64. Ngalamulume, "City Growth," 157.

65. Terence O. Ranger, "Godly Medicine: The Ambiguities of Medical Mission in Southeastern Tanzania, 1900–1945," in *The Social Basis of Health and Healing in Africa*, edited by Steven Feierman and John M. Janzen (Berkeley: University of California Press, 1992), 256–82.

66. L'Abbé Boilat, *Esquisses sénégalaises* (Paris: P. Bertrand, 1853; reprinted, Paris: Karthala, 1984), 5. He left Senegal in 1852 after ten years of missionary work.

67. Ngalamulume, "City Growth," 116.

68. Quoted in Ngalamulume, "City Growth," 157.

69. Nagalamulume, "City Growth," 118.

70. For African healers, see chapter 8. For French physicians tied to miasmatic theory, see ANS\H48, Dr. Grall, "Rapport de la mission sanitaire au Sénégal, Fièvre Jaune, 1900–01"; and M. Courtet, *Étude sur le Sénégal* (Paris: Challamel, 1903), 131.

71. There is a rich and growing literature on the subject. Major studies include two books by John Janzen, *The Quest for Therapy: Medical Pluralism in Lower Zaire* (Ber-

keley: University of California Press, 1978); and *Ngoma: Discourse of Healing in Central and Southern Africa* (Berkeley: University of California Press, 1992). See also Steven Feierman, *Peasant Intellectuals: Anthropology and History in Tanzania* (Madison: University of Wisconsin Press, 1990); and D. M. Anderson and D. H. Johnson, eds., *Revealing Prophets: Prophecy in Eastern African History* (London: James Currey, 1995).

72. Meredeth Turshen, *The Political Ecology of Disease in Tanzania* (New Brunswick, N.J.: Rutgers University Press, 1984), 10–11.

73. Alice L. Conklin, *A Mission to Civilize: The Republican Idea of Empire in France and West Africa, 1895–1930* (Stanford, Calif.: Stanford University Press, 1997), 50.

74. Diop, "Santé," 175–78.

75. Conklin, *A Mission*, 49–50.

76. What she fails to note, however, is that in percentage terms, health expenditures were only 8 percent of the 1903 loan of 65 million francs, and only 3 percent of the 100 million borrowed in 1906. Conklin, *A Mission*, 47–48.

77. The most recent account of Leopold's atrocities is the outstanding work by Adam Hochschild, *King Leopold's Ghost: A Story of Greed, Terror, and Heroism in Colonial Africa* (Boston: Houghton Mifflin, 1998).

78. Conklin, *A Mission*, 50, note 31.

79. Alexandre Kemorgant, *Hygiène coloniale* (Paris: Masson, 1911), 30.

80. Ribot and Lafon, *Dakar*, 160.

81. Dr. Sorel, *Journal d'un vagabond*, 14, cited in Bruno Salleras, "La politique sanitaire de la France à Dakar de 1900 à 1920," (mémoire de maîtrise, Université de Paris X—Nanterre, 1980), 7–8.

82. ANS\2G7\18, Annual Report for Senegal, Dr. Merveilleux.

83. Diop, "Santé," 63–68.

84. Assane Seck, *Dakar, métropole ouest-africaine* (Dakar: IFAN, 1970), 128–32.

85. Alain Sinou, "Idéologies et pratiques de l'urbanisme dans le Sénégal colonial" (Université de Paris, École des Hautes Études en Sciences Sociales, thèse de troisième cycle, 1985), 210.

86. Governor-General Ponty's circular announcement, dated 24 April 1909, in *Journal Officiel du Sénégal*, 211.

87. Diop, "Santé," 267–68.

88. Georges Savonnet, "Une ville neuve du Sénégal: Thiès," *Cahiers d'Outre-Mer* (1956): 74.

89. Diop, "Santé," 69; Savonnet, "Thiès," 81, notes that the densest quarters of Thiès were Randoulène, "Derrière-la-voie-ferrée," and "Bambara."

90. Diop, "Santé," 310, estimates that the mortality rate for Dakar ranged from 40 to 33 per 1,000 between 1902 and 1914, and postulates a birth rate for Senegal in 1910 of 26.7 per 1000. Salleras estimates the overall mortality rate for Senegal for the period 1899 to 1920 at 41.6 per 1,000, compared with a rate of 20 per 1,000 for France in the same period; he provides no sources other than a few census estimates. He may be on firmer ground when he suggests that the European mortality rate for Senegal from 1905 to 1914 was 13.3 per 1,000, since French officials kept careful track of what were, overwhelmingly, citizens from the metropole. Salleras, "La politique sanitaire," 108–9.

91. Diop, "Santé," 308, gives the following estimates: Dakar and Gorée, 19,775; Rufisque, 19,177; Saint-Louis and suburbs, 28,469; and the entire colony of Senegal, 1,070,393.

92. Martin A. Klein, *Slavery and Colonial Rule in French West Africa* (Cambridge: Cambridge University Press, 1998), 199; Bernard Moitt, "Peanut Production and Social Change in the Dakar Hinterland: Kajoor and Bawol, 1840–1940" (Ph.D. dissertation, University of Toronto, 1985), 244–45.

93. Elikia Mbokolo, "Peste et société urbaine à Dakar: L'épidémie de 1914," *Cahiers d'Études Africaines* 22 (1982): 16.

94. C. Jojot, *Dakar. Essai de géographie médicale et d'ethnographie* (Montdidier, France: Grau-Radenez, 1907), 30, stated that the city had grown recklessly and dramatically from 8,700 in 1900 to 18,000 in 1904, and by 1908 included almost 30,000 inhabitants, including the transients. Official statistics listed the Dakar population as 17,000 in 1910. Diop, "Santé," 308.

95. Jojot, *Dakar*, 35–36.

96. Ribot and Lafon, *Dakar*, 81.

97. Ribot and Lafon, *Dakar*, 25, 82.

98. ANS\3G2\159, Minutes of the General Council, Saint-Louis, 1908.

99. Ribot and Lafon, *Dakar*, 138–40. They note some 200,000 francs in compensation was paid out to home owners who lost their property, which averages out at only 200 francs per unit.

100. Seck, *Dakar*, 122.

101. Seck, *Dakar*, 124.

102. ANS\3G2\158, on the 1905 Convention; Seck, *Dakar*, 124.

103. G. Wesley Johnson, *The Emergence of Black Politics in Senegal: The Struggle for Power in the Four Communes, 1900-1920* (Stanford, Calif.: Stanford University Press, 1971), 104, 148.

104. Seck, *Dakar*, 124; Raymond F. Betts, "The Establishment of the Medina in Dakar, Senegal, 1914," *Africa* 41 (1971): 143–49.

105. Diop, "Santé," 277–80.

106. Diop, "Santé," 284–85.

107. Mbokolo, "Peste," 16.

108. Ngalamulume, "City Growth," 261.

109. Iba Der Thiam, " L'évolution politique et syndicale du Sénégal colonial de 1840 à 1936," vol. 3 (thèse d'état, Université de Paris I, Paris, 1982–83), 945–46; Diop, "Santé," 252. On 18 May 1912, Governor Cor of Senegal passed the original legislation, which applied to the four communes, and on 12 December of the same year he extended it to all towns in Senegal where Europeans resided. For the text, see *Journal Officiel du Sénégal*, decree of 12 December 1912, 36–37.

110. Diop, "Santé," 276–77.

111. Bruno Salleras, "La peste à Dakar en 1914: Médina, ou les enjeux complexes d'une politique sanitaire" (thèse de troisième cycle, Université de Paris, École des Hautes Études en Sciences Sociales, Paris, 1984), 50.

112. For a detailed account of the losing battle to secure an adequate and safe supply of drinking water in Saint-Louis, see Ngalamulume, "City Growth," 262–81.

113. Diop, "Santé," 185.

114. Cited in Diop, "Santé," 193–94. One French physician noted that resistance to smallpox vaccination was much stronger in Senegal than in either Dahomey or Côte

d'Ivoire, and attributed this to the Muslim *marabouts*' powerful opposition to vaccination. Papa Amadou Gaye, "La diffusion institutionnelle du discours sur le microbe au Sénégal au cours de la Troisième République française (1870–1940)" (thése de doctorat, Université de Paris VII, Paris, 1997), 209.

115. See Michel Foucault, *The History of Sexuality*, translated by Robert Hurley (New York: Penguin Books, 1976), 126.

116. *Journal Officiel du Sénégal*, 26 March 1904, 164–65.

117. ANS\H11, Dr. Huot to governor of Senegal, 6 May 1913, and 7 March 1914.

118. Excerpt from a letter addressed to the governor-general of FWA by a group of Dakar women on 8 January 1909, quoted in Diop, "Santé," 215.

119. Senegal sent its first deputy to the French Assembly as early as 1848 when Durand Valantin, the Creole mayor of Saint-Louis, was elected. For the early electoral contests, see Johnson, *The Emergence*, 47–55.

120. The Creoles were descendants of European and African unions resulting from the lack of European women in seventeenth- and eighteenth-century Senegal. The African *signares*, mistresses or wives of Europeans resident in the trading post, set the fashion for early town life in Senegal. George Brooks, "The Signares of Saint-Louis and Gorée: Women Entrepreneurs in Eighteenth Century Senegal," in *Women in Africa*, edited by Edna Bay and Nancy Hafkin (Stanford, Calif.: Stanford University Press, 1976), 19–44. For details of the prominent French merchant families, see Rita Cruise O'Brien, *White Society in Black Africa: The French of Senegal* (London: Faber and Faber, 1972), 36, 56–57.

121. For a detailed but uncritical account of his career, see G. Wesley Johnson, "William Ponty and Republican Paternalism in French West Africa, 1866–1915," in *African Proconsuls: European Governors in Africa*, edited by L. H. Gann and P. Duignan (Stanford, Calif.: Hoover Institution, 1978), 134.

122. For legal restrictions, see Richard Roberts, "Text and Testimony in the *Tribunal de Première Instance*, Dakar, during the Early Twentieth Century," *Journal of African History* 31 (1990): 453; for the military, see Joe Lunn, *Memoirs of the Maelstrom: A Senegalese Oral History of The First World War* (Portsmouth, N.H.: Heinemann, 1999), 61. See also Johnson, *The Emergence*, 147–53; and James F. Searing, "Accommodation and Resistance: Chiefs, Muslim Leaders, and Politicians in Colonial Senegal, 1890–1934" (Ph.D. dissertation, Princeton University, Princeton, 1985), 384–88.

123. An autobiography of one of its founders discusses these early years of African activism. See Lamine Guèye, *Itinéraire africain* (Paris: Présence Africaine, 1966); and Johnson, *The Emergence*, 149–53.

124. For Diouf's erratic early political career, see Johnson, *The Emergence*, 118–19, and 146–47.

125. Thiam, "L'évolution politique," vol. 4, 1702; Johnson, *The Emergence*, 147.

126. *La Démocratie*, 13 November 1913.

127. Wesley Johnson is Diagne's quasi-official biographer. Johnson's monograph, *The Emergence*, is largely centered on Diagne, and he has supplemented this with several articles. Although Iba Der Thiam and Amady Aly Dieng have offered a perspective on Diagne in French, their interpretation closely follows Johnson's. Johnson interviewed Diagne's family, and had access to some of Diagne's corre-

spondence. Unless otherwise stated, details of Diagne's life and career are drawn from *The Emergence*, 154–77. See also Iba Der Thiam, "L'évolution politique"; and Amady Aly Dieng, *Blaise Diagne, premier député africain* (Paris: Éditions Chaka, 1990).

128. The governor of French Guyana, Fernand Levecque, acerbically described Diagne as a man who "suffers from assimilation indigestion." Johnson, *The Emergence*, 157–58.

129. French ruling ideology is discussed in Raymond F. Betts, *Assimilation and Association in French Colonial Theory, 1890–1914* (New York: Columbia University Press, 1961); see also Conklin, *A Mission*. Diagne joined the Freemasons early in his career, and established a correspondence and a friendship with two Creole politicians, Senator Alexandre Isaac of Guadaloupe and Gratien Candace, the deputy from Martinique.

130. A full account of the 1914 election and the candidates can be found in Johnson, *The Emergence*, 154–77.

131. Dieng, *Blaise Diagne*, 67.

132. Émile Masson was a long-time employee of Maurel and Prom, the leading Bordeaux trading firm in Senegal. He was closely associated with Fernand Marsat, a Dakar pharmacist who organized Senegal's first political machine. Masson won the election for mayor of Dakar in 1908, and was the incumbent when the bubonic plague epidemic burst upon the scene. Johnson, *The Emergence*, 160.

133. Dieng, *Blaise Diagne*, 61.

134. Johnson, *The Emergence*, 161.

135. Johnson, *The Emergence*, 173.

136. Dieng, *Blaise Diagne*, 76.

137. Johnson, *The Emergence*, 161.

138. For Diagne's "pact" with the Bordeaux houses, see Cruise O'Brien, *White Society*, 61; and Johnson, *The Emergence*, 214.

139. Quoted in Johnson, *The Emergence*, 161.

140. Johnson, *The Emergence*, 170.

141. Johnson, *The Emergence*, 170.

142. Johnson, *The Emergence*, 170–71.

143. Dieng, *Blaise Diagne*, 72.

144. See telegram of complaint by Diagne and Sergent to the Minister of Colonies, 4 May 1914, cited in Johnson, *The Emergence*, 171.

145. Dieng, *Blaise Diagne*, 72–73. In 1909, Diagne had married Odette Villain of Orléans, whom he had met in Paris during one of his leaves. The couple were to have four children, three sons and a daughter. One son, Adolphe, became a physician and entered the French Health Service in Senegal.

146. The breakdown was as follows: Diagne, 2,424 votes (47 percent); Heimburger 2,249 votes (44 percent); and Carpot 472 votes (9 percent). Johnson, *The Emergence*, 172.

PART I

"TAKE [A JOB IN DAKAR] IF YOU WANT TO DIE": THE PLAGUE EPIDEMIC OF 1914

When the year 1914 began, a wide gulf of suspicion and hostility separated French and African perceptions of health and disease. The colonial state had, it is true, imposed new sanitary regulations with good intentions, but the manner of their imposition, and the hardships the health regulations brought to African urban residents, had led to misunderstanding and resistance. On the other hand, not good intentions but a strong will to dominate lay behind the French practice of denigrating African therapies and delegitimating African healers.

By 1914 Dakar had become a powerful magnet attracting people from within Senegal and abroad. Substantial expenditures to modernize the port and build the federal capital's infrastructure provided work for new immigrants from the interior and attractive positions in the expanding colonial bureaucracy for French arrivals from Europe and for a small but growing African elite. By the year's end, however, Dakar had become a city many chose to avoid, a hecatomb where bubonic plague and arbitrary, sometimes risky, sanitary control measures were combined specters. It had also become a city where the idea of relocating Africans into segregated neighborhoods for allegedly sanitary reasons was gaining ground.

The experience of one potential immigrant to Dakar illustrates the dangerous reputation the city had acquired by 1914. In that year, Hélène Senghor, who became the wife of René, and sister-in-law of Léopold Sédar Senghor, the man who would lead Senegal to independence half a century later, was a young woman residing in Saint-Louis. In 1914, she became one of the first African women to complete secondary school. Offered a teaching position at an elementary school in Dakar, Hélène was ready to begin her career in the federal capital when a friend of the family wrote: "It is a fine post Hélène. Take it if you want to die." With little hesitation, Hélène wrote the inspector of education and turned down the otherwise attractive position.[1]

The four chapters which make up Part One examine this transformation of Dakar against the backdrop of a devastating bubonic plague epidemic. They enable the reader to follow the plague's arrival, progress, retreat, and consequences in rich detail. It will be seen that political rather than epidemiological concerns underlay the friction between French rulers and African subjects. At issue throughout the 1914 epidemic was whether Dakar would be a typical colonial city characterized by residential segregation separating ruler from ruled and white from black. Unique to Senegal was the additional question as to whether the colony's seat in the French National Assembly would remain under the control of French and Creole elites. Finally, a careful assessment of the French medical response offers the reader a portrait of early public health in the colony. We begin with the plague's outbreak.

NOTE

1. Janet G. Vaillant, *Black, French and African: A Life of Léopold Sédar Senghor* (Cambridge: Harvard University Press, 1990), 27.

3

OUTBREAK, APRIL–MAY 1914

A forty-two-year-old government clerk named Iba Ndiaye had reason to be proud of his accomplishments as he reviewed his situation in early May 1914. Born in Saint-Louis on 15 October 1871, into a Wolof family with sufficient means to educate him at the French secondary school in that city, he had entered the colonial service as a clerk in the Treasury Department soon after his graduation in 1893.[1] Two years later, Iba Ndiaye was seconded as an interpreter to the French Army of Conquest of the Sudan, under the command of Colonel de Trentinian. While the army was on campaign, his talents were noted by a young French administrator named William Ponty, and in 1898 he joined Ponty's administration in the Sudan.[2] As Ponty's star rose rapidly in the colonial service, his young African protégé benefited as well. When Ponty returned to Dakar in 1908 to become governor-general of FWA, he brought Iba Ndiaye with him. By 1914 Ndiaye had risen to the rank of *adjoint principal*, or senior clerk in the Native Affairs Bureau of the federal government, with an annual salary of 2,400 francs.

Iba Ndiaye, an *originaire* by birth but doubly qualified to be an elector by his social and economic status, was keenly interested in the elections for deputy which were then taking place. Yet, despite the fact that Blaise Diagne was a fellow African and civil servant, Iba Ndiaye is said not to have supported the ambitious young Senegalese politician, preferring instead the Ponty administration's favored candidate, the Parisian lawyer Henri Heimburger.[3]

With his position in the civil service came a salary that enabled Iba Ndiaye, his wife, and his sixteen-year-old son to live comfortably, considerably above the standard experienced by the majority of Africans in Dakar. The entire Ndiaye household, including relatives and servants, numbered close to twenty people. All were housed in a several-storied building of

European construction at 27, rue Thiers, between Blanchot and Raffenel streets, on the "Plateau," the area of central Dakar inhabited by the majority of Europeans in the colony.[4] The Plateau in 1914 was segregated neither by race nor by class. Some less privileged Africans, searching for scarce accommodation in the crowded city, were to be found living in squalid housing within a stone's throw of the Ndiaye residence, or even close to the governor-general's palace and other sparkling new edifices on the Plateau.

Despite his relatively comfortable surroundings, Iba Ndiaye was surrounded by visual and oral evidence that something was seriously wrong in his quarter. Rumors were making the rounds that some of his African neighbors were succumbing to a particularly virulent form of pulmonary infection which was killing off its victims in as little as two or three days from the onset of symptoms. While the cooler *hivernage* or winter months from December to February heightened the risk of pulmonary infection, it seemed odd that bronchial infections were persisting now that the days and nights of April and May had brought with them warmer weather.[5]

Not all of those infected with the mysterious ailment were poor. One of the victims of this lethal infection was a man described by the press simply as "Arthur . . . , a devoted employee of Maison Peyrissac."[6] A clerk in the Maison Peyrissac's retail outlet, Arthur was so well thought of that his employer, M. Soulier, visited him on his sick bed. Iba Ndiaye visited Arthur on Monday, 11 May 1914. The day before, when he had cast his ballot in the run-off election, Iba Ndiaye had been in the best of health. But when he awoke on the morning of Tuesday, 12 May, the day after his visit to Arthur's sick bed, Iba Ndiaye himself had fallen seriously ill, with shivering, vomiting, headache, giddiness, intolerance to light, aching limbs, and a badly swollen lymph node, or egg-like bubo, in the groin. Perhaps, Iba Ndiaye may also have had a blackish rash or "rosie" on the leg, where he had been bitten by a plague-infected flea.[7] As the day progressed, the bubo grew larger still, and excruciatingly painful; the patient probably grew delirious, and produced sweat, excrement, and spittle so fetid as to be overpowering to those trying to attend to him. No doubt his alarmed family had by this time gone from concern to panic as his condition worsened hourly. A French physician was summoned, and he had Iba Ndiaye rushed to the Colonial Hospital, where he died the next day, 13 May.

On Thursday, 14 May, Iba Ndiaye was given a state funeral, with Governor-General Ponty presiding, and with Mayor Émile Masson and most municipal councillors present. Ponty's speech paid tribute to this loyal servant of France, and implied that he had succumbed to his fatal illness as a result of having visited his sick friend Arthur.⁸ The governor-general promised to care for Iba's family and to see that the son was sent to the Lycée d'Alger "in order to make him into a good Frenchman."⁹ The Ndiaye family did not simply accept Ponty's words as idle promises. Iba's brother, Idrisse, wrote the governor-general on 24 June, explaining that he had tried to see the governor-general to no avail, that Idrisse was now responsible for raising his nephew to maturity and looking after his widowed sister-in-law, and that he needed financial help, and so he asked Ponty to give him five minutes of his time. The letter is on file, without any reply from the governor-general. Nevertheless, Ponty may have felt obliged to help Iba's son because the boy was admitted to the *École Normale* in 1916.¹⁰

The medical authorities should have been alarmed by the highly contagious and lethal nature of Iba Ndiaye's case, even if they gave no such indication in the reports which described the medical events of 1914. They did not appear to be aware that the city of Dakar in the month of April 1914 had experienced a rate of mortality at least double that of the previous year, according to the official register.¹¹ A third peculiarity which went unremarked at the time was the high concentration of deaths in a five-block rectangular zone of the Plateau defined by Thiers, de Grammont, Blanchot, and Vincens streets.¹² Some time later, after the bubonic plague emergency had been declared, the Navy physician Dr. André Marcandier conducted detective work on the mysterious April pulmonary infections in a search for the index case, the first human to have contracted the plague. His informants indicated that in a building of European-style construction on Thiers Street, at the corner of Blanchot, a man described only as "Alioun N'D.," a public works employee, had died within four days of "galloping pneumonia," according to the physician who had treated him.¹³ A woman who nursed him told Marcandier how fearful she was of the rapidity of the illness's progress, and of how, a few days before, three or four others had died at the same locale in a similar manner. Marcandier learned that two other casualties had been immigrant laborers from Saint-Louis, while a third was described as a sailor who had come from a southern port. Finally, Marcandier discovered that the Dakar Health Service had disinfected the building some time after 17 April, but apparently without suspecting that the disease involved was anything other than pneumonia. He was forced to conclude, however, that no particular index case could be located.¹⁴

Marcandier's honest account stands in contrast to the official medical reports by the officials charged with public health in Dakar. These officials later blamed their delayed response to the plague outbreak on

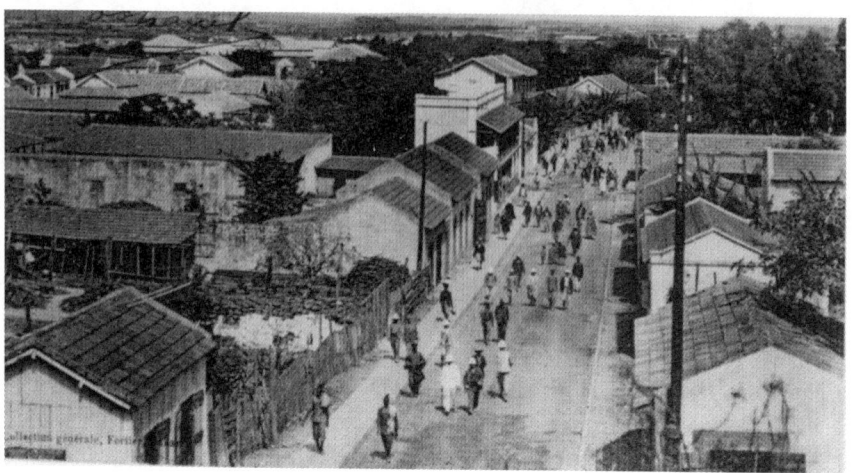

Photo 3.1 Vincens Street, Dakar, c. 1910. Cement construction dominates in this postcard, but note the open courtyard and ramshackle housing (lower left). Courtesy of the Archives Nationales du Sénégal. All rights reserved.

Africans who had concealed the epidemic from them. The evidence, however, makes it clear not only that an early African case, treated by a French physician, had been misdiagnosed, but also that the Dakar Health Service had failed to recognize that plague was spreading right under their noses.

Iba Ndiaye was one of the earliest, but not the first, plague victim to come to the attention of the French medical community. By a remarkable coincidence, on that fateful 10 May, the very Sunday when Diagne was winning the run-off election, Dr. Barros, a physician employed by the Dakar Health Service, was setting in motion a train of events which would lead to the declaration of the bubonic plague emergency. For Barros, politics was undoubtedly not his prime concern that Sunday evening. According to his account of events, he had become alarmed at the high number of recent pulmonary deaths, and had determined that he would have blood samples taken by the recently established Bacteriological Laboratory of French West Africa (BLFWA) for any of his patients with serious lung infections.[15] He testified that, on Sunday night, 10 May, he visited the laboratory, bringing with him blood samples from two African women who were his patients, and who are identified in the historical record only as Aissatou B. and Coumba B. Barros requested a report from Dr. André Lafont, Director of the BLFWA, as quickly as possible.

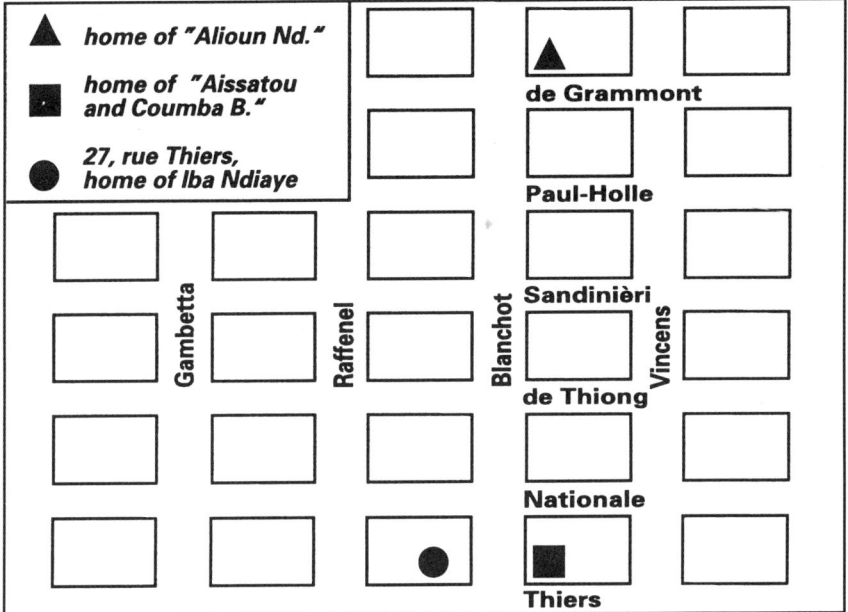

Map 3.1 Streets of Dakar Infected by Plague, 1914. This map has been adapted by the author from data in ANS\H55, Dr. Huot, "Rapport d'ensemble."

As was to be the case in so many of the events during the 1914 plague epidemic, the narrative reconstruction of events becomes murky at this point. Dr. Lafont's published account of events differs dramatically from that of Dr. Barros.[16] According to Lafont's version, Dr. Barros never visited the BLFWA on Sunday evening. Instead, Barros had intended to send his two patients by ambulance on Monday morning, 11 May, to the Central Hospital. But the ambulance in error transported the two sick women to the BLFWA instead. Lafont took the blood samples before letting the ambulance continue with them to the hospital. In Lafont's account, which is much less self-serving than Barros's version, the BLFWA's role in sounding the plague alarm was accidental. Lafont's account reveals the confusion surrounding the medical handling of the early stages of the epidemic.

The accounts of Lafont and Barros come together again for the events which unfolded on Monday, once Lafont had communicated his findings to Barros. The blood samples and sputum of the two women revealed a bacillus resembling *Yersinia pestis*, the causal agent of the dreaded bubonic plague, but additional work was required to obtain full confirmation.[17] Dr. Barros then set in motion a formal chain of events that marked the first official response to the Dakar medical emergency. He despatched a telegram to his medical superior in Saint-Louis, Dr. Huot, director of the colony of Senegal's Health Service, and ended his message with the ominous words, "PLAGUE POSSIBLE."[18]

Meanwhile, Dr. Barros's patients, admitted to hospital with temperatures of 40 degrees Celsius and coughing up red sputum from their lungs, continued to decline. When the younger woman died thirteen hours after being admitted, an incision in a blister she had developed revealed numerous live bacilli. The older woman died during the night; her body was free of buboes, but her sputum revealed the presence of plague bacilli.

Medical accounts did not provide many details about the first two officially declared plague victims. It was noted that they had lived in the area around de Grammont and Blanchot streets, only five blocks from Iba Ndiaye's residence, and had been under Barros's care for two days previously.[19] They and their neighbors were described as being "relatively affluent," dispelling the myth that plague was exclusively to be found among the poor.[20] In fact, within less than a month after the discovery of plague, the first sixteen to eighteen declared cases, all of them fatal, came from two African families and their neighbors in the same comfortable quarter.

Meanwhile a third victim, a male, came to Dr. Barros's attention. This patient's sputum showed the *Y. pestis* bacillus, alive and in a state approaching purity.[21] Now the cautious Dr. Barros was able to send a second telegram to Dr. Huot in Saint-Louis. Once again his message contained only two words, but these were unequivocal: "PLAGUE CONFIRMED."[22]

Two days later, on 13 May, the governor of Senegal, acting on the advice of the Dakar Health Committee, declared the native quarter of Dakar contaminated by plague. On that same day the city's Health Committee met to discuss emergency measures.[23] At last, both medical and civil authorities had come to recognize that Dakar was in the middle of a plague epidemic. The inefficiency of the colonial health system and, as will be seen, the silence of the African community had combined to give the plague a foothold in Dakar and an open road into the villages of the surrounding countryside.

NOTES

1. ANS\1C\1922, Personnel File of M. Iba Ndiaye.
2. *L'AOF*, obituary, 16 May 1914.
3. ANS\1C\1922. Personnel File for M. Iba Ndiaye. He is described as an "assiduous and methodical worker."

4. For the description of the building, see André Marcandier, "La peste à Dakar (1914–15)," *Archives de Médecine Navale* 106 (1918): 129.

5. Marcandier, "La peste," 129.

6. *L'AOF*, "Dakar en quarantine," lead headline and story, 16 May 1914.

7. In the absence of a clinical report on Iba Ndiaye's case, this reconstruction is based on typical case histories.

8. *L'AOF*, obituary, 16 May 1914. In fact, Iba N'Diaye had been exposed to *Yersinia pestis* before visiting his sick friend, since the incubation period for bubonic plague is a minimum of three days.

9. *L'AOF*, obituary, 16 May 1914.

10. ANS\1C\1922, Personnel file of M. Iba Ndiaye for a copy of the letter, and evidence of the son's admission to school.

11. Marcandier, "La Peste," 127, notes that civil registers showed a large increase in death rates beginning with the period from 29 March through 10 April. April death figures from 1909 through 1913 had averaged 46, but in 1914 they more than doubled to 106.

12. Marcandier, "La peste," 129.

13. Marcandier's description places this house only half a block from Iba Ndiaye's home on Thiers Street, but there is no suggestion that the two men might have been related. To preserve anonymity, it was conventional medical practice not to give the complete family name of patients in published literature. Alioun "N'D"'s family name could have been Ndoye or Ndiaye. Even in the latter case, this is a common patronymic and does not necessarily imply a close family tie. What is clear, however, is that the district around Thiers Street had become infected with *Y. pestis* before Iba Ndiaye fell ill.

14. Marcandier, "La peste," 129–30.

15. Dr. Barros's account of his activities are to be found in Dr. L. Huot, Director of the Health Service of Senegal, "Rapport d'ensemble sur l'épidémie de peste 1914–1915," Dakar, 3 March 1915, ANS\H55 (hereafter cited as Huot, "Rapport d'ensemble").

16. André Lafont, "Une épidémie de peste humaine à Dakar (avril 1914–février 1915)," *Bulletin de la Société de Pathologie Exotique* 8 (1915): 660.

17. Lafont, "Une épidémie," 661, gives a full description of the laboratory analysis.

18. The full text reads as follows: "High mortality among blacks for several days. Many in the same building. Showing all symptoms pneumonia. Illness lasts three days. Today I sent two patients to hospital for [eventual] autopsy to establish certainty. Plague possible." Huot, "Rapport d'ensemble."

19. Huot, "Rapport d'ensemble."

20. Lafont, "Une épidémie," 662, reconstructed details of this first plague center after the fact. All the victims were said to have contracted the lethal pulmonary form of plague.

21. Marcandier, "La peste," 126. Once plague was confirmed, it became clear that one woman suffered from pulmonary plague and the other from bubonic.

22. Huot, "Rapport d'ensemble."

23. Huot, "Rapport d'ensemble."

4

PLAGUE'S PROGRESS IN DAKAR, MAY–NOVEMBER 1914

This chapter examines the political response to the sustained plague epidemic of 1914. Two distinct phases of the epidemic can be discerned (see Chart 4.1). The first phase began in May, when the official declaration was made at the very moment when Blaise Diagne and his supporters were celebrating his stunning electoral triumph. This phase ended with an ill-considered political decision to declare the medical emergency over in July, despite still rising death rates. The second phase began with the renewed medical and political emergency of early August and ended with what proved to be the temporary retreat of *Yersinia pestis* in January 1915. Like the first phase, the epidemic's second phase was marked by a major political conjunction. This time the event was the outbreak of the First World War in Europe.

These remarkable conjunctions in 1914 are dramatic illustrations of how the Dakar medical epidemic was constructed and deconstructed. Diagne's controversial election provided additional reasons for many to view the declaration of the plague emergency as a punitive political action. The outbreak of hostilities in Europe helped convince the highest French political authorities in Dakar and especially in Paris to soften the unpopular anti-plague control measures, whether or not the epidemiological evidence justified such a course. In combination, the heady mix of plague, war, contested elections, general strikes, and massive street demonstrations would mark 1914 as arguably the most eventful year in the entire history of colonial Senegal.

THE MEDICAL EMERGENCY

The emergency meeting of the Dakar Health Committee on 13 May sent shock waves through the European and African communities of

Plague's Progress in Dakar, May–November 1914 59

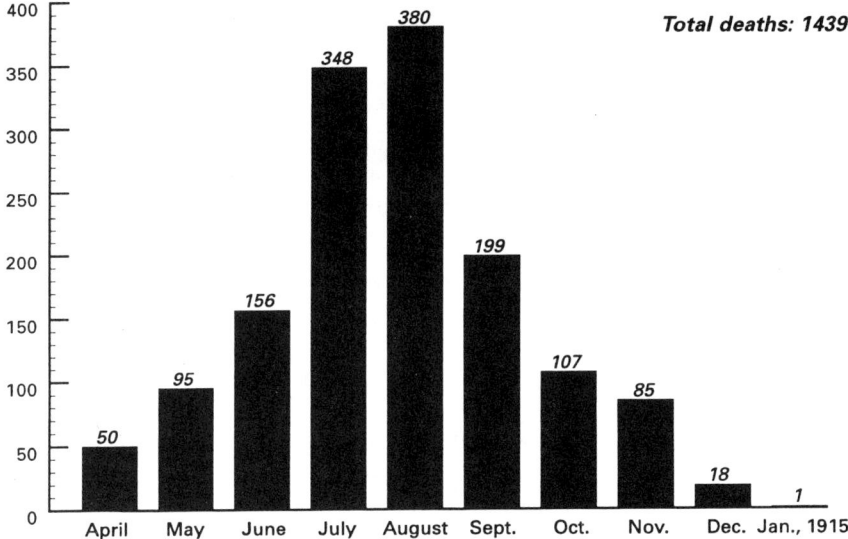

Chart 4.1 Dakar Plague of 1914, Monthly Mortality. From ANS\H55, Dr. Huot, "Rapport d'ensemble."

Senegal. The committee's decision to declare Dakar contaminated and to grant sweeping powers of intervention to health officials was not only warranted, it was probably several weeks late in coming. In fact, the day before the meeting, all military personnel had been confined to barracks. Now the committee was ordering the port quarantined, part of the city isolated by means of a *cordon sanitaire*, houses burned by the hundreds, schools closed as of the next day at noon, and temporary shelters erected at the racetrack for Africans undergoing medical treatment.[1]

Committee members, even if they expected some mild protests from both Europeans and Africans in Dakar, must have been dismayed at the heated response their declaration of an emergency provoked. The first public record of reaction came when the Dakarois awoke on 16 May to a front-page headline in *L'AOF* which read, "Dakar under Quarantine."[2] Hoping not to alarm readers, the lead article emphasized the control measures which were being put in place. Although there had been many "native" deaths over a period of roughly two months, these had been attributed by medical authorities to the chilly nights. Recently, however, two Dakar physicians had become alarmed at the severity of their patients' illnesses, and Dr. Lafont at the Bacteriological Laboratory had confirmed the presence of bubonic plague. The newspaper went on to reassure its primarily European readership that the epidemic had not affected whites and had been localized in the native quarter, which was being sealed off to the west of Vincens Street by a *cordon sanitaire* manned by the military. The paper reported this segregation of the city without commentary, and only the most perceptive readers might have wondered why the *cordon* did not include areas east of Vincens, a residentially mixed area of the Plateau where some of the first cases had developed. On page two of the same issue, *L'AOF* published the emergency decree declaring only the African residential quarter of Dakar contaminated by plague.

While this news was supposed to reassure readers, they may have been less comforted by an additional item in the front page story. They learned that the wife and son of the governor of Senegal, Henri Cor, had departed for France from Saint-Louis just before the emergency had been declared in Dakar. Governor Cor had also left the country, but after the emergency had been declared, *L'AOF* was quick to add. The article asked rhetorically whether he should have left during the emergency. Readers were informed that Governor-General Ponty himself had approved Cor's departure, with the proviso that he should return by the quickest means at his disposal if the epidemic had not ended within a few days, as all hoped.

THE FIRST WAVE OF AFRICAN PROTESTS

The response of the African public to the medical emergency was much more dramatic. A day after the declaration, on 14 May, the sanitary brigades burned a group of twenty-three dwellings where the first cases had been found. The action was "very badly received" by the public.[3] By 16 May, the press was reporting that the health squads were burning African dwellings "by the hundreds."[4] For five days beginning on 20 May, Africans responded with mass street protests and arguably the first general strike in Dakar's history. Trouble began on 20 May when a crowd of angry Lebu citizens, estimated at 1,500, gathered in front of the Dakar City Hall to protest the draconian measures of the Health Committee.[5] There they were said to have roughed up Mayor Masson and other members of the Municipal Council, and to have clashed with the Tirailleurs Sénégalais, who had been hastily summoned to protect the municipal officials.[6] One demonstrator is reported to have cried out: "They have chosen to burn straw huts while respecting the houses of Europeans. We have had enough of the whites' manner of doing things."[7]

To calm people down, Ponty agreed to see a delegation of Lebu notables. He patiently explained the history and severity of plague and its great dangers. He showed that the plague could potentially spare no one, pointing to the deaths of a white like the Syrian merchant Amin Gaouy, or Africans like the government clerk Iba Ndiaye, or old Arthur, the Maison Peyrissac employee.[8] Ponty confirmed that sanitary control measures would have to continue for the good of all, but they would now come under the direction of Delegate Vidal rather than Mayor Masson. Indemnities would be paid quickly, within twenty-four hours, to all property owners who had lost their houses. Finally, Ponty noted that the next Chargeurs Réunis ship to arrive in Dakar would bring with it 10,000 doses of serum to fight the plague.[9]

Ponty's soothing words could not avert a more peaceful but effective challenge to French authority, the market hold-up which began on 21 May and was to last until 25 May. Truck farmers, fishermen, poultry sellers, and market women united to keep their produce away from the daily Dakar market. This effectively closed the market down and aroused the concern of the various French interests. *L'AOF* attempted disingenuously to argue that the boycott was most harmful to wives of Tirailleurs Sénégalais and other "foreign" Africans living in Dakar who were without family networks through which to obtain food elsewhere.[10] Ponty, on the other hand, was more candid, and could not conceal his surprise over the complete success of the action. In his lengthy twenty-one-page report to Paris, which was labeled "highly confidential," he observed: "The market stayed deserted and the Blacks in the villages refused to sell their vegetables, eggs and chickens, or their fish to Europeans or to their employees. This strike was extremely well organized, and was a complete success. It is the first manifestation of this type which I in my experience had ever witnessed in these regions."[11]

In addition to the market hold-up, there is other evidence that the local economy was feeling the impact of the plague outbreak. *La Démocratie* reported on 6 June that with all the rebuilding required after the burnings, merchants were exploiting the situation by raising the price of building materials by 40 to 50 percent. In retaliation, the truck farmers and the fishermen were doubling the prices of their products.[12] A week earlier, the Diagnist newspaper had argued that the strike was an entirely justified response to what had occurred earlier, during the election campaign, when the large firms had threatened to suspend credit to Africans and to deny them supplies of merchandise if they chose to support Diagne.[13]

Reprisals for the strike were not long in coming. A day before it ended, on 24 May, Demba Aita, a Lebu notable, was arrested and charged with having persuaded a market woman, initially inclined to challenge the boycott, to close her stall and leave. Delegate Vidal was persuaded by the anti-Diagne faction to sentence Demba Aita to ten days in jail for having interfered with the woman's right to work.[14]

Other Diagne backers were also being harassed. Schoolteacher Amadou Duguay-Clédor was said to have received a disciplinary rebuke for having shown too strong a sympathy for Diagne in the election campaign. He was defended surprisingly by *Le Petit Sénégalais*, a paper that had opposed Diagne in 1914, in its issue of 6 June.[15]

THE DEPUTY AND THE GOVERNOR-GENERAL: DIAGNE AND PONTY

Alerted to these events at his home in Rufisque, Diagne nevertheless waited until two weeks after the formal declaration of the medical emergency to intervene on behalf of his supporters. Not until the day after Demba Aita's arrest did he go over Vidal's head and cable Governor-General Ponty directly. Diagne charged that the arrest of Demba Aita was an act of reprisal against the Lebu leadership which had supported him, and was orchestrated by his political opponents Escarpit and Lavie. Unless Demba Aita were released immediately, Diagne promised to extend the boycott to include the French firms Maurel et Prom and Buhan Teisseire. Noting that Demba Aita had never used force, Diagne attacked the judicial system for what he argued was a purely political sentence.[16]

Diagne's intervention may have forced Ponty's hand. Ponty decided to cut back on the intrusive sanitary measures and take a more conciliatory approach to the Lebu, if not yet to Diagne. On 30 May, before an emergency session of the Municipal Council, and in the presence of a delegation of Lebu chiefs, Ponty announced that there would be no property expropriations, that all the victims of sanitary cleansing operations would be compensated fairly, and that their dwellings would be rebuilt solidly in cement with the financial and technical help of the government. Most significantly, he ordered Demba Aita released from jail.

In his report to the minister of colonies in Paris, Ponty sought to place responsibility on everybody but himself. He insinuated his disapproval of medical and municipal officials by using terms such as "excess of rigor," and "panic," and argued that the sanitary measures had been applied "somewhat precipitously." He accused both the Diagnists (but not Diagne directly) and the anti-Diagne French faction of playing politics by deliberately using "rumors" to mislead the Lebu, "whose credulity is similar to that of all natives," into believing that only Muslim electors and their families had been infected by the plague, as "a punishment from Allah for the way they had voted."[17]

To be sure, both the Diagnists and their opponents saw the emergency medical measures in political terms. When Ponty strove to portray himself as the neutral arbiter, he managed to displease both sides. Most vocal among the Diagnists was Jean D'Oxoby, editor of *La Démocratie*. A thorn in the side of the colonial administration and of big business interests, he had been harassed continually and had spent fifteen days in jail on one occasion on a charge of endangering the public peace.[18] D'Oxoby, Jules Sergent, and the other Diagnists never wavered in their attack on what they regarded as a manufactured medical crisis. On 23 May, in a piece entitled "Things Come to a Head," D'Oxoby singled out the Devès family as orchestrators of the anti-Diagne movement, and noted that although arbitrary searches, gratuitous burnings of entire districts, and a general climate of injustice and discrimination had marked the application of the *cordon sanitaire*, not "a single rat cadaver" had been found.[19] Two days later, Sergent penned a stinging attack entitled "To Emile Masson and his Counselors," stating that the mayor and his henchmen had provoked the so-called "anarchy" of 20 May, and predicting that political disorder would not end until Masson and his clique left Dakar.[20]

Émile Masson and his deputy mayor, Caland, were both long-time employees of Maurel et Prom. Masson was also president of the Chamber of Commerce and was therefore, to all appearances, the voice of French business interests in Dakar. The honorary president of the Chamber was M. Fourmeaux, director of Maurel et Prom for over twenty years. Initially, the Masson team spoke with one voice. As the crisis gathered steam after 20 May, Masson and his supporters tried to pressure Ponty to stay firm. The mayor and several of his supporters visited the governor-general in the middle of the night and reminded him that agents of the Health Service had been physically threatened and jostled.[21] The next day, Mayor Masson wrote Ponty urging him to declare a state of siege, advice Ponty wisely rejected.[22] After Ponty announced his conciliatory proposals to the Lebu on 30 May, the entire municipal team viewed this as capitulation and threatened to resign en masse, along with several influential members of the Chamber of Commerce. Ponty persuaded them to back down.[23] Perhaps not coincidentally, that same day *L'AOF* reported without comment that Masson was about to take his vacation and return to France.[24] One Senegalese historian, Iba Der Thiam, speculates that Maurel et Prom had come to feel that Masson was too emotionally involved in local politics, had placed the firm at some economic risk, and was therefore being recalled. The hypothesis makes good sense, even if it cannot be documented. *L'AOF* also reported that Fourmeaux too was leaving Senegal to begin his retirement in France.[25] Whether the departure had been planned long before, or was precipitated by the risks of living through a plague epidemic, cannot be established.

Diagne's most formidable opponent at this time was Raphaël Antonetti, the acting governor of Senegal. On 10 June he wrote Ponty blaming Diagne for all of the political troubles surrounding the plague emergency, and suggesting that this was but one symptom of a distorted electoral system that allowed Africans to vote. Antonetti's remarks linking epidemic disease and politics amounted to racist invective:

> We are excluded from the direction of public affairs, and by whom? By our porters, our copyists, by fishermen, by people of another race, ignorant, fanatical, 90 percent illiterate. Tomorrow the thousand Muslim Lebu electors can elect in Dakar, an important European city, a port of war and an international port, a Lebu municipal council made up of ignorant, fanatical, illiterate blacks. The same blacks who forcefully resist the removal of plague victims will be in charge of applying the sanitary and hygienic regulations against which they have continuously protested. Tomorrow they will be in charge of the police with which they are in constant conflict and they will be able to use armed force against us. If this is the result of political liberty in Senegal, it would be better to abolish the deputyship and even the municipal councils.[26]

Claiming that Diagne's victory was tainted and that he should be denied the deputyship, Antonetti's rash suggestion was that Ponty should either buy off Diagne, perhaps with a high administrative post in France, or, if that could not be arranged, simply "get rid of him."[27] Ponty was too clever even to comment on such extreme proposals, let alone forward them to Paris. Instead, he wrote Paris urging a change in the electoral system, and claimed that since Diagne had not been a registered voter in the communes, he was ineligible for office.[28]

One of the most intriguing elements in the drama of 1914 was the evolving relationship between the newly elected deputy and the powerful governor-general. Ponty had been forced to reassess his position in the light of strenuous African resistance to the emergency health measures. He showed some willingness to treat the Lebu more gently, while remaining critical of both the Diagnist and the Masson camps. No admirer of Diagne at this stage, Ponty was also keenly aware that his task of governing the French West African Federation would become next to impossible should Diagne remain as deputy and attempt to exploit every political crisis to his advantage. It is not surprising, therefore, that while Diagne's claim to the deputyship was still undecided, Ponty would report back to Paris in unfavorable terms. The minister of colonies, nevertheless, must have been taken aback to read that Diagne was charged not only with political irresponsibility but with cowardice as well:

> M. Blaise Diagne, the newly elected Deputy for Senegal, who should have been with the Lebu population, since they were almost unanimous in being strongly attached to his candidacy, only made a brief appearance in Dakar, the day after his election, and then left town almost as soon as the epidemic was announced, never to reappear since. He has kept himself wisely and prudently in Saint-Louis or in Rufisque, but always far enough away from the foyer of the epidemic and from the milieu of his electoral campaign, little concerned by how the means employed have blindly and profoundly overexcited his milieu.[29]

THE CONSPIRACY AGAINST DIAGNE

This far removed from events, recollections of those fateful days immediately following Diagne's election are shrouded in myth and conspiracy theory. Diagne contributed to the confusion in no small measure by remaining in seclusion, possibly in his home base of Rufisque, for most of the period following his election on 10 May until he secretly set sail for France from an unknown Senegalese port roughly seventeen days later. There is evidence of only two public appearances by Diagne in the dramatic two weeks before he left Senegal. On the 11th, the day after the election, he appeared in Dakar.[30] Exactly one week later he was in Saint-Louis when the commission charged with counting the ballots announced the definitive results of the run-off election.[31] More to the point, Ponty had been correct in drawing attention to Diagne's low visibility. While his leading supporters Sergent and d'Oxoby were prominent during the five days of disturbances which followed 20 May, Diagne was nowhere to be seen. The only written record of Diagne's activity comes from the article which bore his signature in *La Démocratie* of 23 May, and from his cable to Ponty two days later from Rufisque defending Demba Aita.[32]

Why was Diagne so reclusive? His supporters would later claim that Diagne feared for his personal freedom of movement, and even his life, in the unstable period during which his election was being legally challenged by his enemies, and at a time when the medical emergency in Dakar had dramatically curtailed civil liberties.[33]

One dramatic theory even has it that Diagne's enemies were prepared to use medical techniques to eliminate him if all else failed. The final revenge of the whites would be to inject Diagne with a fatal dose of the plague bacilli, since vaccination had now been made compulsory for noncitizens (and the legal challenge against Diagne's election turned in part on whether Diagne was a citizen), on or before the moment he was to sail for France.[34]

Some sixty years after the events, Iba Der Thiam consulted an eyewitness and *griot*, Ndéné Mbaye. Mbaye was the personal *griot* of Galandou Diouf, the Rufisque politician and a Diagne supporter at the time of the plague epidemic.[35] Mbaye tells this story: Diagne was at Rufisque when Demba Aita was arrested on 24 May. Diagne did not take his telegram in person to the Rufisque post office. Galandou and all of Diagne's other supporters had learned in effect that if Diagne were so imprudent as to show himself in public, the Health Service people were surely going to inoculate him, under cover of the obligatory vaccination regulation, with a lethal dose of plague bacilli. Diagne therefore had to be hidden in a secret locale. Galandou then arranged with some of his friends in the port of Rufisque to contact the captain of the steam vessel *Ariane*, then docked there but about to leave for Nantes with a cargo of peanuts belonging to the Maurel et Prom firm. The Dutch captain was given a large sum of money to take on a passenger who wished to leave the colony incognito. Diagne was then dressed up in African clothes, made entirely unrecognizable, and taken during the night by dug-out canoe to the *Ariane* just before it departed for France.

Clearly, Diagne's reclusive behaviour did not go unnoticed by his opponents. Ponty, as has been seen, criticized Diagne for not being available to help calm his supporters, and observed caustically that Diagne was being "prudent" in staying away from Dakar and thus protecting himself from plague.[36] The anti-Diagnist press displayed no such subtlety. Roughly one month after Diagne had arrived in France, Georges Ternaux, editor of *L'AOF*, in an article called "The Elected One and the Plague," proclaimed that Diagne "feared for his precious black skin" and had "bravely fled the scourge to Rufisque, then Saint-Louis, and finally Paris without ever setting foot again in Dakar." Ternaux went on to note that Diagne had been very actively courting the French press since his arrival in the metropole, giving interviews describing the corrupt and unscrupulous opposition to him of big business, the Creoles, and the colonial administration, and the manner in which the plague epidemic was being exploited by Masson and his friends to persecute Diagne's loyal followers, who loved France and were totally devoted to the cause of colonialism.[37]

In one respect, Ternaux was correct. Diagne was indeed lobbying furiously in France. His claim to the deputyship was being adjudicated by a parliamentary committee, and his career hung in the balance. Thiam is also on sound ground in arguing that Diagne had no choice but to hurry to France to defend himself, and to curry support with the Republican Radicals. Indeed, on 7 July 1914, the ruling came down from the Parliamentary Credentials Committee declaring the election valid and Diagne the recognized deputy from Senegal.[38] One month later, France would be at war with Germany, and the first African deputy from Senegal would begin to play his part as a great patriot and an enthusiastic supporter of African military conscription.

If the rumor that the French were prepared to use assassination if necessary to "get rid of Diagne" seemed far-fetched, there was nothing surprising or irrational about the conviction among his supporters that the emergency health measures were, in Ponty's words, "nothing but vengeance invented by the party hostile to the newly elected M. Blaise Diagne."[39] Even if they have obvious medical components, all epidemics are politically constructed, as Charles Rosenberg has persuasively argued.[40] Indeed, the inhabitants of Senegal had several rational arguments for viewing the medical emergency of 1914 as an orchestrated campaign of reprisals against the African electors. For one thing, Dakar had experienced yellow fever epidemics in the past without such extreme measures having been invoked. Second, Europeans and their property were exempted from control measures, even when some of their housing was, to all appearances, substandard. Third, the *cordon sanitaire* was applied only to African residential neighborhoods. Fourth, anti-plague vaccinations were voluntary for Europeans, but compulsory for West Africans, Moroccans, and Syrians, impeding the free movement of traders and merchants who were in competition with the French. Lastly, leading members of the Dakar Health Committee, the people involved in declaring the emergency, had bitterly opposed Diagne's candidacy. Indeed, it is hard to imagine how the political character of the medical situation could have been more explicit.

Whether Diagne's people were correct in believing that a French physician would seek to poison Blaise Diagne is more problematic. Clearly, however, there is good evidence for arguing that the perception that Diagne's life was in danger was widely shared. From a Western biomedical perspective, the poisoning of Diagne through an overdose of anti-plague serum would have been too reckless a flouting of the Hippocratic oath. It would also have further deterred the community's acceptance not only of the vaccine but of the entire Western medical dispensation. On the other hand, passions and conspiracy theories ran high on both sides in the charged postelection atmosphere. Had not the acting governor himself not imprudently suggested to Ponty that Diagne should be "gotten rid of"? It is entirely possible that this correspondence could have leaked. It should also be recalled that the African majority had by no means accepted Western biomedical rhetoric about how public health officials were dedicated to the well-being of the entire public. Too often in their experience, public health had become a code word for the health of Europeans, not Africans. Instead, for many, a different, reductionist ideology prevailed. Disease causation and life-and-death issues were part of a primordial struggle between the forces of good and evil. The perception could easily arise, therefore, that a French physician, brandishing a syringe laced with toxic liquid, was either a sorcerer himself, or else a sorcerer's apprentice.[41] Given the highly charged atmosphere of Dakar in May 1914, the fear that Diagne's enemies sought his death should be taken seriously as an indication of the political temperature of the times.

REPEAL AND RESTORATION OF CONTROL MEASURES IN JUNE–JULY 1914

With the departure of Masson and Diagne to France, and with a temporary decline in the number of reported plague deaths in late June, Ponty had reason to believe that he had weathered both the medical and the political crisis. What he hoped would be the retreat of bubonic plague turned out, however, to be only a pause between the first and second phases of a continuing crisis.

Ponty, at this stage, had taken full charge of the emergency. At his urging, the Dakar Health Committee met on 12 June and agreed to repeal the health emergency decree of 13 May, bringing a halt to the severe control measures that had aroused such opposition.[42] Two days later, the French Navy lifted its orders confining personnel to barracks,[43] and later in June, spokesmen for the French business community declared the crisis over. For example, the *Bulletin du Comité de l'Afrique française*, published by Auguste Terrier, happily announced to its influential French readership interested in colonial affairs that the precautionary health measures taken when plague had been discovered in Dakar had produced "some emotion in the black population," but, thanks to the skilful efforts of Mayor Masson and Governor-General Ponty, responsible "natives" now understood that the measures had been taken in their interest.[44]

Ponty received somewhat more mixed news on political matters during this period, when, on 7 July, the Credentials Committee in Paris issued their long-awaited ruling declaring Diagne's election valid and proclaiming him deputy.[45] Although Ponty may have wished for a different decision, at least the matter was resolved. He may even have hoped that Diagne was sincere in stating that he sought cooperation and not confrontation with the colonial administration.[46]

Unfortunately, events were unfolding in Europe and in Senegal which would dash Ponty's hopes. Those concerned with military tensions among the Great Powers were alarmed at the news coming out of Sarajevo, Bosnia. There, on 28 June 1914, while Diagne was lobbying for support in France, an assassin was bringing down Archduke Ferdinand of Austria. One month to the day after the bloodshed in Sarajevo, Austria would declare war on Serbia and set in motion hostilities which would involve the entire world.

Meanwhile, in Senegal, the plague's alleged retreat turned out to be wishful thinking. Plague cases and deaths began to rise again, and medical authorities now acknowledged that they had been deceived into thinking the epidemic had abated only because so many Africans had been concealing their sick and their dead.[47]

As the death toll in Dakar rose in July, pressure to restore emergency sanitary measures came not only from the medical professionals but from the diplomatic community, whose doyen was the British consul, Charles Braithwaite Wallis. Responding to this pressure, on 16 July, the Dakar Health Committee once again declared the Port and the city contaminated and reintroduced the emergency control measures.[48] Soon afterward, the colonial administration took two further steps which were not prescribed in the international protocol against plague, and which would further inflame African passions. On 24 July, Governor-General Ponty passed a law making sanitary segregation legal,[49] and on August 2nd, he made the anti-plague vaccine compulsory for Africans, but voluntary for Europeans.[50]

SANITATION AND RESIDENTIAL SEGREGATION: THE DAKAR MÉDINA

The story of plague in 1914 is inseparable from the issue of residential segregation. As we have seen, medical arguments to rationalize racially inspired urban residential segregation were widely used in colonial Africa. In Senegal the call for residential segregation was closely linked to the so-called Lebu land question, the strongly contested issue of who actually owned much of the prime real estate in the heart of the city of Dakar. When plague broke out in 1914, considerable social engineering of the residential map of the city had already occurred. Early removals were conducted through a variety of means, such as private purchase, expropriation, and annexation by the state. During the yellow fever epidemic of 1900 several villages,

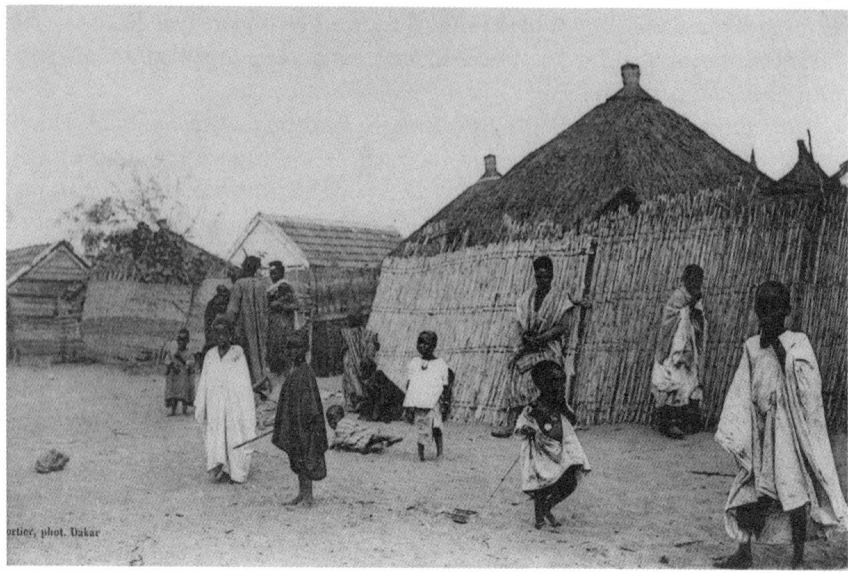

Photo 4.1 Village of Hock, c. 1910. This scene shows the predominance of straw dwellings on the sandy soil typical of Dakar and the Cape Verde peninsula. No doubt, villages such as Yoff and Cambérène, where plague was to cause such devastation, were similar in appearance. Courtesy of the Archives Nationales du Sénégal. All rights reserved.

such as Hock and a part of the village of Kaye, were moved. By 1905, almost all the original Lebu villages of the southeast corner of the city had been displaced and were now relocated to the north and west of the rue Vincens.[51]

These relocations, while they did tend to congregate the poorer Africans to the north, did not produce a fully segregated residential pattern according to a preconceived plan. In fact, during the medical crisis of 1914, it was discovered that no official definitions, let alone demarcations, existed for any of the city's districts or neighborhoods. Nevertheless, by 1910, there had emerged what might be called three distinct zones: a rich European town concentrated in the south and southwest, an African town to the north, and a mixed quarter of European workers and middle-class Africans in the center.[52]

In 1914, there was still unoccupied land in the sectors that became known as Niay-Tioker and the marshes of Rebeus. The new segregation village created in July–August 1914, soon to take the name of Médina, continued the process of transferring old Lebu villages from their earlier sites to less desirable ones further from the port and the city center.[53] Located some 3 to 4 kilometers out of town, the Lebu place name for the locale had been "Tilène, the region frequented by jackals."[54] Lebu elders recounted that the area had become taboo because, when it had been inhabited in the past, it had been found to be unhealthy.[55]

The issue of residential segregation came up as soon as the medical emergency had been declared. At its critical session on 13 May and at three further meetings that month, the Dakar Health Committee discussed the creation of an African segregation village, consisting of between 60 and 70 hectares, to be established on the Ouakam road to the northwest of Dakar.[56] At its meeting of 7 July, during the quiet time between the first and second phases of the plague epidemic, the committee forcefully stated its conviction that residential segregation was both indispensable and urgent:

> The committee declares that segregation of the native population at a place some distance from the European city and the destruction of all shacks and huts incapable of being disinfected constitutes the only measure capable of stopping the current epidemic and preventing the return of others which have periodically desolated the city.
>
> The committee repeats its view that this measure be immediately brought into effect.[57]

Clearly, a more powerful force was holding back the immediate implementation of residential segregation. Though the record is silent, everything points to Governor-General Ponty. Realizing that formal segregation would trigger widespread resistance, Ponty had not yet become convinced that this step was required. The surging case rates of plague in July probably convinced him to act. On 24 July 1914, his decree laid down precise plans for the new African segregation village.[58] Once the legislation for the sanitation village was in place, the pace of destruction of housing in Dakar accelerated, peaking in October even though the plague epidemic had reached its apogee two months earlier, as Chart 4.1 illustrates.

The new segregation village started its existence as wooden barracks, each divided into four compartments to provide temporary shelter for four families while they made preparations for more permanent housing of their own devising.[59] In short, Africans would be freed from European construction standards, although it was recognized that some who purchased their

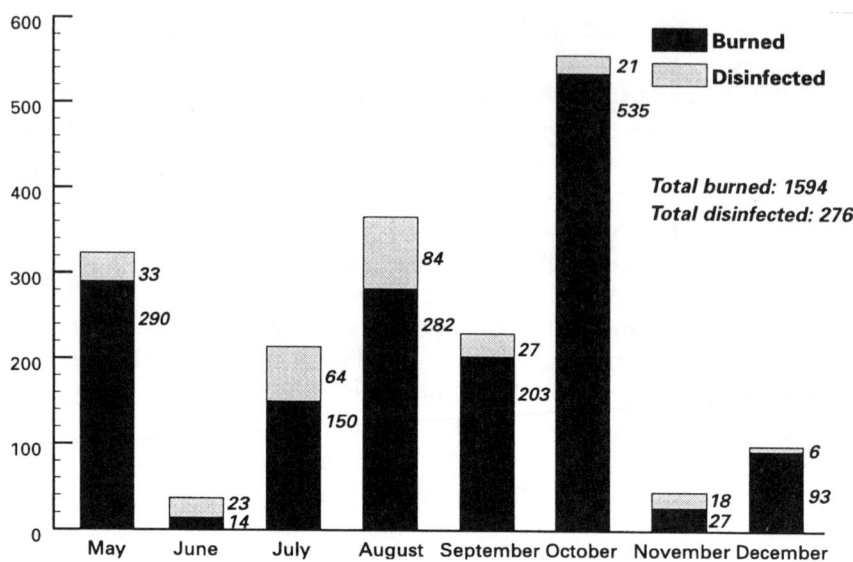

Chart 4.2 Dakar Dwellings Burned or Disinfected, 1914. Adapted from Elikia Mbokolo, "Peste et société urbaine à Dakar: L'épidémie de 1914," *Cahiers d'Études Africaines* 22 (1982): 39.

land "could be authorized eventually to rebuild according to European norms."[60] Police were assigned to the village from the start to make sure there were no escapes to the old contaminated neighborhoods of Dakar, as well as to prevent the introduction of objects which had not been disinfected. Inhabitants of the new village who could produce vaccination papers were issued cards allowing them access to Dakar during working hours from 6 A.M. to 6 P.M. Thereafter, Dakar was off-limits to Africans, who were obliged to return to the segregation village. A doctor was assigned to the new camp to maintain sanitary control of garbage removal, organize the distribution of drinking water, and conduct campaigns against insect larvae.[61]

The authorities recognized that it would have been more desirable to prohibit all building materials from contaminated sites from being recycled in the new locale. But the acute shortage of building materials left them no choice but to tolerate the recycling of disinfected wood, straw, and other items.[62]

Despite the high-sounding health concerns expressed in the legislation, in reality, the new segregation village was quite insanitary. When the segregation camp opened in August, in great haste, there was no effective sewage system, no electricity, and no clean water.⁶³ The Lebu had clear reason to regard sanitation rhetoric as a device to remove them from the Europeans' urban space. Two months later, when haste was no longer an excuse, Acting Governor Antonetti, in his public address at the opening of the General Council, made clear the prevailing segregationist mind-set, using language only slightly more moderate than he had used in his correspondence with Ponty:

> It was not a question of race but of health, pure and simple. There is a danger and a mutual annoyance in letting two groupings who have their ways of living that are so completely distinct cohabit. . . . It is far more desirable to have on the one hand the European city with its full demands based on modern hygiene, and on the other, the native town with full liberty to build in wood or in straw, to beat the tam-tam all night and to pound millet at 4 o'clock in the morning.⁶⁴

The reaction of the African population to the destruction of their homes can be heard in the plaintive words of a petition which survives from 1916, when these hygienic control measures were resumed:

> These decisions have caused us great concern. They have forced us to abandon the places where we were born, where our parents lived and died, and where we had hoped to remain ourselves. Moreover, this is a question not only of feelings but of interests: for all who, with much difficulty, have realized sufficient savings to allow them to construct a small house or a shack where they and their families have taken shelter, it was ruination.⁶⁵

Raymond Betts has best understood the importance of the Médina in the urban and social history of Dakar. He recognizes that while it may have been a "cheap answer to a growing housing need" during an emergency, it was also a major failure, "ill-conceived and equally ill-received."⁶⁶

WAR IN EUROPE AND FRENCH WEST AFRICA

In France, July 1914 was a difficult month.⁶⁷ As the month ended, mobilization became the frightening reality. On 31 July, just as the French cabinet prepared for war, news arrived that the great Socialist leader Jean Jaurès had been assassinated by a crazed young man who resented Jaurès' antiwar stance.

Both the German and French General Staffs assumed the war would be short. The French High Command's Plan XVII was silent regarding the role of the overseas colonies, though it did provide for the transfer of troops from Algeria and Tunisia to France.[68] Even before mobilization in France was completed, however, Governor-General Ponty saw an opportunity to display his patriotism and have his colony play a greater role in the coming struggle. On 29 July, he offered Paris no less than thirty-three companies (6,600 men) within twenty-five days. No doubt pleasantly surprised, the French government accepted the offer "with appreciation" and asked Dakar to send eight battalions to Morocco as quickly as possible to replace units of the Occupation Army, which could then be called back to France.[69] Thus, as Marc Michel makes clear, when war did break out, FWA had become involved without having been formally requested to participate.[70]

Ponty did not stop there. Claiming that Africans were "enthusiastic" about the war and would be even more so if they were allowed to fight in France, he requested that Tirailleurs be permitted to fight there.[71] Again, Paris was pleased to respond affirmatively, and three battalions were rushed immediately to the metropole. All told, in the first six months of the war, FWA would send 11,000 men abroad. By November 1915, the total was roughly 34,000 men, with 7,500 in Cameroun, 13,500 in Morocco, and over 12,000 in the metropole.

All of this quickly became a heavy burden for the population. Nor was the expectation of easy recruiting fulfilled. Mobilization of reservists was disappointing; they were difficult to trace, of uneven quality, and hard to retrain. The regimental stations were not overwhelmed by volunteers; less than 5,000 had come forward by October 1915. The result was that the colonial administration had to approve three emergency levies in a twelve-month period beginning in September 1914. Nothing like this had ever been seen before under French rule and it took its toll politically.[72]

Most of the Senegalese recruits did not willingly go off to a war that was not theirs. By the beginning of 1915, resistance to military recruitment ranged from self-mutilation and organized evasion to escape from FWA across the border into British Gambia or Portuguese Guinea. In the *cercle* of Thiès, among the Lebu of the Cape Verde peninsula, and among the Tukolor in Matam, entire villages refused to present their young men to the recruiters. In Bawol, among Sereer minorities in the *cercle*, scuffles broke out between villagers and the agents of the canton chiefs.[73]

If the war was unpopular once oppressive recruitment had been imposed, it is more difficult to assess attitudes in the early days. Censorship in August had been severe, since the French commander in chief, Marshal Joffre, believed civilians should be told nothing, and he prohibited the presence of journalists at the front.[74] If the general public in France, let alone Dakar, was kept in the dark, Ponty and Diagne, on the other hand, were well placed to know the seriousness of the situation. Both would express their patriotism by expanding on the military role Africans were to play in the First World War.[75] All the ingredients for an understanding between Ponty and Diagne were in place if they could only agree on how to control bubonic plague politically.

Thus, just as the outbreak of plague had coincided with a political event of great importance, the victory of an African in the election for deputy, so too a second conjuncture arose in August: the renewal of the bubonic plague emergency at the same time as the guns began firing in western Europe. For the first time but not the last, war and plague would come together to politicize events in Dakar. As will be seen, higher political considerations would once more have their impact on the strictly medical aspects of the epidemic.

THE DIAGNE-PONTY PACT OF AUGUST 1914

On 11 August 1914, Blaise Diagne wrote a long letter to Ponty offering his considered opinion on how urban tensions between the Lebu and the municipal administration had become inflamed, and how the situation could be set right.[76] This important intervention marked a major turning point, the moment at which, with war already raging in Europe, Diagne and Ponty would begin to arrive at an understanding that would carry Senegal through the twin crises of pestilence and war.

Diagne began by alluding to a letter dated 28 July, which he had received from a "franco-native" friend. The letter indicated that the Lebu were determined to stand firm on the lands they occupied and owned, and would refuse to be transferred to the new so-called "public domain" which had been legislated into existence the day before. Next, Diagne assured Ponty that, despite the slings and arrows thrown his way by Ponty's "friends," "all my actions proceed from a desire to serve the cause of a true and just colonialism." He continued:

> My sentiments regarding the successive expropriations, of which the Lebu of Dakar and Rufisque have been victims since the Guy Convention,

under your misguided predecessor, are known to you. It is a patent illegality, and has only served to benefit speculators, whether they are natives or Europeans.

If you again revive these expropriations, you risk ugly incidents from the people of Dakar and Rufisque. You will bring them to a deplorable resistance, however justified.

The municipality, aided by the delegate of the Governor of Senegal, have acted in bad faith. What have they done? They have distanced the natives from the city, installing them in an area with neither electricity nor water, without sewers or latrines. They have been subjected to the brutality of native sanitary agents recruited from among races hostile to them, and under the control of amateur Europeans with little knowledge of sanitation themselves. Such were the beginnings of the plague of which even the physicians were ignorant. No wonder we still have unhappy natives who have no choice but to support anarchy and chaos.

It is perfectly clear that if the administration has the duty to eliminate the plague by all the means at its disposition, its role stops there. It should not, in opposition to the law, expropriate the lands of the Lebu community in order to enrich speculators.

What should be done? The municipalities, with or without budget assistance from Senegal and from FWA, should construct inexpensive housing the way this is done in the metropole. The natives would preserve the right to buy these buildings after a certain period of time, during which they would pay an annual rent. Whether the municipalities do the building, whether the natives in cooperatives do it, or whether private enterprises take up the task, this is the only solution. My friend, M. Joucla, currently the second-ranking official in the Ministry of Colonies, and a former *chef de cabinet* of the governor-general, has already done a study along these lines which you will find in your files.

I would also add that such a system could be extended to European settlers of modest means.[77]

Obviously, other considerations were now at work persuading Diagne to make peace with Ponty and put the plague issue to rest. In the middle of August, Diagne wrote his assistant, Galandou Diouf, from Paris, urging him to convey to the young electors of Senegal that they must enlist immediately in the armed forces so as to consolidate their voting privileges, and ultimately, their right to citizenship: "War has been declared and I urge young Senegalese to enlist. At an hour when France is playing a huge role against German brutality, all Senegalese must, based on their time-honored history of loyalty, unite as good Frenchmen. We will pay in this way for the honor of having our own representation in Parliament now and forever."[78]

Ponty did not respond to Diagne's overture for over a month.[79] When he did so, he was both conciliatory and unapologetic, and probably resentful of Diagne's intrusion into matters of high colonial policy. Yes, it was true that the high cost of rentals had led to serious overcrowding and then to an overreaction by health authorities. But he personally had explained his administration's position to two Lebu delegations on 19 and 21 May, and had authorized generous compensation. He also insisted that he had already anticipated Diagne's solution of subsidized housing and that he had always been an opponent of the *concessionnaire* system. One week later, Ponty followed up his letter to Diagne with a communication to Lebu village elders repeating his promises about compensation and vowing not to tolerate any land speculation at their expense.[80] In short, despite the governor-general's haughty tone, it could be said that Ponty and Diagne had come to see the plague emergency through the same political prism.

Evidence of an actual understanding emerging between Diagne and Ponty appeared in the press in early September. *La Démocratie* ran a story describing Diagne's conversation with Louis Pasteur's successor as the director of the Pasteur Institute, Dr. Émile Roux. Roux was introduced as an eminent yet disinterested authority because he was not attached to the colonial administration. When Diagne asked what needed to be done to stamp out the plague in Dakar, Roux recommended three steps: (1) less overcrowding and better ventilation in dwellings; (2) more masonry construction; and (3) the destruction of animal and insect vectors of plague.[81]

While Diagne was extending the olive branch to Ponty in early August, and Ponty was deciding how he would respond, the plague raged on. Indeed, mid August proved to be the apogee of the epidemic, while in the month as a whole 380 deaths were recorded. Burnings and relocations also went forward, as did construction work in the new segregation village. On 25 August, the new village was ready to receive its first residents. Meanwhile, tensions continued to rise as Ponty's conciliatory ideas were not yet accepted by the French government in Paris. On 29 August, the minister of colonies wrote Dakar calling for "energetic measures" to put down the disturbances caused by the epidemic.[82]

THE SECOND WAVE OF AFRICAN PROTESTS: AUGUST TO NOVEMBER 1914

The decision to restore the medical emergency, this time with residential segregation and compulsory vaccination, was bound to inflame tensions.

Soon after anti-plague vaccination became mandatory on 2 August, a group of seventy-one artillery workers employed near Ouakam Mamelles as masons, carpenters, painters, and unskilled laborers refused to be inoculated. Raphaël Antonetti, now governor of Senegal, through Delegate Vidal, immediately ordered the men arrested. The procurator-general, however, probably acting on Ponty's orders, refused to prosecute and ordered all the men released.[83]

Some sense of how the war in Europe affected health measures in Dakar during the plague can be gleaned from the testimony to the Procurator-General's Office of the eighty-year-old Samba Guèye, chief of the village of Ouakam. Guèye's remarks also shed light on the dilemma faced by local chiefs in the face of the special privileges offered to certain members of the population:

> From the start of the epidemic which rages at this moment in Dakar, I have recommended that my subjects prohibit access to the village of any native coming from Dakar or from Yoff.
>
> The administration, seeing the epidemic's spread from Yoff, judged it necessary to isolate the village, and to this effect a *cordon sanitaire* was established around it. But after the declaration of war, the *cordon* was completely lifted, and the inhabitants of Yoff were able to circulate freely to Ouakam and to contaminate it. At that point I wrote to the delegate of the government at Dakar to ask him what measures I should take to avoid contagion in my village, and I directed M. Amadou Yadda to go to Dakar to deliver the letter, a copy of which I attach here.
>
> Amadou Yadda was received by M. Mouroux[?] who said: "You tell your chief that there's a war on, and I no longer have any Tirailleurs available to man a *cordon sanitaire*; let him use his own villagers to do surveillance work." But of course we cannot stop native employees of the administration who have full freedom to travel. I have never prevented anybody from freely taking the vaccine if they wanted to. Ask them.[84]

Also pertinent were the statements to the police of two miltary employees from the Ouakam site, Aly Guèye, a forty-four-year-old carpenter who lived in Ouakam, and Assane Niar, a mason at the site. Both men objected strenuously to vaccination. Niar noted that two of his uncles at Yoff had died of plague, even though they had been vaccinated earlier, and that as a married man and the sole supporter of his widowed mother, he could not take the risk. Aly Guèye's actual testimony has survived:

I do not want to be vaccinated because two brothers of mine, one in Dakar, one at Yoff, died after having been vaccinated. I would be prepared to go to war, but I do not want to die from an injection, because I have five children whom I have to raise.

I insist on this right by myself, and not because I am afraid of, or influenced by, anybody else.[85]

The month of September had brought some diminution in plague deaths, but the total of 199 was still substantial. It became clear by the end of the month that tensions remained high in the community. On 26 September, twenty-nine notables, speaking on behalf of the inhabitants of ten neighborhoods and villages in the Dakar area, petitioned Governor-General Ponty.[86] At issue was the segregation village, and who was behind it. By now, the African community completely mistrusted City Hall and the governor of Senegal, and looked to Diagne for support, and ultimately to Ponty for redress. There was the hint of a threat in their remarks:

The only motive for our letter is to know exactly from which source our expropriation originates since the subject seems to be passed from one authority to another. The entire matter is completely unclear, and we want to know as quickly as possible who is the original source. In this manner we will be entirely clear on this point and know how to act in the circumstances. It has been about a month now since the epidemic has ceased to ravage the population, in any case, and that has been noted by the doctors. There are only three or four deaths daily in a city of 40,000 people, counting the strangers.[87]

It was indeed the case that plague deaths were diminishing by this time; the toll went from 199 in September to 107 in October. The African community in Dakar had reason to wonder why expropriations and other control measures remained so severe. As later statistics would reveal (Chart 4.1 above), the plague was indeed burning itself out, though none could know this before the fact.

Ponty, aware of the danger that the possibility of another massive African protest represented now that the war was raging in France, replied to the Africans' petition the next day. This time he made two new and remarkable concessions. First, he declared that removals to the segregation village were only temporary measures. Second, when the villagers returned to their original locales where new homes would be built for them, they would continue to own the dwellings in the segregation village.[88]

If Ponty hoped to buy off the notables with this largesse, the strategy failed. In October, the burnings carried out by the sanitation squads continued. The entire Santiaba district was put to the torch, and the Parc à Fourrages neighborhood was destined to receive the same treatment. On 28 October, however, a sharp confrontation took place there as the inhabitants refused to allow their goods to be moved and the burnings to begin. Ponty was forced to intervene; he granted a delay of two days. But since this would interfere with the forthcoming Muslim feast of Tabaski, the delay was extended until 9 November.[89]

On that day, the worst confrontation of the entire 1914 plague epidemic took place. Despite the fact that a back-up company of Tirailleurs Sénégalais was standing by, and a group of European agents from the Dakar Health Committee was present, the chief commissioner of Dakar was unable to carry out the Health Committee's orders at Parc à Fourrages. Even the presence of four African notables who supported the health measures was insufficient to prevent the confrontation. The commissioner's report to Governor Antonetti in Saint-Louis graphically described the events:

> I sent Elimane Médoune Diène to preach calm and resignation. He was unceremoniously told to go away with the *toubabs*. . . . As soon as the torch was put to the first huts, our *cordon* of agents and police was quickly overrun. Threats and cries were sounded, a variety of weapons, including revolvers, came out, and the first group of protesters was reinforced by natives pouring out of all the huts and alleys of the village: the forces of law and order were confronted with a full-fledged riot. And on Gambetta Avenue, we had to face 3,000 to 4,000 natives who were only waiting for the order to take the offensive. All the Lebu had their boubous tied at the waist, all their *gris-gris* outside, and were armed with the inevitable native dagger, clubs, axes, old trade guns, without counting hidden revolvers. It was at that point that the order came from the governor-general to withdraw.[90]

Desperate for calm to be restored, Ponty must have been delighted at this stage to receive a cable the next day from Blaise Diagne in Orléans. It read: "In solidarity with your efforts in the interests of the population and if you think my presence useful [I] am ready to come to assist you."[91] Ponty's reply showed clearly that he and Diagne were in agreement. "[I] thank you sincerely for your proposal and your steps taken in the interest of the Dakar population. Strongly hope our common efforts will succeed and will permit me soon to announce good news to you. Will keep you posted."[92]

By this time, Ponty was well aware of Diagne's efforts to make his constituents comply with all the sanitary measures dictated by the plague, while at the same time opposing extremists like Antonetti and insisting that Lebu property rights be respected. As Ponty indicated in a telegram to the minister of colonies on 28 October, he had read an exchange of cables between Diagne and one of his representatives in Dakar, Bamar Guèye, when the Parc à Fourrages troubles were beginning. Guèye had alerted Diagne to the refusal of the inhabitants of the Parc and six other villages to relocate. Guèye's cable to Diagne also stated that, while the Lebu knew that Diagne wished them to accept vaccination, they also believed that the deputy did not support removals. Guèye ended by remarking, "Troubles are likely. Please state your views again."[93] Diagne's reply was unequivocal: "If natives desire us to serve them usefully they must follow my counsel and accept vaccination *and* removals."[94]

Diagne had been kept abreast of the events of 9 November. On that day he fired off another cable to Bamar Guèye urging cooperation with Ponty: "Galandou [Diouf] and Crespin have cabled that the population is refusing evacuation contrary to my latest cables and my letter expedited yesterday. Urge you to insist on compliance or will not be able to do anything further for compatriots, whose rights have been guaranteed by the government."[95]

Despite his understanding with Diagne, Ponty nevertheless faced a serious crisis. With Governor Antonetti in Saint-Louis urging him to declare a state of siege, Ponty apparently was prepared to do so, and, presumably, to use military force to bring about the evacuations.[96] While the minister of colonies reluctantly gave Ponty permission, he made it very clear that the war effort took priority over local health considerations in an epidemic that seemed to be running its course. He remarked: "I approve of your actions and your project to place Dakar in a state of siege—but I remind you how dangerous it would be at this moment to have a bloody conflict with Muslim Lebu—the affair would risk being exploited against us by Germany and Turkey in Muslim circles which until now have remained very loyal in all French and British colonies."[97] Clearly the French government was strongly urging an end to the medical emergency on political grounds.

The next day, Ponty wrote back to the ministry, this time with a new request from the Lebu elders. Explaining that the elders would only deal with him personally, and that Diagne had been an enormous help during the latest emergency, Ponty stated that, if the Dakar Health Committee would agree, he wished to allow all those who had accepted three doses of the anti-plague vaccination to be exempt from having to relocate in the segregation village.[98] Reassuring Ponty that he was doing a "great job," the minister hastened to reply the next day that he thought this an excellent idea and also hoped the Health Committee would be agreeable.⁹⁹

The general counselor, Galandou Diouf, at this period still a strong Diagnist, was also lending his cooperation to the new initiative. On 15 November, Diouf notified Ponty that the Lebu were aware that the governor-general's meeting with the medical people would take place the next day, and that the authorities were very "hopeful" that positive results would follow.¹⁰⁰

Faced with this pressure, it is not surprising that the Dakar Health Committee agreed. To all intents and purposes, this last Ponty compromise ended the political crisis. The medical crisis was also winding down. The last planned removals of Africans never took place. The number of victims declined daily and the emergency decrees ceased to be applied after mid November. Officially, the city of Dakar was declared plague-free on 25 January 1915. The only medical writer to comment on the political dimensions of plague, Marcandier, observed that the authorities were forced to back down in the face of the strong show of force by the Africans of the Parc à Fourrages, and that in December, there still remained roughly 200 condemned dwellings which were never destroyed.¹⁰¹

PONTY'S FINAL COMPROMISE

There can be little doubt that the Great War had played a large part in Ponty's decision making in November 1914. His willingness to accept Governor Antonetti's recommendation that he declare a state of siege evaporated once he had received the stern message from Paris that "a bloody conflict with the Muslim Lebu" might have terrible repercussions for French and even British colonialism and the war effort. Yet it should not be concluded that Ponty's choice was simple. Throughout the medical and political crisis of 1914, he had been pushed by French interests in Senegal and especially by Acting Governor Raphaël Antonetti to take a firmer stand against the Diagnists and the Lebu. Antonetti's angry letters to Ponty reveal a hard-line administrator prepared to go to extreme lengths to maintain French control. His strongest views were expressed immediately after the November confrontation.¹⁰² He urged the governor-general to show no leniency to the Lebu protesters. The Lebu of Dakar were responsible for spreading plague to forty villages outside Dakar and Rufisque, with over 2,500 dead. "Entire regions have been devastated by the epidemic, and it could spread further, to the rest of Senegal, even to all of FWA. It would be in the tens of thousands that we would count the dead and Senegal would be ruined for twenty years."[103] For that reason alone, a firm show of force in Dakar was required "to reassure those who are devoted to us, and to frighten those who are hostile."[104]

Blaming "hostile *marabouts*" for the rural resistance, Antonetti urged Ponty to adopt three recommendations: first, a state of siege would be declared in all recalcitrant villages; second, civilian authorities would resume health control measures there with the help of the army; and third, in each case, civil lists would be established, the population disarmed, and people sent to trial immediately. Antonetti added confidently that after one week of this and thirty stiff sentences, all resistance would end. He concluded by stating that Commander-in-Chief General Pinaud, whom he described as "an old Africa hand," endorsed these views.[105]

Although Antonetti's suggested response was extreme, there is no doubt that, based on the reports he was receiving in Saint-Louis, the security situation for the French in Dakar and in the regions of Thiès, Bawol, and the Casamance was a major concern. As the chief commissioner of Dakar had written on 13 November, "for some time now, persistent rumors have spread that the war had obliged us to recall many Whites, many troops and that our means of maintaining order have been significantly reduced."[106]

After months of wavering, Governor-General Ponty, pushed by the Lebu reaction and the signals he was receiving from Paris, finally and firmly rejected Antonetti's strong-armed option. In a strong letter twelve days after the Lebu confrontation, Ponty reprimanded Antonetti for his mishandling of the plague emergency.

Noting that he had personally promised that "each proprietor of burnt huts would be immediately indemnified for his losses," it now turned out that, to Ponty's embarrassment, only 130,000 francs had been paid out in indemnities because the colony's treasurer had exhausted his credits. As a result, many Lebu were left without resolution to their claims. Antonetti was remiss not to have informed Ponty earlier, since the governor-general would have found additional funds immediately. Ponty concluded that this breach of promise "greatly attenuates the responsibility of the Lebu for the serious error they made in opposing the sanitary measures on the 9th of November." Force should be used against the population only when all other steps had been exhausted. At this point, however, since France appeared to have broken its word, conciliation was needed.[107]

In reviewing the course of events in 1914, the political construction and deconstruction of the plague epidemic stands out sharply as one of the most dramatic episodes in Senegal's colonial history. Ultimately, it was the highest political authority in the colony, acting under the watchful eye of his minister in Paris, who determined not so much when the medical emergency had begun as when it had ended, whether or not medical officials agreed with him. At several junctures, Governor-General Ponty had sufficient reasons to justify his actions. Not only did the two phases of the plague emergency correspond with Diagne's election and with the outbreak of war in Europe. Along the way the epidemic generated the most militant popular opposition the young colony had ever experienced, including the first general strike in its history, and several massive street demonstrations, the most serious of which was the confrontation between approximately 4,000 Dakarois, some of them armed, and the forces of law and order. For good measure, the plague emergency was also partially responsible for the popular perception that a plot existed to assassinate Blaise Diagne, and for the creation of the Médina, Dakar's first encounter with formally sanctioned residential segregation.

NOTES

1. Dr. L. Huot, Director of the Health Service of Senegal, "Rapport d'ensemble sur l'épidémie de peste 1914-1915," Dakar, 3 March 1915, ANS\H55 (hereafter cited as Huot, "Rapport d'ensemble").
2. *L'AOF*, 16 May 1914, 1.
3. André Marcandier, "La peste à Dakar (1914–15)," *Archives de Médecine Navale* 106 (1918): 192.
4. *L'AOF*, 16 May 1914.
5. *L'AOF*, "The Riot," 23 May 1914.
6. Elikia Mbokolo, "Peste et société urbaine à Dakar: L'épidèmie de 1914," *Cahiers d'Études Africaines* 22 (1982): 40.
7. Anonymously cited in Iba Der Thiam, "L'évolution politique et syndicale du Sénégal colonial de 1840 à 1936" (thèse d'état, Université de Paris I, Paris, 1982–83), 1647.
8. Thiam, "L'évolution politique," vol. 4, 1649.
9. Thiam, "L'évolution politique," vol. 4, 1649. Marcandier, "La peste," 192, asserts that the protests led Ponty to suspend house burnings, despite the spread of the epidemic in June. The measures were only resumed after mid July.
10. Thiam, "L'évolution politique," vol. 4, 1655.
11. ANS\H55, Ponty to Minister of Colonies, 27 May 1914.
12. *La Démocratie*, 6 June 1914.
13. *La Démocratie*'s headline on 30 May 1914 proclaimed: "Starve those who wish to starve others. For major wrongs, major remedies."
14. Thiam, "L'évolution politique," vol. 4, 1667–68.
15. Cited in Thiam, "L'évolution politique," vol. 4, 1673.
16. ANS\20G\21, Diagne to Ponty, from Rufisque, telegram of 25 May 1914.

17. ANS\H55, Ponty to Minister of Colonies, 27 May 1914. *La Démocratie* of 6 June 1914 reported on Ponty's actions in an unsigned article entitled "A Nice Gesture."
18. Thiam, "L'évolution politique," vol. 4, 1706–07.
19. *La Démocratie*, 23 May 1914.
20. *La Démocratie*, 25 May 1914.
21. Thiam, "L'évolution politique," vol. 4, 1650–51.
22. Thiam, "L'évolution politique," vol. 4, 1656.
23. Thiam, "L'évolution politique," vol. 4, 1652.
24. *L'AOF*, 30 May 1914.
25. Thiam, "L'évolution politique," vol. 4, 1671.
26. ANS\20G\21, Antonetti to Ponty, 10 June 1914.
27. ANS\20G\21, Antonetti to Ponty, 10 June 1914. It is astonishing that such a high colonial official suggested political assassination in writing. It must be assumed that other eyes had access to this letter.
28. ANS 20G\21, Ponty to Minister of Colonies, 24 June 1914. As Johnson points out, the argument was specious since Heimburger was not registered either. G. Wesley Johnson, *The Emergence of Black Politics in Senegal: The Struggle for Power in the Four Communes, 1900–1920* (Stanford, Calif.: Stanford University Press, 1971), 175.
29. ANS\H55, Ponty to Minister of Colonies, 27 May 1914.
30. ANS\H55, Ponty to Minister of Colonies, 27 May 1914. Ponty's report gave the clear impression that Diagne was in hiding.
31. Thiam, "L'évolution politique," vol. 4, 1675. Thiam adds that Diagne was in Saint-Louis between 21 and 25 May when the acting governor, Antonetti, announced that Diagne had given him his personal assurance that he would attempt to calm his partisans in Dakar. But there is no evidence that Diagne met Antonetti face-to-face to communicate this assurance. The fact that Antonetti did not stipulate a date would suggest that they did not meet.
32. *La Démocratie*, 23 May 1914; and ANS\H55, 25 May 1914, Diagne cable to Ponty.
33. Thiam, "L'évolution politique," is the only author to discuss Diagne's disappearance in the three weeks following the election. He strongly defends Diagne for having gone to ground to protect himself.
34. Thiam, "L'évolution politique," vol. 4, 1674.
35. Thiam identifies Ndéné Mbaye as his source for these events not in vol. 4 of "L'évolution politique," where the aftermath of the election is discussed, but in vol. 9, index, 356. Thiam states that the interview took place in 1974 in Mbaye's home in the Médina district of Rufisque. Mbaye's reconstruction of events has to be treated with some caution, and so too does Thiam's use of this evidence. While Thiam accepts Mbaye's version of the plot against Diagne as gospel in vol. 4, 1674, in vol. 5, 2000, Thiam takes issue with Marc Michel for having accepted Mbaye's criticism of Diagne regarding military recruitment in 1918. For Mbaye's version of Diagne's activities after the election, see Thiam, "L'évolution politique," vol. 4, 1674–79.
36. ANS\H55, Ponty to Minister of Colonies, 27 May 1914.
37. *L'AOF*, 27 June 1914.

38. Johnson, *The Emergence*, 176.
39. ANS\H55, Ponty to Minister of Colonies, 27 May 1914.
40. Several have put forward this argument but none better than Rosenberg. See Charles Rosenberg, "What Is an Epidemic? AIDS in Historical Perspective," *Daedalus* 118 (1989): 1–17.
41. Two articles by Luise White invite comparisons with African discourse in East Africa. See "Vampire Priests of Central Africa: African Debates about Labor and Religion in Colonial Northern Zambia," *Comparative Studies in Society and History* 35 (1993): 746–72; and "Tsetse Visions: Narratives of Blood and Bugs in Colonial Northern Rhodesia," *Journal of African History* 36 (1995): 219–45.
42. Mbokolo, "Peste," 25.
43. Marcandier, "La peste," 139.
44. *Bulletin du Comité d'Afrique française*, June 1914, 272.
45. Johnson, *Emergence*, 176–77. The committee did not at this time decide whether Diagne was a citizen, but accepted the historic tradition of voting rights among the *originaires* of Senegal.
46. Thiam, "L'évolution politique," vol. 4, 1741.
47. Huot, "Rapport d'ensemble."
48. Marcandier, "La peste," 139.
49. The leading authority on the creation of the Médina, Dakar's monument to sanitary segregation, is Raymond Betts. He has written on the subject in the following works: "The Problem of the Medina in the Urban Planning of Dakar, Senegal," *Urban African Notes* 4 (1969): 5–15; "The Establishment of the Medina in Dakar, Senegal, 1914," *Africa* 41 (1971): 143–52; and "Dakar, ville impériale," in *Colonial Cities: Essays on Urbanism in a Colonial Context*, edited by Robert Ross and Gerard J. Telkamp (Dordrecht, Holland: Martinus Nijhoff Publishers, 1985), 193–206.
50. Thiam, "L'évolution politique," 1741.
51. Assane Seck, *Dakar, métropole ouest-africaine* (Dakar: IFAN, 1970), 129, 131, and map, 130. The community of Hock was divided into two new locations some distance apart, Hock-Fann and Hock-Colobane.
52. Roger Pasquier, "Villes du Sénégal au XIXe siècle," *Revue Française d'Histoire d'Outre-Mer* 47, nos. 168/69 (1960): 419.
53. Seck, *Dakar*, 131. The name "Médina" was not immediately attached to what the French first called simply "the segregation village." Sylla states that the plan was to call it "village William Ponty" after Ponty's death in 1915, but the Lebu objected, and, on the advice of Al-Hajj Malik Sy, chose "Médina" instead. Assane Sylla, *Le peuple Lébou de la presqu'île du Cap-Vert* (Dakar: Les Nouvelles Éditions Africaines du Sénégal, 1992), 74.
54. Armand-Pierre Angrand, *Les Lébous de la presqu'île du Cap-Vert, Essai sur leur histoire et leurs coutumes* (Dakar: La Maison du livre, 1946), 124.
55. ANS\H55, Dr. Guyot to Governor-General, 24 April 1916.
56. Collomb, Huot, and Lecomte, "Note sur l'épidémie de peste au Sénégal en 1914," *Annales de Hygiène et de Médecine Coloniales* 19 (1921): 63. The official decree was not promulgated until 18 August.
57. ANS\H57, Minutes of the Dakar Health Committee, 7 July 1914.

58. Mbokolo, "Peste," 38. Salleras regards this 24 July legislation as the most important in the history of Dakar because it made segregation legal. At the same time, he offers the conservative view that "the creation of the Médina was a voluntarist and coherent response to the structural and conjunctural difficulties that the colonial administration faced." Salleras, "La peste," 12, 115.

59. Collomb, Huot, and Lecomte, "Note," 69.

60. ANS\2G14\20. "Rapport sur l'épidémie de peste," circa July 1914.

61. Collomb, Huot, and Lecomte, "Note," 69.

62. Marcandier, "La peste," 193.

63. Betts, "The Establishment of the Medina," 148.

64. Raphaël Antonetti, Acting Governor of Senegal, Address at the opening of the General Council on 1 October 1914, in *Conseil Général, procès verbal des délibérations, session of October 1914* (Paris and Saint-Louis: Imprimerie du Gouvernement, 1915), 12–21 (Hereafter cited as Antonetti, "Address").

65. ANS\3G2\160, 4 May 1916 Petition to the Governor-General of FWA.

66. Betts, "The Problem of the Medina," 6. Betts adds that, although it was begun as a "planned ghetto," the Médina grew haphazardly, and at the end of the 1920s housed only 8,000 of the 20,000 Africans living in Dakar.

67. For example, the newspapers were full of the scandal associated with Madame Caillaux, who had shot the editor of *Figaro*, and whose murder trial daily revealed "unpleasant irregularities in finance, the press, the courts, the government." Barbara W. Tuchman, *The Guns of August* (New York: Dell, 1962), 107.

68. Marc Michel, *L'appel à l'Afrique: Contributions et réaction à l'effort de guerre en AOF, 1914–1919* (Paris: Publications de la Sorbonne, 1982), 41.

69. Ponty to Reynaud, on 29 July 1914, and Reynaud's reply on 31 July 1914 in Michel, *L'appel*, 43–44.

70. Michel, *L'appel*, 43–44.

71. Ponty to Doumergue, 27 August 1914, in Michel, *L'appel* 43. Doumergue had just replaced Reynaud as minister of colonies.

72. Michel, *L'appel*, 44–45. Senegal's share of these levies: for the first recruitment period in September–October 1914, 1,400 men out of 8,000 (17 percent); for the second levy in February, 1915, 1,000 out of 10,000 (10 percent); and for the third levy, May–September 1915, 800 out of 5,500 (14.5 percent). Overall, Senegal contributed 3,200 out of 24,500 men, or 13 percent. Senegal's high share of the total contingent was attributed to the unrest and other recruitment problems in such recently conquered territories as Mauritania and Niger. For an extensive analysis of Senegalese recruitment, see Joe Lunn, *Memoirs of the Maelstrom: A Senegalese Oral History of the First World War* (Portsmouth, N.H.: Heinemann, 1999).

73. Michel, *L'appel*, 51.

74. No names of generals or regiments were given out, and no casualty figures released. In the absence of concrete news, foolish optimism prevailed. It was widely reported that the Belgian forts at Liège had held out for two weeks in August whereas in reality the German advance had been delayed by only two days. Tuchman, *Guns*, 214, 218–20.

75. For full accounts of African participation in the First World War, see Myron Echenberg, *Colonial Conscripts: The Tirailleurs Sénégalais in French West Africa*,

1857–1960 (Portsmouth, N.H.: Heinemann, 1991); Michel, *L'appel*; and Lunn, *Memoirs*.

76. ANS\H55, Diagne to Ponty, 11 August 1914. The letter was in stencil form, suggesting that Diagne wanted the letter widely distributed among his supporters in Senegal and in France.

77. ANS\H55, Diagne to Ponty, 11 August 1914.

78. The letter was dated 17 August 1914 and was published on 9 September in *La Démocratie* as part of a front-page article on the war.

79. ANS\H55, Ponty to Diagne, 16 September 1914.

80. ANS\H55, Ponty to Lebu elders, 27 September 1914.

81. *La Démocratie*, 9 September 1914. Significantly, Ponty's letter to Diagne a week later cited the newspaper piece about Roux, suggesting not only that Ponty was reading the hostile press carefully, but that he recognized that Diagne and the Diagnists were willing to back reasonable sanitary control measures.

82. ANS\H55, Minister of Colonies to Ponty, 29 August 1914.

83. ANS\H55, Vidal to Procurator-General, 3 September 1914, calling for "sanctions without mercy" against the men. When it became clear that the courts were not going to come down hard, Antonetti wrote Ponty protesting the procurator's "laxity," and arguing that it was "more necessary than ever to apply the law rigorously." ANS\H55, Antonetti to Ponty, 1 October 1914.

84. ANS\H55, 8 September 1914, Minutes of the testimony of M. Samba Guèye, eighty years of age, village chief of Ouakam, to the Procurator-General's office.

85. ANS\H55, 8 September 1914, declaration to police.

86. ANS\H55, Petition to Governor-General Ponty of 26 September 1914. The locales were listed as Hock, Parc à Fourrages, Tiedème, Mbott, Yaghoul, Dièko, Gouye Salane, Souf, Kaye Guelh, and Thiérigne.

87. ANS\H55, Petition to Governor-General Ponty of 26 September 1914.

88. ANS\H55, Ponty's reply to the petition, Dakar, 27 September 1914.

89. Mbokolo, "Peste," 41.

90. ANS\ H55, 13 November 1914, Chief Commissioner of Dakar to the Governor of Senegal.

91. ANS\H55, Cable from Diagne to Ponty, 10 November 1914.

92. ANS\H55, Cable, Ponty to Diagne, 11 November 1914.

93. ANS\H55, Undated excerpt from cable sent by Ponty to the Minister of Colonies, Dakar to Bordeaux, 28 October 1914.

94. ANS\H55, Undated excerpt from cable sent by Ponty to the Minister of Colonies, Dakar to Bordeaux, 28 October 1914.

95. ANS\H55, Diagne cable to Bamar Guèye, 9 November 1914.

96. Ponty's communication to the minister of colonies requesting approval of his decision to place Dakar in a state of siege was probably sent on 10 or 11 November, but it is missing from the record. We do have the minister's reply granting approval on 12 November. ANS\H55, Minister of Colonies to Ponty, Bordeaux to Dakar, 12 November 1914.

97. ANS\H55, Minister of Colonies to Ponty, Bordeaux to Dakar, 12 November 1914.

98. ANS\H55, Dakar to Bordeaux, Ponty to Minister of Colonies, 13 November 1914.

99. ANS\H55, Minister of Colonies to Ponty, 14 November 1914.
100. ANS\H55, Diouf to Ponty, 15 November 1914.
101. Marcandier, "La peste," 192.
102. ANS\1H79\163, Antonetti to Ponty, 15 November 1914.
103. ANS\1H79\163, Antonetti to Ponty, 15 November 1914.
104. ANS\1H79\163, Antonetti to Ponty, 15 November 1914.
105. ANS\1H79\163, Antonetti to Ponty, 15 November 1914. Three days later, Antonetti wrote General Pinaud requesting 100 to 200 soldiers to back up his medical and civilian personnel in the Thiès region. ANS\H55, Antonetti to the Général Commandant Supérieur, Saint-Louis to Dakar, 18 November 1914.

106. ANS\H55, Chief Commissioner, Dakar, to Governor, Saint-Louis, 13 November 1914.

107. Ponty's final remarks were sheer sophistry: "I realize you know too well the mentality of Blacks not to share with me the knowledge that the first rule of native policy for a leader is to keep promises made to them, without the slightest exception, regardless of the circumstances." ANS\H55, Ponty to Antonetti, 21 November 1914.

5

THE MEDICAL RESPONSE

The last two chapters of Part One examine the medical aspects of the plague emergency. The present chapter investigates the medical personnel involved and the four types of control measures they implemented. The following chapter measures the demographic and financial costs, the gender, ethnicity, and occupation of the plague victims, and plague's diffusion into the interior of Senegal. Part One ends with a general overview of epidemic plague and Senegalese society between 1914 and 1918.

THE MEDICAL PERSONNEL

The French physicians and researchers involved in combating plague in Senegal formed an important but overlooked component of what Michel Foucault has called a "power-knowledge regime." Just as Frederick Cooper has shown how French and British labor inspectors in colonial Africa articulated the knowledge upon which their claims to power lay, in similar fashion and in a crisis of dramatic proportions, French biomedical experts in Dakar exercised power based upon their claims to knowledge.[1] On the one hand, the medical specialists were concerned to stress their expertise versus that of the civilian authorities. Yet at the same time, both civil and medical officials were determined to use medical knowledge to justify their continuing rule over Africans, whose forms of knowledge were either irrelevant, or worse, distorted and harmful to the public good.[2] Both groups of French decision makers brought with them cultural baggage which denigrated Africans, while at the same time permitting facile generalizations about a complex continent. As Valentin Mudimbe has put it, various forms of "invented Africa" were fundamental to the colonial experience.[3] During the Dakar medical crisis of 1914, such constructions took the place of wisdom and understanding.

The medical experts who played a major role in the 1914 epidemic exemplified what was becoming an important division in twentieth-century biomedicine, the practicing physician versus the medical researcher. In Dakar, the biomedical researchers operated out of the new Bacteriological Laboratory of French West Africa (BLFWA).[4] It was headed in 1914–15 by Alexandre Lafont, who had succeeded André Thiroux, the laboratory's first director. During the epidemic, Lafont was aided by two energetic assistants, an old Africa hand, Dr. Alexandre Kermorgant, and Dr. Ferdinand Heckenroth, who would serve as acting director in 1915 and 1916.[5]

The practitioners outnumbered the researchers and had far more decision-making power. The colony of Senegal's Health Service was almost exclusively composed of clinicians, and only they represented the medical community on the Dakar Health Committee in 1914.[6] Clinicians in early twentieth-century Senegal were almost entirely state employees, and members of a branch of the military, the Health Corps of the Colonial Army, having been trained in tropical medicine at the École de "Pharo" in Marseille after completing medical school either at the army's medical school in Lyon or the navy's in Bordeaux.[7] Military physicians in French West Africa treated both military and civilian personnel, depending on their commissions, and far outnumbered civilian doctors.

Five medical authorities have left written records of the 1914 Senegalese plague epidemic, and together, their works constitute important source material. Their accounts all share certain assumptions couched in medical language, for example, their belief in residential segregation for sanitary reasons.[8] On the other hand, a careful reading of their work shows considerable disagreement over the medical community's handling of the epidemic.

Not surprisingly, Dr. L. Huot, chief of the Senegal Health Service, whose writings include a massive document entitled "Rapport d'ensemble sur l'épidémie de peste 1914–1915," was extremely defensive about his service's performance.[9] At the BLFWA, Alexandre Kermorgant went on record in praise of Western biomedicine, and blamed Africans in general and Muslims in particular for refusing to cooperate with public health officials.[10] The director of the BLFWA, Alexandre Lafont, was more balanced in his assessment, perhaps because, as a recent arrival in Senegal, he was relatively free from strong biases against the local population. What distinguished Lafont from Huot and Kermorgant was his willingness to probe more deeply into the lived experience of the 1914 epidemic. Like Lafont, the navy physician André Marcandier was new to Dakar.[11] His account of the plague was similarly balanced, as well as being the only one that displayed a sense of compassion for all those who suffered during this terrible time, perhaps because Marcandier had personally conducted interviews with Africans as part of his inquiry into the origins of the plague.[12] The fifth account, and the most devastating critique of health officials' handling of the 1914 epidemic, was penned by an obscure physician with a sharp ax to grind, Dr. Paul Rousseau.[13] His general tone can be discerned from his angry assertion that in Senegal, "medical assistance to natives is a myth, and as for sanitary prevention and defence I have shown it is nonexistent."[14]

QUARANTINE AND *CORDONS*

Quarantine was the oldest control measure known to European health officials, with its roots dating back to medieval times. Though it predated germ theory and disease specificity by centuries, it was a method not without merit for diseases in which humans were the main carriers. Isolation of index cases, suspects, and so-called "healthy carriers" remained an important control measure in smallpox and typhoid epidemics, when disease could spread directly from person to person. Quarantine was ineffective, however, for diseases with insect vectors, such as yellow fever, malaria, or bubonic plague. While it isolated some humans thought to be infective from others, it had little or no effect on the main vehicle of infection, the biting insect.

Such an analysis, however, presumes not simply an awareness of the insect vector, but a penetration of epidemiological theory into sanitary practice. That would require at least a generation, until newly trained specialists and their techniques displaced earlier personnel and practices. In 1914, as in 1900, when the third pandemic made its way round the world, quarantine and isolation, together with the establishment of *cordons sanitaires* enforced by the military, remained standard practice.

Officials regarded quarantine and *cordons sanitaires* as their best means of containing the plague outbreak of 1914. Quarantine was initially declared on 13 May, and a *cordon* immediately established between Hann and Cambérène in an attempt to separate the Cape Verde peninsula from the rest of the colony. On 18 May, the Dakar Health Committee established a second *cordon* inside the city in an effort to isolate the Africans living in and around Blanchot, Thiers, and Grammont streets from the wealthier section of town to the south. But the economic requirements of life in Dakar exempted many Africans whose labor was indispensable, and so many thousands of *laissez-passers* were issued that any possible value of such a *cordon* was compromised. The language of the Health Committee, apart from being discriminatory, was in fact an indication of how commercial interests, which were well represented on the committee, were reluctant to see their employees pre-

The Medical Response

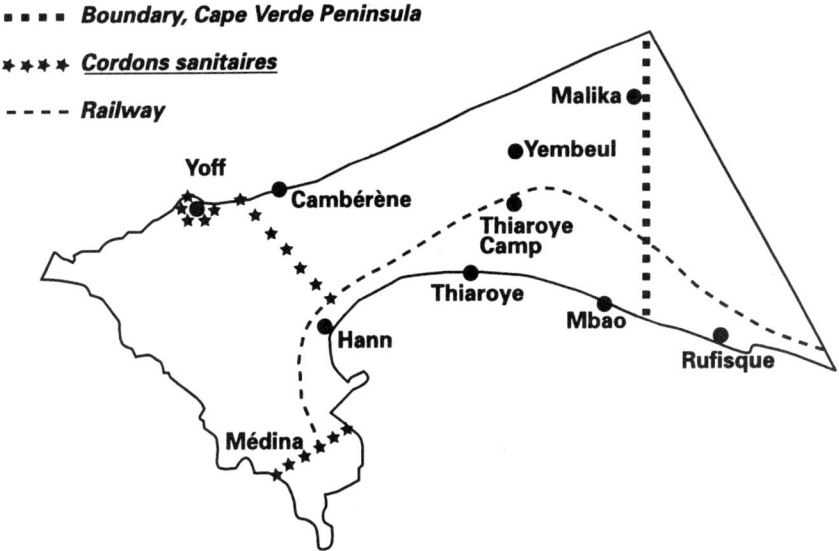

Map 5.1 *Cordons Sanitaires* Established in 1914. This map has been adapted by the author from data in ANS\H55, Dr. Huot, "Rapport d'ensemble."

vented from traveling to work. "The Europeans are authorized to travel everywhere freely. Those natives regarded as indispensable to the material life of Dakar, employees of the commercial houses, of the administration, those involved in the cleansing of buildings and streets, will be supplied with a travel permit upon request from their employers."[15]

The soldiers who manned the *cordons* were usually illiterate and often allowed through individuals who showed any sort of written documentation. Not surprisingly, *Yersinia pestis* easily leaped over these initial barriers and was soon rampant in newly infected districts, such as the customs area on the border of the Avenue Faidherbe.[16] By 20 May, there were enough cases outside the *cordon sanitaire* to show that the entire city was contaminated.[17] Nevertheless, the authorities were reluctant to apply emergency regulations to the entire city, including the mixed and European quarters. The *cordon*, in short, had been designed to isolate infected Africans, but not necessarily infected rats, and certainly not Europeans. Not until 24 July did officials extend the plague regulations to include the entire urban area of Dakar, as defined by a line from the sea to the racetrack.[18]

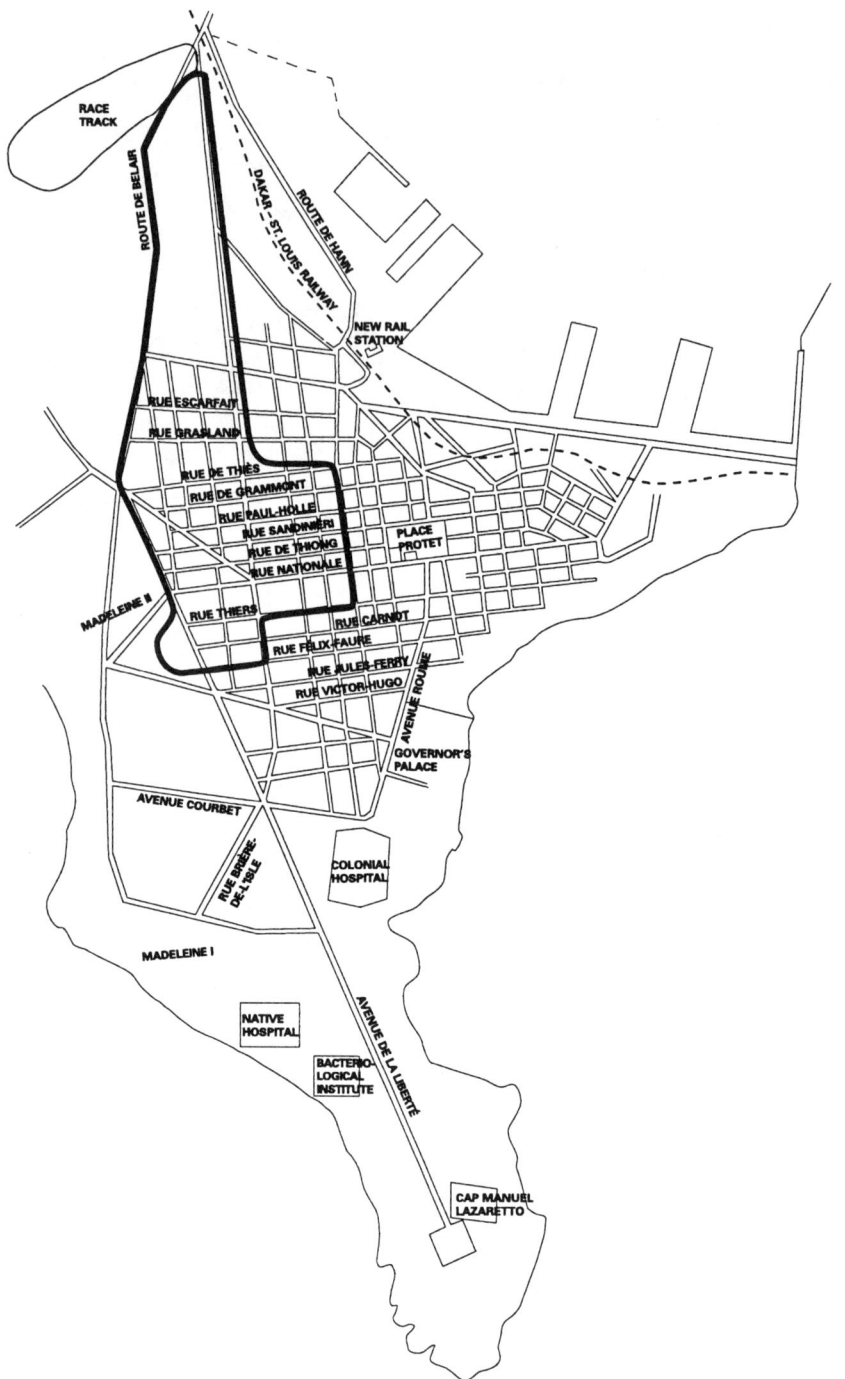

Map 5.2 Plague Zone in Dakar, 1914. This map has been adapted by the author from data in ANS\H55, Dr. Huot, "Rapport d'ensemble."

Included in the quarantine system was the creation of isolation camps, called lazarettos, for the temporary housing of "suspects." Suspects included all relatives and friends who had been in contact with a plague patient at any time during his or her infection. Since such people might be carrying *Y. pestis*, they were to be kept under observation for a prescribed period in the lazarettos. When plague began in Dakar, the city found itself with a single lazaretto with a capacity of only 700 to 800 people.[19] The 13 May emergency decree called for five days of isolation. But on 22 May, two Africans who had been discharged from the lazaretto three days previously died of plague. Judging that five days was too short a period, officials doubled the period of isolation in the lazaretto to ten days.[20] Between 13 May and 1 June, some 405 individuals passed through the lazaretto. During the epidemic's hiatus in mid June, when authorities felt free to lift the emergency regulations, the lazaretto closed its doors to the general public and was converted into a medical center for African troops. The closure of the original lazaretto created a pressing need for a new isolation camp once plague surged again in July and was a strong motive for the creation of the new segregated village, which would solve two problems at once for the Dakar Health Committee. The new isolation camp was built to the north, near Hann, and consisted of a barracks and huts, with one doctor, a couple of African medical assistants, and a nurse in attendance. The ten-day isolation period allowed the staff to complete vaccinations, disinfect the goods and clothing of the suspects, and send them on their way to the new village.[21]

By 25 August, authorities were finally able to state that the new lazaretto at Bel-Air and the new segregation village on the Ouakam road (it was not to acquire the name "Médina" until the following year) were both in operation. Some 2,900 people, the entire population of Santiaba quarter next to the railway depot, and the most ravaged of all neighborhoods by the epidemic, were evacuated, with everybody residing in the new lazaretto for ten days before continuing on to the new village. All the straw huts were burned save those capable of being transported to the new village after thorough disinfection.[22] At a rate of some fifty to sixty persons each day (the process took two months to complete), people were transferred to the new lazaretto, which had three large barracks in wood, divided into twenty compartments, each receiving six persons. To these were added twenty-five straw huts, each large enough to lodge eight or ten Africans. Each set of barracks or huts formed a district isolated from the others, each with its own kitchen and toilets. The lazaretto housed a large disinfection chamber where the inmates' possessions were subjected to sulphur fumes for twenty-four hours.[23]

In contrast to the civilian sector, the navy took the epidemic seriously from the outset and was able to establish a much tighter security net around its perimeter. The navy's arsenal was located in the north of the city between the Hann road and the Dakar-Saint-Louis rail line.[24] On 12 May, the navy declared the contaminated districts of the city off-limits to all European sailors and *laptots*. Night leave was canceled and crews restricted to the barracks and navy yards. Women, who until then had brought meals to *laptots*, were now forbidden entry to the barracks or to the arsenal area. Their calabashes were deposited at a designated door, where the interested parties could claim them. On 19 May, with health conditions in the town worsening, this privilege of receiving food was withdrawn; from that point onward, *laptots* were fed within the arsenal in the same manner as the European sailors. All communication with persons outside the naval perimeter was now prohibited.

Other navy measures were directed at civilian workers. All, including domestics, were subjected to a compulsory medical examination, the home address of each was noted, and an inquiry was made every time one of them missed work. The hiring of new workers was suspended.[25]

When it was realized that domestic inquiries were impossible due to the uncertainty of addresses and what Marcandier called "the bad will" of Africans, the base commander ordered the firing of all African workers and apprentices whose absence from morning call was noticed. Finally, as of 18 May, all workers and apprentices whose tasks were not urgent were let go. After 22 May, the entire navy basin was closed except for emergency repairs, and an interior fence was erected to keep workers in the commercial port away from the navy basin. Yet another high fence was erected to the north to keep Africans from the Parc à Fourrages neighborhood from entering a navy housing area by walking beside the sea. European sailors were permitted morning and afternoon leave in town on Sunday, but sailors of all ranks and races were confined day and night the rest of the week. Once vaccinations began on 29 May, *laptots* were allowed to communicate with their families from a distance, but had to avoid close contact. Only in early June, when conditions in town were officially declared improved, were Africans permitted some contact, but only if their entire families had been vaccinated. Night leave, however, remained in suspension, and access to certain quarters of town "rigorously forbidden."[26] Permission to attend funerals of parents was given only after an inquiry into the cause of death. Leave to locales outside Dakar was denied until an inquiry into their sanitary situation had given these locales a clean bill of health.

With the resurgence of plague in July, the navy restored its strict controls. Not until Africans had received two more vaccination shots were they permitted some freedom of movement. Civilian workers who had not received their third shot by 26 July (they were given three days' notice), were fired immediately. Even if some movement off the base was permitted, night leave was not allowed, with the exception of noncommissioned officers and married sailors who could certify that their families had been installed in the new segregation village.[27] The navy did not lift its quarantine controls until 11 February 1915. Marcandier stated afterward that this rigor kept the navy yards and its personnel plague free. The navy's closest call was the detection in August of plague-infected rats on the premises of a school for apprentice mechanics of FWA in the naval yards. The area was totally evacuated, the students were sent to barracks, and they were allowed to return to their school only after it was completely disinfected and Marcandier was confident that the epizootic was completely over.[28]

Writing after the epidemic, Lafont was particularly critical of the whole *cordon sanitaire* exercise. In his view, the Dakar experience demonstrated the futility of a *cordon* when the epidemic was detected so late, and when the African and European towns were tightly interwoven. In such instances, not only did the entire city have to be quarantined, but sanitary defence had to be preplanned and launched automatically, not hastily put into place, as in Dakar. Lazarettos and segregation villages had to be ready for occupancy at the first signs of an outbreak, and equipped with disinfection agents. Also required was surveillance of neighboring colonies and updated documentation on the history of prior epidemics. Clearly, Dakar authorities had failed to take any of these precautions.[29]

Not only did *cordons* fail to do any good, they can actually be said to have done harm. The decision to encircle the Lebu fishing village of Yoff, located on the Cape Verde peninsula some 12 kilometers from Dakar, was perhaps the most terrible blunder in the entire 1914 epidemic. The village's fate in 1914 evokes comparison with that of earlier bubonic plague hecatombs such as Eyam, Derbyshire, in 1665, or Marseille in 1721.[30] As early as May, isolated cases began to occur in Yoff, although the medical authorities did not become aware of this until 27 June.[31] The illness was probably brought in by fishermen going to and from Dakar to sell their catch. It was later determined from oral accounts that casualties had risen daily from the beginning of May until they reached the staggering rate of fifteen to twenty a day in this village of 2,000 inhabitants. By the end of June, over 600 people had died of plague and the number would continue to rise.[32] Yoff was an ideal incubator for plague with its closely clustered straw huts and its women and children in constant contact with the sick, amidst generally unsanitary conditions.³³ Before the plague burned itself out in September, Yoff had doubled its death rate to reach the staggering total of 550 deaths per 1,000.

The hecatomb at Yoff had human as well as natural causes. When they discovered the epidemic raging in Yoff in late June, French medical authorities threw a military *cordon* of 150 Tirailleurs Sénégalais around the village. Authorities provided a daily ration of 500 grams of rice, 50 grams of oil, 40 grams of salt, and 250 grams of fish or meat per person. Presumably, this diet was inadequate because several villagers developed beriberi. The weakened condition of the inhabitants of Yoff may very well have contributed to the progress of the plague epidemic because daily casualty rates soared to as many as twenty-five or thirty, with no improvement until August when the survivors were transferred to a new location.³⁴

The health authorities, alarmed by the deteriorating conditions at Yoff, finally responded with a few measures. To combat the food shortages which had led to beriberi outbreaks, Dr. Huot ordered the *cordon* widened so that villagers could have access to their manioc and potato fields some 2 kilometers from Yoff. He also ordered Haffkine vaccinations for the entire village.³⁵ Nevertheless, the death rate declined only temporarily to twelve in early July before doubling to a high of twenty-five as the month wore on. French health officials were to complain later that Yoff villagers refused a second vaccination and would only accept with the greatest reluctance the isolation of the sick and the disinfection of their goods. The same report acknowledged that one good reason for the Yoff villagers' reluctance to see their houses destroyed was that the seaside village was built on sandy soil and no new building material was available. The French found themselves obliged to allow villagers to rebuild their village with straw materials that had been disinfected, at a new site some 500 meters away from the original one. Almost immediately, the death rate in the old village fell to four or five a day; by 15 August the epidemic was declared ended.³⁶ Because the Yoff epidemic raged continuously from May until August or even later, some authorities suspected that it might have been responsible for reinfecting Dakar in July.³⁷

Even if Yoff is set aside as an honest if terrible mistake, the attempts to control plague by means of quarantine, *cordons*, and travel restrictions were doomed to failure. The physical geography of the Cape Verde peninsula provided innumerable water routes used by all manner of small fishing boats and other vessels. Blaise Diagne's alleged flight first to Rufisque and then to France was in part achieved by water, although, in fleeing to Rufisque, he may not have been escaping plague at all, since the disease quickly traveled there as well. Discriminatory regulations prejudiced the trading activities of Syrians, Moroccans, and the African majority, many of whom were competing with French trading houses for the lucrative peanut crop. The losses of the majority population in manpower, livelihood, and morale far outweighed any benefits that might have accrued from such draconian control techniques.

DISINFECTION, INCINERATION, AND BURIAL

In addition to quarantine, disinfection or incineration of dwellings and property and insistence on specific burial practices constituted a second category of what might be termed classic epidemic control measures. The physicians of the Health Service were in charge of the sanitary squads which carried out these measures. They made the initial determination of which homes were capable of being disinfected, and which should be burned. That same day, the "Commission on Unsanitary Buildings" performed an evaluation for purposes of later compensation. Official statistics registered the disinfection of 280 buildings and the burning of 1,594 dwellings, a total far in excess of the 120 homes burnt during the minor yellow fever epidemic of 1912.[38]

The disinfection method for dwellings consisted of spraying with the Clayton apparatus and cleansing with a creosote solution. The French navy went further in the disinfection of its property, using sulphuric acid for all buildings inhabited by crews, including the barracks, the infirmary, the jail, and the sleeping quarters of tugs and sailing vessels. Hammocks, sleeping bags, and other bedding were all treated with strong chemicals. All Africans, including apprentice mechanics, were required to bathe in a solution of creosote, and the Europeans' barracks were washed with the same product.[39]

The literate inhabitants of Dakar, who were very largely French, were also encouraged to disinfect their homes. The makers of one commercial antiseptic manufactured in Paris with the brand name of "Aniodol," hoping to capitalize on fears of plague sweeping Dakar in May 1914, changed their advertisement in *L'AOF* at that time to include plague among the long list of "microbes" which their product could "instantly destroy."[40]

The first burnings were authorized by the emergency legislation of 13 May, which made no provision for where Africans might live during and after the destruction of their homes, nor exactly how their compensation would be determined. In July, however, the legislation was made slightly more precise, indicating that compensation would be paid to owners, not renters, and that in certain circumstances, those Africans

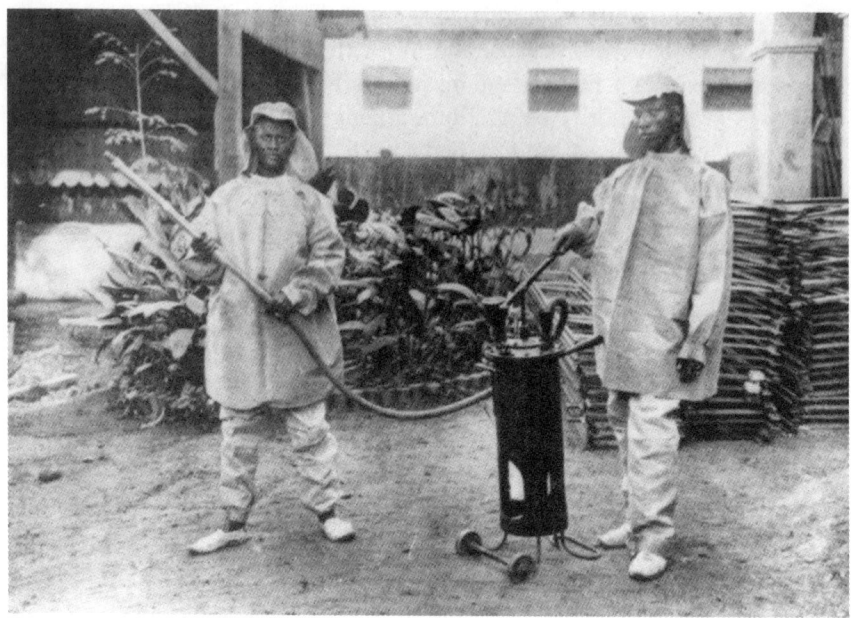

Photo 5.1 Disinfection Crew, Dakar Health Service, c. 1908. From Georges Ribot and Robert Lafon, *Dakar. Ses origins, son avenir* (Bordeaux: G. Delmas, 1908), 149.

who had clear title to their land and wished to rebuild in the European manner would be permitted to do so.[41] The Municipal Council's plan was to move the overwhelming majority of Africans into segregated housing in the planned new village. Only two councillors protested against total segregation, arguing that some Africans, presumably *originaires*, should be allowed to rebuild on their own land.[42]

Incineration measures had mixed results. The burnings did destroy infected fleas, larvae, and even rats, although they may also have caused some individuals who were already incubating bubonic plague to escape and spread the disease.[43] On the other hand, these control efforts destroyed public morale, raised serious issues of fair compensation for lost property, and, most significantly, contributed to overcrowding. The issue of providing shelter for the dispossessed seems to have been entirely ignored during the days immediately following the official declaration of the outbreak. Perhaps the authorities assumed that the epidemic would be minor, and the numbers of uprooted people small. The decision to halt emergency measures provided a respite in June. But when incineration resumed in intensity in July and August, people had no choice but to crowd into existing housing or, in some cases, to rebuild their straw huts in quarters of town relatively lightly touched to that point. One such neighborhood was the Parc à Fourrages, where overcrowding became pronounced with the arrival of more dispossessed people. Plague, however, followed people to the Parc à Fourrages; it was one of the most seriously infected quarters when the Dakar epidemic reached its peak in mid August.[44] The failure of the authorities to make available adequate alternative housing was yet another serious blunder.

The heavy precipitation of the rainy season toward the end of August and September called a halt to the burnings, but they resumed once more in October. It was the fierce opposition to their dispossession in late October and early November that precipitated the angry Lebu protests that once more caused Ponty to give ground. When the plague was dying out in December, some 200 condemned dwellings had yet to be put to the torch.[45] Only those medical authorities who were in touch with the African community, like Marcandier, commented on the housing problem. Even Marcandier failed to note that Africans had little choice but to recycle building materials. The demand for straw was very high, the small supply was quickly exhausted, and no new straw could be made available for two to three months, when the straw could be harvested and dried.[46]

Little evidence has survived regarding compensation procedures. One eyewitness in Diourbel in 1914, Dr. Rousseau, observed that the destruction or the sparing of certain areas and dwellings was a function of the influence of the proprietor, or simply the size of the indemnity the local officials would be obliged to pay out.[47] The official report on plague in 1915 stated that disinfection was carried out on all suspect buildings in which Syrians, Moroccans, and West Africans lived, implying that French proprietors were not subjected to these regulations.[48]

Burial procedures during the 1914 epidemic were also spelled out in the 13 May emergency legislation. As soon as a plague death was determined, the corpse was transported to the cemetery in a closed vehicle.[49] The grave was dug to a depth of one and a half meters, the body having been immersed in lime or a creosote solution.[50] Although sources do not specify this, it is likely that multiple if not mass burials were carried out. Lafont actually recommended cremation, but perhaps fearing the strong objections Muslim clerics would raise to such a practice, the French authorities in Dakar did not use cremation in 1914.[51]

Plague burials and other control practices differed in rural Senegal. Not only were isolation and incineration widely practiced, but entire villages were sometimes destroyed. The medical authorities argued that because the Africans had buried their previous plague dead inside the villages, even the noncontaminated neighborhoods had become unsafe. The officials dictated where the new dwellings were to be located. Then the abandoned villages, isolation camps, and cemeteries were destroyed by vast fires, and the ashes encircled with tree trunks and roots to prevent any attempt to rebuild homes or to grow crops on these sites.[52]

These provisions for disinfection, incineration, and burial left deep scars among the African population. The control of village space was one dramatic intrusion into everyday life. The damage or destruction of the personal property of dead plague victims also prohibited lineages from transferring symbolic goods to the next generation, and thus intruded on important cultural practices designed to ease the pain of bereavement. Muslims were distressed that their practice of washing corpses, wrapping them in expensive textiles, and maintaining a vigil over them, were all ruled out by authorities. Multiple burials in lime were anathema as well. In rural Senegal, people have preserved lurid memories of African public health workers wearing masks and gloves, dragging corpses with ropes attached to the ankles for mass burial in lime pits. Such graphic images help explain the traumatic nature of the epidemic and also the deep resentment felt by African communities toward the medical authorities and their "bogeymen" enforcers.

VACCINATION

If quarantine and cleansing represented old public health measures with deep roots in the European past, vaccination was the prize by-product of the new discipline of immunology. In this new field, France took particular pride of place, since Louis Pasteur was the leading practitioner. To French physicians, nothing better illustrated the superiority of their biomedicine over African and Islamic alternatives than the hostility directed by the Senegalese toward the concept of immunological protection through inoculation.[53]

The vaccination story is one of the best documented aspects of the 1914 Senegalese epidemic, largely as a result of the efforts of André Marcandier, the leading practitioner of vaccinations in Dakar in 1914. At the Naval Arsenal he personally supervised some 37,000 of the roughly 45,000 inoculations performed with the Haffkine vaccine during the course of the epidemic.[54] Additional vaccination clinics were held at City Hall, where roughly 7,300 vaccinations were performed; unspecified numbers were also carried out at the Colonial Hospital, the Bacteriological Laboratory, and the segregation and isolation villages and camps. Approximately half of the vaccine batches were prepared at the Pasteur Institute Laboratory in Paris, and half by Dr. Lafont in Dakar.[55]

The Dakar Health Committee approved the Haffkine anti-plague vaccine at its first emergency meeting on 13 May, but the vaccination program was delayed until the beginning of June because of a mix-up in the despatching of the vaccine from Paris.[56] As the vaccinations began on 29 and 30 May, Marcandier expressed concern about how the Senegalese naval personnel in particular would accept them.[57] The response was sufficiently encouraging that on 3 June, the navy informed the *laptots* that their families could also receive preventive inoculations. The families of the noncommissioned officers set the example, and many neighbors and friends followed. Marcandier received permission from the Naval Command to establish a public vaccination clinic, and a building near the infirmary on the arsenal grounds was assigned to the project. The site proved much more popular than the City Hall vaccination center, perhaps because of the encouragement of the noncommissioned officers, and the confidence people had in Marcandier.[58]

The injections were invariably given on the arms of patients. When abdominal injection was attempted, not only did patients object, but it was found that belts rubbed against the mark and produced painful abscesses. Control over vaccination certificates caused concern. Marcandier was told that on the black market certificates could fetch from 5 to 10 francs. In an effort to prevent trafficking, signs that would aid in the identification of the certificate holder were added, and lost or stolen cards were not replaced. The clinic was exceptionally busy on Dakar market days, with lineups stretching onto the Hann road. Often as many as 1,000 people lined up, though the maximum number that could be vaccinated in a long day stretching into the evening was 750 or 780 at most.[59]

African resistance to the vaccine generally appeared to diminish over time. Marcandier noted that even the residents of the Parc à Fourrages neighborhood, which had resisted health control measures so forcefully in early November, had become convinced of the protection vaccinations afforded. As a result, November was the navy team's busiest month, with 10,879 vaccinations carried out. In December, the entire village of Thiaroye requested protection from the navy clinic, and this helped bring the December total number of vaccinations to 7,597.[60]

By today's standards, the Haffkine vaccine was dangerously potent and even toxic.[61] In Senegal in 1914, it produced a wide variety of side effects ranging from mere soreness at the point of inoculation and low-level fever to painful swellings of the lymph nodes in the groin or armpit. Frequently, large and painful abscesses formed, some of them persisting for a month or more.[62] These numerous side effects forced Marcandier to reduce the dosage of vaccines and to use only the batches which had been imported from France. Only later was the local Dakar laboratory able to produce vaccines which resulted in lower incidences of abscesses. Other general reactions, whether to one strain of the Haffkine vaccine or both is not clear, were diarrhea and insomnia. Finally, breast-fed children were found to have vomited the night following the inoculation of their mothers.

Marcandier honestly admitted that despite precautions, on days when the volume of patients was heavy, it was not possible to examine each recipient carefully. Perhaps, then, poor screening may have been responsible for inducing more serious illness among those subjects already incubating plague. A few who were inoculated were indeed already incubating bubonic plague. Marcandier gave specifics of the fatalities from the vaccine, naming names, in one of the rare examples of such a practice in the clinical history of the 1914 epidemic.[63] Marcandier noted that in the month of August, of the 380 deaths from plague, 95 were those of people who had received only one vaccination, indicating to him that one injection simply did not provide sufficient protection.

In his assessment of the effectiveness of the Haffkine vaccine, Marcandier candidly admitted that most of the vaccinations had taken place toward the end of the epidemic. Of the 4,000 to 5,000 Africans who received all three injections, all were residents of the new segregation village near Dakar, which reduced their exposure to the bacilli. Marcandier also admitted that the 7,000 to 8,000 single-shot vaccinations performed in late May and June had not prevented the epidemic from gathering momentum in July and August. Finally, the numbers of deaths began to diminish in September, before the booster and third inoculations had been given to most of the potential recipients. What Marcandier did conclude was that giving three vaccinations possibly shortened the declining phase of the epidemic and probably prevented its reawakening the following year.[64] Lastly, he conceded that his confidence in the Haffkine vaccine stemmed from anecdotal rather than clinical evidence.[65] He accepted that no true controls existed, that there was no accurate total population census for Dakar, and that there was no precise counting of the plague dead.[66]

Not all practitioners attempted to be as even-handed as Marcandier. Kermorgant, for one, refused to admit that serious side effects were ever a problem and asserted that even the youngest children, those eighteen months and older, "handled successive vaccinations very well." He would

The Medical Response 105

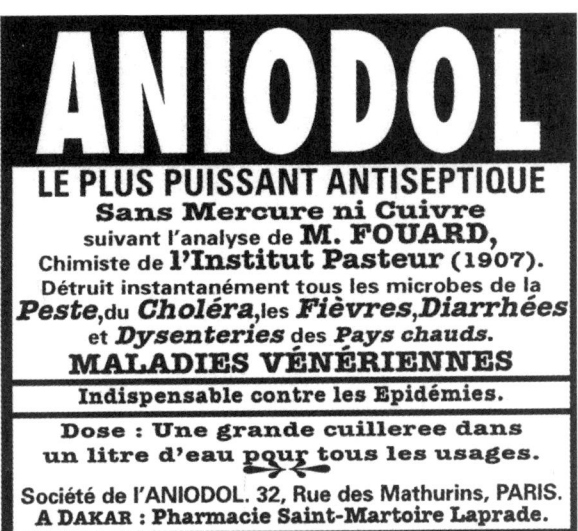

Photo 5.2 Advertisement for the Antiseptic "Aniodol," Dakar, 1914. The text informs readers that a chemist of the Pasteur Institute had determined that the antiseptic "Aniodol" did not contain any mercury or copper (but note that neither the chemist nor the Pasteur Institute were endorsing the product), and that it was "indispensable against epidemics," including, in addition to plague, "cholera, fevers, diarrhea and dysentery found in tropical countries, and venereal diseases." The advertisement mentioned plague for the first time in the Dakar newspaper *L'AOF,* 30 May 1914.

only concede that those with tuberculosis had some difficulty, and rheumatoid arthritis sufferers experienced increased pain following their injections.[67]

Africans, however, had legitimate reasons for resisting the Haffkine vaccine. Too many vaccinated people took sick with plague and died for wide public confidence to develop. The painful side effects, and the dangers to children in particular, alarmed many. Most tellingly, the European community lacked confidence as well, and insisted that anti-plague vaccination remain voluntary for European's throughout 1914 and beyond.

The only product in which some of the Europeans had confidence was an antiseptic with the brand name of "Aniodol," developed by a Parisian chemist at the Pasteur Institute in 1907. In the middle of the Dakar epidemic, *L'AOF* began running advertisements indicating that Aniodol would kill plague "microbes" with the same facility that it attacked those responsible for cholera, diarrhea, dysentery, and venereal diseases. One tablespoon in a liter of water was said to be "indispensable against epidemics."[68]

VECTOR CONTROL

Not surprisingly, vector control measures received very low priority in the Senegalese epidemic. Dr. Huot and the health officials below him never fully appreciated the role played by rats and fleas in spreading bubonic plague. Toward the very end of the epidemic, when it was too late, authorities did organize "rat hunts" using traps and poison, and paid what they regarded as the substantial bounty of 25 centimes per rat; yet in their view, the African population "showed little enthusiasm" for rat hunting.[69] The most reliable reporting on rodents came from Lafont and the staff of the Bacteriological Laboratory at Dakar, since they were the ones who did the examinations. Lafont noted the difficult circumstances in which he was required to function. An acute shortage of personnel meant that rats could neither be captured daily nor examined properly.[70] Of 143 rat cadavers examined, 65 could not yield any reliable results because the rodents had been dead too long. Of the remainder, 53 proved to be free of plague, 19 were found to be infected, and 6 suspected. In May and June, no infected rats were found; but beginning in July, evidence of an epizootic became clear from rat cadavers found in such dispersed areas as the navy yards, the port neighborhoods, and the storehouses of M. Caland, the deputy mayor.[71]

Lafont complained that the municipal authorities in Dakar did not begin to become concerned about the destruction of rodents until the epidemic was at its height, and then they quickly abandoned the effort because of its cost. "Some even claimed that there were no rodents in the city," whereas in fact, Lafont asserted, they were plentiful. He viewed it as fortunate that the rodents did not succeed in spreading the plague more extensively.[72] The Africans were not the only ones, Lafont added, to conceal the presence of rodents. "Certain commercial warehouses, where a certain number of dead rodents were found, carefully concealed this fact."[73] Yet, he continued, it was only through systematic rodent control, employing a variety of means, ranging from bounties paid to the population, traps, teams, chemical poisons, and gas to the use of dogs such as terriers imported from Europe, that Dakar would gain the upper hand in its ongoing battle to improve the city's public health.

It is revealing that few observers mentioned the true vector of *Yersinia pestis*, the humble flea, and that no one distinguished among the potential varieties of fleas to be found in Senegal.[74] Lafont was the only researcher to note that the straw huts of many Dakar residents were infested with fleas and their larvae, and for that reason had to be "destroyed without pity by fire."[75] In the countryside, in certain villages of Kajoor during the hot season, the sandy soil literally "bubbled with the agitation of millions of swarming fleas," and people were on occasion actually driven from their homes by them.[76] The countryside was a concern to Lafont for another reason. It was the habitat of the giant rat, *Cricetomys gambiae*, which was abundant in the bush and a terrible menace to granaries. Africans took preventive measures against this pest, but ate its flesh in times of severe food shortage. Calling for more research on the subject, Lafont speculated that this wild rodent might be a vector of plague in Africa just as tarabagans were in Manchuria.[77]

Not surprisingly, the only medical reporter to describe efforts at rat control in any detail, and with compassion for Africans, was the naval physician André Marcandier. The following account reveals both this sense of compassion and the difficulties of determining plague causation. On 5 July, an eleven-year-old boy named Bernard Senn carried a dead mouse in his hands to the Bacteriological Laboratory in return for a 25 centime payment. At first, he hid from authorities the locale where the mouse had been captured, but he later revealed that it was the cellar of a house on the rue Grasland, in a plague-contaminated neighborhood. When the rodent tested positive for *Y. pestis*, medical authorities interviewed a woman who was the wife of Niaki Senn and a relative of the little boy. Madame Senn noted that she had found fourteen to fifteen dead rats around her premises, and had observed the rats going out into the open to die in broad daylight. Others had observed the same phenomenon as well, but Madame Senn had been told not to mention these facts to medical authorities and not to send the rat cadavers to the laboratory.[78] Madame Senn stated that despite being vaccinated, her husband had contracted bubonic plague and only recovered after a long illness. But little Bernard, meanwhile, fell ill twelve days after visiting the laboratory and passed away on 20 July.[79] Marcandier claimed his success in keeping his perimeter relatively rodent free was due to his prompt actions from the beginning of the plague outbreak in May. The navy used traps and sulphuric acid and then, in July, stepped up its efforts by offering a bonus of kola nuts to each *laptot* who brought in a rat, found dead or alive, in the navy yards. European sailors and *laptots* were warned of the dangers of touching rodent cadavers, while tugs and ferries were ordered to remain at a distance from the navy quays. In addition, the navy joined with the Dakar municipality in offering a bounty of 25 centimes per rat carcass.[80] Marcandier confessed, however, that the bounty produced poor results because the Africans feared that discovery of an infected rat would bring down on their property and their homes the fire and brimstone of the sanitary brigades.[81]

Marcandier was an important exception to the otherwise mediocre performance of the medical authorities. Perhaps because they are required to manage their confined environments carefully, naval officers have always had a strong sensitivity to the ordering of space. Within a controlled environment, or perimeter, to use the more technical term, it was possible for Marcandier to seal off his men and their dependents from civilian society in Dakar in a manner that probably offered them some protection from plague infection. Second, because he was newly arrived in the colony when the outbreak began, Marcandier did not share other Europeans' acquired prejudice toward the African population. His inquiries taught him that entire families were wiped out by the plague, that often children were orphaned and had to be taken in by relatives and neighbors. He devoted himself to the care of his naval charges, European *and* African, and he interpreted his obligations toward his men to include their dependents as well.

While the period concluding in 1918 witnessed significant strides in public health in France, very little of this scientific and technological advance was transferred to Senegal.[82] The French authorities cited financial constraints, yet they often invoked blatantly racist opinions in order to blame the main victims of infectious disease, the African population. In reality, however, like other colonial powers in the initial stages of imperial rule in Africa, the French medical authorities saw their task as protecting French officials and their dependents from the unhealthy African masses, who were expected to cope with both familiar and newly introduced pathogens through their own efforts. Few, if any, among the French medical authorities appreciated the degree to which the Senegalese disease environment had changed as a result of direct French rule.

It cannot be said that the health authorities in Senegal were operating in a colonial backwater. Bubonic plague in Dakar and its hinterland cannot be compared to a rural outbreak, for example, in desert-edge Morocco, or, let us say, the sleepy port of Grand Bassam in the Ivory Coast. This is not to argue that suffering and death anywhere from the scourge of bubonic plague can be dismissed. Rather, the point is that Dakar was the nerve center of France's empire in Africa. Epidemic plague there had wide political and economic implications. Were the outbreak

The Medical Response   109

to spread throughout a large part of the federation, as had happened in British India only two decades earlier, the costs would have been colossal. Nevertheless, apart from the presence of a Bacteriological Laboratory in Dakar, medical and colonial circles in the metropole seemed to leave their wards in Senegal to fate. In the end, the First World War was probably a restricting factor, but no additional personnel or resources were sent from France during the medical crisis, and no *mission d'inspection* was ever sent to assess performance, as had been done immediately after the yellow fever scare in 1900, for example. In the final analysis, colonizer and colonized were fortunate that natural constraints on the spread of *Y. pestis* kept the medical crisis from becoming a catastrophe.

NOTES

1. Frederick Cooper, *Decolonization and African Society: The Labor Question in French and British Africa* (Cambridge: Cambridge University Press, 1996), 15–16.

2. Diana Wylie makes this point forcefully when she demonstrates that medical experts in southern Africa condemned Africans as a people without science, and, therefore, doomed to perpetual domination by their superiors. Diana Wylie, *Starving on a Full Stomach: Hunger and the Triumph of Cultural Racism in Modern South Africa* (Charlottesville: University Press of Virginia, 2001).

3. Valentin Y. Mudimbe, *The Invention of Africa: Gnosis, Philosophy, and the Order of Knowledge* (Bloomington: Indiana University Press, 1988).

4. In 1913, the laboratory had been moved from its previous locale in Saint-Louis. It would change its name to the Institute of Biology in 1920, and to the Pasteur Institute of Dakar in 1924. Each change in institutional title brought improved funding and greater responsibility and prestige. Constant Mathis, *L'oeuvre des Pastoriens en Afrique noire, Afrique occidentale française* (Paris: Presses Universitaires Françaises, 1946), 20–21.

5. Later directors in succession were André Léger (1916–19), Fernand Noc (1919–21), Marcel Léger (1921–24), and Constant Mathis (1924–37).

6. A review of the eight medical men who sat together with seven laymen on the Dakar Health Committee in 1914 shows that the Senegal Health Service had four representatives: the chief of the service, Dr. L. Huot; his assistant, Dr. Vassal; and two additional medical employees, Drs. Barros and Pichard. The French army and navy each had one physician on the committee, Drs. Sautorel and Marcandier respectively, responsible for health and sanitation within the military bases. The Municipality of Dakar was represented by Dr. Gontier, who may have been a civilian. The eighth member, Dr. Maignal, was clearly identified as a private clinician. The other seven members of the committee were three appointed officials, Mayor Masson, his assistant, Caland, and Vidal, the governor of Senegal's delegate in Dakar; two clerks; and one veterinarian and one engineer from Public Works. It is striking that no representative

of the federal government or bacteriologist from the laboratory served on the committee. Salleras, "La peste à Dakar," lxiv.

7. The official name of the "Pharo" ("Lighthouse") school was l'École d'Application du Service de Santé des Troupes Coloniales. No full study of this program has been undertaken, but in a general essay Marc Michel suggests that many of the military medical students came from the northwest, especially Brittany, that they were from families of modest means, and that they had chosen military medical schools because their education was paid for by the state. Some no doubt were enthralled with the idealistic and adventurous image of the Colonial Health Corps, inspired by some of its outstanding members such as Albert Calmette, who invented BCG, Alexandre Yersin, who first isolated the plague bacillus, and Paul-Louis Simond, who discovered the flea vector of bubonic plague. Simond was the assistant director at Pharo and professor of bacteriology in the school's first years. He taught there for six years, and counted among his students Jamot in 1910 and Sicé in 1911. Marc Michel, "Le Corps de Santé des troupes coloniales," in *Histoire des médecins et pharmaciens de marine et des colonies*, edited by Pierre Pluchon (Paris: Editions Privat, 1985), 185, 191, 212.

8. Huot cited the precedent of the French Pacific colony of New Caledonia in 1912–13, where health officials moved entire villages and transferred them to new sites. Marcandier called for "the complete separation of the natives from the Europeans and their isolation in a special village." Lafont and Kermorgant used virtually identical language. Huot, "Rapport d'ensemble"; André Marcandier, "La peste à Dakar (1914–15)," *Archives de Médecine Navale* 106 (1918): 218; André Lafont, "Une épidémie de peste humaine Dakar (avril 1914–février 1915)," *Bulletin de la Société de Pathologie Exotique* 8 (1915): 677; and Alexandre Kermorgant, "L'épidémie de peste qui a sévi à Dakar et au Sénégal d'avril 1914 à février 1915", *Bulletin de l'Académie de Médecine*, 76 (1916): 133.

9. ANS\H55 contains this report, cited as Huot, "Rapport d'ensemble." While it numbers 253 pages, the majority of which deal with plague, the report also includes several pages on general sanitary matters and statistics. These data were required for the Annual Medical Report of the colony of Senegal, which the chief medical officer had to submit six months after the end of each calendar year.

10. Kermorgant, "Épidémie," 126–33. This published report on plague was the text of an address he delivered on 22 August 1916 to the Academy of Medicine in Paris. Kermorgant was an old hand in Africa, with numerous research publications to his credit from 1899 to 1916 on such diverse diseases as tuberculosis, yellow fever, sexually transmitted diseases, malaria, and plague. In 1910 he published one of the first medical texts in the newly emerging specialty of colonial public health, with the major Paris publisher, Masson. See Alexandre Kermorgant, *Hygiène coloniale* (Paris: Masson, 1911). For a complete list of his publications, see René Collignon and Charles Becker, *Santé et population en Sénégambie des origines à 1960: Bibliographie annotée* (Paris: Institut National d'Études Demographiques, 1989).

11. Marcandier, "La peste," 125. He reported hearing rumors of a "disease that struck like lightning" in the second half of April, a few days after his arrival in the city to take up his post as physician in charge of naval personnel. He also stated that he had penned his report from memory, without access to a medical library, in

an unnamed city which had experienced frequent bombardment during the First World War.

12. Marcandier, "La peste," 127.

13. Little is known about this individual, but from his writings he appears to have been a disgruntled member of the Colonial Health Service who had been passed over for promotion, and who was assigned as physician in the rural region of Diourbel in 1914. His medical understanding remained closely tied to miasmatic theories. Paul Rousseau, "Au sujet de la peste du Sénégal," *Journal des Praticiens* 31 (1917): 738–44.

14. Rousseau, "La peste," 744.

15. Huot, "Rapport d'ensemble."

16. Marcandier, "La peste," 191.

17. Marcandier, "La peste," 135.

18. Diop, "Santé," 269.

19. Collomb, Huot, and Lecomte. "Note sur l'épidémie de peste au Sénégal en 1914," *Annales de Hygiène et de Médecine Coloniales* 19 (1921): 67.

20. Collomb, Huot, and Lecomte, "Note," 67. As Marcandier politely remarked, this trial-and-error approach resulted in yet another blunder by medical authorities. Marcandier, "La peste," 192.

21. Marcandier, "La peste," 193.

22. Collomb, Huot, and Lecomte, "Note," 67–68. The reason given for allowing this recycling was the acute shortage of straw and other construction material.

23. Collomb, Huot, and Lecomte, "Note," 68.

24. Marcandier, "La peste," 195.

25. Marcandier, "La peste," 195–96.

26. Marcandier, "La peste," 197.

27. Marcandier, "La peste," 198. He stated that it was navy policy to "encourage the peopling of the new village."

28. Marcandier, "La peste," 198.

29. Lafont, "Une épidémie," 673–74.

30. For Eyam, see chapter 2 above. For Marseille, see Charles Carrière, M. Courdurié, and F. Rebuffat, *Marseille, ville morte: La peste de 1720* (Marseille: Éditions Jean-Michel Garcon, 1988).

31. Collomb, Huot, and Lecomte, "Note," 47.

32. Collomb, Huot, and Lecomte, "Note," 48.

33. Huot, "Rapport d'ensemble," 145.

34. Huot, "Rapport d'ensemble." Collomb, Huot, and Lecomte, "Note," 48, state that the death rate reached twenty-five at its peak.

35. Huot, "Rapport d'Ensemble."

36. Collomb, Huot, and Lecomte, "Note," 48, state that the vaccination strengths were 2 cc. for adults, 1 cc. for children under 10, and .5 cc. for infants.

37. Marcandier, "La peste," 137.

38. Collomb, Huot, and Lecomte, "Note," 67 for the statistics; Diop, "Santé," 275, for the comparison with 1912.

39. Marcandier, "La peste," 195.

40. *L'AOF*, 30 May 1914.

41. Huot, "Rapport d'ensemble," 61.

42. Mbokolo, "Peste," 38.
43. Lafont, "Une épidémie," 674.
44. Marcandier, "La peste," 140.
45. Marcandier, "La peste," 192.
46. Diop, "Santé," 294.
47. Rousseau, "La peste," 743.
48. Huot, "Rapport d'ensemble."
49. Collomb, Huot, and Lecomte, "Note," 67.
50. Kermorgant, "Épidémie," 128.
51. Lafont, "Une épidémie," 676.
52. Collomb, Huot, and Lecomte, "Note," 69–71.

53. Kermorgant, for example, explicitly accused "the *marabouts* and a few agitators of inciting the population to avoid vaccinations." Kermorgant, "Épidémie," 130.

54. Marcandier specifies some 17,400 initial inoculations, 14,868 boosters, and 12,953 third injections, making a total of 45,221. Marcandier, "Les vaccinations," 592.

55. Lafont acknowledged "difficulties" related to the climate and the fact that the atmosphere was saturated with dust, which was scattered by strong, even violent winds. He strenuously denied that vaccination produced serious side effects, and the only death from the Dakar vaccine he would acknowledge was that of a young woman from Haut-Sénégal-Niger who was treated at the Dakar Laboratory. His most serious admission, however, was that his team only followed up on its subjects for one day after the injections. Lafont, "Une épidémie," 671–72.

56. Someone inadvertently ordered the *Lutétia*, the vessel carrying the vaccine, to pass by Dakar; instead, the vaccine was off-loaded at Tenerife in the Canary Islands. *L'AOF*, 23 May 1914; and Marcandier, "La peste," 200. François Devès, a member of the Colonial Council, understandably criticized the director of the Senegalese Health Service for this bungling and argued that, following the experience of the most recent yellow fever epidemic, medical authorities should have acted more promptly. Minutes of the Colonial Council for the session of 5 November 1914, 153.

57. Marcandier, "La peste," 200. As has been noted previously, vaccinations were not mandatory initially, but travel outside Dakar was not permitted without a vaccination card. On 2 August, the Health Committee ruled that vaccinations were to be compulsory for all Syrians, Moroccans, and "natives," whether they wished to travel or not. For Europeans, the vaccinations remained discretionary. Huot, "Rapport d'ensemble"; Collomb, Huot, and Lecomte, "Note," 63.

58. Marcandier, "La peste," 200.
59. Marcandier, "La peste," 202–3.
60. Marcandier, "La peste," 203.

61. Thomas C. Butler, *Plague and Other Yersinia Infections* (New York: Plenum Medical Book Co., 1983), 199.

62. André Marcandier, "Note sur les vaccinations contre la peste faites pendant et après l'épidémie de Dakar (1914–1915–1916)," *Bulletin de la Société de Pathologie Exotique* 9 (1916): 597. He graphically described one as being as the size of an orange, another as being the size of a large egg, and the worst case, a seven-month-old abscess, as being the size of an infant's head! When lanced, the abscess secreted yellow pus which ran like oil, but the bacteriological examination revealed it to be aseptic, with quite harmless bacteria.

63. For example, 31-year-old Abdoulaye Silla, a laborer at the Compagnie des charbonnages, received his first shot on 17 June; two weeks later, feeling ill, he left work and hurried to receive a second shot, thinking it would cure him. He died of pulmonary plague three days later. Maram Diop, aged 27, was vaccinated on 28 October, but died of plague the next week; 26-year-old Abdoulaye Diaye was vaccinated first on 19 June, again on 21 September, and succumbed ten days later; 46-year-old Diabaye Touré was first immunized on 28 October and died the following week of bubonic plague; 29-year-old Isaac Boume was vaccinated on the 19 and 26 October and died two days later. Marcandier, "Les vaccinations," 596–98.

64. To support this conclusion, Marcandier cited the case of Thiaroye. His team vaccinated the entire village in December 1914, but a mild epidemic of bubonic plague broke out again there in July 1915. Since seven months had elapsed, he jumped to the conclusion not only that the protection had lasted close to six months, but also that the vaccinations might have helped provide some immunological protection even to those who developed mild cases. Marcandier, "Les vaccinations," 599.

65. As an example, he cited the case of Yacine Diop, an eighty-year-old who died of plague on 23 January 1915. Because of his advanced age he had not been vaccinated. His daughter, son-in-law, and grand-daughter, with whom he lived in a neighborhood where plague was rampant, had all been vaccinated three times; none contracted plague. Marcandier, "Les vaccinations," 600.

66. The question of whether the confidence of Marcandier and others in the Haffkine vaccine was justified must be placed in historical context. By later twentieth-century standards, the Haffkine vaccine would have been unacceptably dangerous. But in 1914, as is the case today, the question about vaccines was whether the risk accompanying the acquisition of protection offset the risk of the disease itself. Clearly for those health workers exposed daily to rats, fleas, and sick people, the vaccine would be essential. For the rest of the population, its value may have resided only in protection preceding potential exposure by more than two weeks, not in a situation where individuals might have been incubating plague.

67. Kermorgant, "Épidémie," 132.
68. See, for example, the advertisement in *L'AOF*, 30 May 1914.
69. Collomb, Huot, and Lecomte, "Note," 66.
70. Lafont, "Une épidémie," 671.
71. Lafont, "Une épidémie," 667.
72. Lafont, "Une épidémie," 676.
73. Lafont, "Une épidémie," 676.
74. Only a decade or more later would French researchers begin to study Senegalese flea varieties. See Mathis, *Pastoriens*, 283.
75. Lafont, "Une épidémie," 677.
76. Lafont, "Une épidémie," 679.
77. Lafont, "Une épidémie," 678–79. Lafont was moving closer to an understanding of the plague cycle, but, his labeling of the giant rat as a "vector," reveals that he did not fully grasp that it was potentially a permanent reservoir of *Yersinia pestis*, a host in which plague could remain for years, and from which it could be transferred by flea vectors during times of perturbation to other, less resistant mammal hosts. Only a decade later did Léger suggest that the African wild rodent, *Crocidura stampflii*, might be a reservoir of plague. Mathis, *Pastoriens*, 66.

78. Madame Senn was interrogated at the Dakar Laboratory and only reluctantly revealed this information. Lafont, "Une épidémie," 664.

79. Marcandier, "La peste," 138. Sufficient time had elapsed between the illnesses of Niaki Senn and Bernard that the vaccination can be ruled out as the primary cause.

80. Marcandier, "La peste," 199.

81. Marcandier, "La peste," 194.

82. See Alice L. Conklin, *A Mission to Civilize: The Republican Idea of Empire in France and West Africa, 1895–1930* (Stanford, Calif.: Stanford University Press, 1997), 141–42, for a discussion of advances in French public health.

6

MEASURING THE IMPACT OF THE 1914 EPIDEMIC

THE STATISTICAL IMPACT OF BUBONIC PLAGUE

Before the epidemic burned itself out in January 1915, plague deaths in Dakar, Rufisque, and rural Senegal had reached an official total of 3,686, a number well below the reality.[1] Dakar alone, with 1,439 recorded deaths, lost more than 5 percent of its population from this single disease, a grisly reminder to perceptive physicians of the lethal power of bubonic plague. Tables 6.1 and 6.2 give the size of the Senegalese losses in 1914, and comparative urban losses to plague in selected cities at the turn of the twentieth century.

The actual death toll was undoubtedly much greater than the official figures suggested. First, the medical authorities missed the beginning of the epidemic and could only guess at the deaths which occurred in the weeks before 11 May. Second, even after the declaration of the medical emergency, no registry of epidemic deaths was opened at the mayor's office until July. Only then did the official statistics acquire some basis in reality.[2] Third, the official figures of deaths from plague included only those of cadavers brought to the attention of the authorities. To avoid official sanctions and control, as the official report put it, "numerous cadavers were buried clandestinely during the night."[3]

Well into the epidemic, most people died at home, out of sight and control of Western medical authorities. One measure of this can be obtained from hospital figures. Claiming that the native hospital was a new concept which had not yet been understood and appreciated by native custom, the young French naval physician, André Marcandier, stated that only thirty declared cases of plague were admitted to Dakar hospitals in August, at the height of the epidemic, of whom fourteen died, leaving 366 deaths outside the medical system.[4] Finally, misdiagnosis of plague

Table 6.1 1914 Plague Epidemic in Senegal

Locale	Deaths	Population	Deaths per 1,000
Dakar	1,439	6,000	55
Yoff	1,100	2,000	550
Cambérène	230	300	767
Thiaroye	30	b.600	50
Cape Verde peninsula	2,799	c. 24,524	114
Rufisque	144	a. 12,873	11
Keur-Gallo-Isser (Pout)	76	115	660
Other Pout villages	277	1,185	234
Rufisque area	497	c. 14,173	35
Guélor	115	e. 1,000	115
Ham (Tatène)	8	230	122
Ndiaganiao	137	2,000	69
Thiomboledj	56	e. 1,000	56
Thiès cercle	336	4,230	79
Diourbel	7	a. 2,192	3
Kaolack center	11	500	22
Kaolack suburbs	36	d. 954	38
Kaolack totals	47	a. 1,454	32
Totals:	3,686	c. 46,573	79

Source: All data from Collomb, Huot, and Lecomte, "Note sur l'épidémie de peste au Sénégal en 1914," *Annales de Hygiène et de Médecine coloniales,* 19 (1921), 38-72, unless specified.

a. ANS\22G\50, tables.
b. My estimate based on mention of the two Thiaroye villages, Thiaroye-Plage and Thiaroye-Bâ.
c. Totals are only for locales known to be infected with plague.
d. My extrapolation from ANS\22G\50. Medical reports used figure of 800.
e. My estimates.

Measuring the Impact of the 1914 Epidemic

Table 6.2 Plague Death Rates in Selected Cities, 1894–1914

Locale	Year	Plague Deaths	Estimated Population	Deaths per 1,000
Dakar	1914	a. 1,500	26,000	58
Hong Kong	1894	2,710	250,000	10.84
Bombay	1896	1,936	850,000	2.3
Alexandria	1899	45	300,000	.15
Cape Town	1901	389	150,000	2.6

Sources: for Dakar, Collomb, Huot, and Lecomte, "Note"; Hong Kong, Carol Benedict, Bubonic Plague in Nineteenth-Century China (Stanford, Calif.: Stanford University Press, 1996), 142; Bombay, Bruce Low, Reports on Public Health and Medical Subjects, no. 3: The Progress and Diffusion of Plague, Cholera and Yellow Fever throughout the World, 1914-1917 (London: Ministry of Health, 1920), 21; Alexandria, A. W. Wakil, The Third Pandemic of Plague in Egypt: Historical Statement and Epidemic Remarks on the first Thirty-Two Years of its Prevalence (Cairo: Egyptian University, 1932), 41-42; Cape Town, Elizabeth van Heyningen, "Cape Town and the Plague of 1901," in Christopher Saunders, Howard Phillips, and Elizabeth van Heyningen (Cape Town: University of Cape Town, 1981), 77.

a. Rounded up from the official figure of 1,439.

---

no doubt occurred, especially since laboratory confirmation of plague was not always provided.[5] In the earliest stages of the epidemic, plague deaths may have been incorrectly ascribed to pneumonia. Later on, however, the reverse could have occurred as lung or glandular infections may have been erroneously diagnosed as bubonic plague. In short, French officials were well aware of the inaccuracy of the plague statistics. The official report admitted candidly that "it has not been possible, either in Dakar or in other contaminated centers, to gain a precise idea of the number of plague cases."[6]

Had plague been confined to Dakar and the surrounding Cape Verde peninsula, its impact would have been tragic enough to warrant concern from the authorities, and strong reactions from the population. But plague spread rapidly from Dakar and its environs, raging in the Rufisque area, spreading selectively to the contiguous and largely rural *cercle* of Thiès, and even making a brief appearance in the more distant town of Kaolack in southern Senegal. Worse, *Yersinia pestis* went to ground among wild rodents, thus establishing a reservoir that would doom Dakar and its hinterland to an entire generation of endo-epidemic plague. Whether prompt action by the Dakar health authorities in the outbreak's early stages would have prevented this dreadful result is a question that can never be answered. Located on a peninsula, and with avenues of escape by water beckoning, Dakar was probably not a city where even the prompt establishment of a *cordon sanitaire* could have succeeded in preventing the entire population, together with any unwelcome vectors hidden in their baggage, from fleeing the region. Still, the fact remains that official negligence made an already difficult situation worse.

Underreporting of deaths and nonexistent census rolls make biostatistical measurement of plague in the countryside an even more haphazard exercise than is the case for Dakar itself. Authorities neglected to mention what they based their estimates on, but since no formal mechanism existed for recording plague deaths, it can be assumed that the totals were based on compilations from a variety of sources, some of them medical, some of them not.[7] Dr. Huot and his colleagues in their official report placed the overall Senegalese toll at 3,686, the lowest of any of the estimates.[8] Lafont cited a figure of 4,000 deaths for all of Senegal, while conceding that the number was too low.[9] Marcandier's estimate of 5,000 deaths included 1,500 for Dakar and 3,500 for the rest of the colony.[10] Kermorgant added an additional 5,000 deaths to the official figure and arrived at a total of 8,686.[11]

My own figures in Table 6.1 above break down the official deaths, and correlate them with population to suggest magnitudes of mortality per 1,000. When this is done, it becomes immediately evident that several smaller locales such as Cambérène and Yoff just outside Dakar in the Cape Verde peninsula, and the village of Keur-Gallo-Isser, near Pout in the Rufisque region, suffered losses approximating two-thirds of their entire population. Overall, I estimate a minimum of 79 deaths per 1,000 for locales known to be infected by plague.

GENDER, ETHNICITY, AND OCCUPATION OF PLAGUE VICTIMS

No analysis of race, gender, ethnicity, or occupation of the Senegalese plague victims was ever undertaken, but fragments of information can be gleaned from the historical record. Ironically, prior to the Dakar epidemic, some medical authors had ignorantly asserted that Africans were immune to plague, despite their obvious vulnerability in other parts of sub-Saharan Africa.[12] Such tales were quickly dispelled when the great majority of the victims in Senegal proved to be Africans. Of the 3,686 officially recorded plague victims, only 7 were described as "European," and one as "Syrian."[13] Noting that four of these cases, and two deaths, occurred very late in the epidemic, in November 1914, Marcandier attributed this to the Europeans having been weakened by the *hivernage* season and by their long residence in the colony without home leave in France.[14]

Whether the 1914 plague discriminated on the basis of gender or age remains unknown. Dr. Alexandre Kermorgant, who treated plague patients in Dakar during the epidemic, claimed that women, and adults generally, were more severely affected. He observed that among children, cases tended to be more benign, with better prospects of recovery.[15]

Many of the Dakar victims were Lebu, the original inhabitants of the Cape Verde peninsula, and no doubt still a majority of the Dakar population in 1914. On the other hand, Soninke and Tukolor speakers were among the new migrants flooding into Dakar from the Upper Senegal Valley, and forced to accept overcrowded and sometimes squalid housing. Without extended families to care for them when ill, or hide their corpses and bury them secretly if they died, new residents of Dakar were probably more vulnerable to plague both in real terms as well as in the official statistics of reported deaths. When new residents of Dakar succeeded in fleeing to their villages, and to towns such as Thiès, Diourbel, and Kaolack to escape plague, to seek a treatment, or to die, they helped spread the epidemic.[16]

One group which must have been occupationally vulnerable to plague consisted of the sanitary workers charged with inspection, fumigation, and destruction of contaminated housing, but no record of their mortality rates survives. African soldiers of the Tirailleurs Sénégalais were charged with manning the *cordons sanitaires* and enforcing the quarantine generally, and there is some indication of their exposure to plague. Soldiers and their dependents were among the first, and the very last, victims of the epidemic. The first cases among the military occurred on 22 May, and involved two soldiers who had manned the original *cordon*. On 24 January 1915, the last officially recorded victim was the wife of a Tirailleur who was serving in Morocco. The woman, who was living in a house in the Abattoir quarter of Dakar, succumbed quickly to pneumonic plague.[17] Some fifty-four soldiers were admitted to the colonial hospital with plague between May and December 1914, and roughly half of them died.[18]

A few individual profiles of plague victims have survived. They are all from the pen of Dr. Marcandier, who stated that he made a point of talking to patients in order to acquire some sense of the impact of the epidemic.[19] The first case he treated personally was an African *laptot* or sailor named Boy "N'Di.," who had been a member of of the guard detail at the Navy Arsenal. He had fallen ill on 29 June with all of the typical bubonic plague symptoms. The sailor was treated with intravenous injections of Yersin's serum. His convalescence lasted forty-five days, perhaps, Marcandier speculated, because his blood showed the presence of malarial parasites; in the end, he recovered.

Others were not so fortunate. In mid July, Marcandier treated an African with pneumonic plague who had been found by a navy patrol, suffering alone in an abandoned hut on the edge of the sea. The man had been put ashore by the crew of a coastal vessel which could not be traced. The patient succumbed within twenty-four hours. Marcandier also discovered that in some cases, entire families were destroyed by plague. In one such instance, the surviving children were adopted by neighbors.

Late in July, Marcandier reported on an African woman, thirty years old and the wife of a *laptot*. She arrived at the navy clinic with the following story. At the beginning of June, along with other *laptot* families, she had received an anti-plague vaccination. Roughly a month later, she developed a bubo the size of an orange under her left arm. She was nursed by her brother, who died soon afterward, having an inflamed bubo in his left groin. The woman had personally incised her bubo with a knife, and a significant scar remained. Her general condition was described as "mediocre."

DIFFUSION OF PLAGUE TO THE INTERIOR OF SENEGAL

As the fate of the fishing village of Yoff demonstrates, plague did not long remain confined to the port of Dakar. Yoff was not the only Lebu village in the Cape Verde peninsula to be seriously infected. Nearby Cambérène, with an estimated population of 300, became plague-ridden sometime in June, but kept this information hidden from medical authorities. By the time the epidemic had burned itself out in September, the plague in Cambérène was estimated to have taken its highest toll in all of Senegal, with some 230 victims claimed in the village. Among the seventy to eighty survivors, French medical authorities noted many convalescing with large scars from recently healed buboes and concluded that the entire village at one time or another had been sick with plague.[20] Three nearby villages, Yembeul, Thiaroye-Plage, and Thiaroye-Bâ, had cut off contact with Cambérène and were less severely infected, although each was said to have experienced a couple of deaths daily at the height of the epidemic in August. If Dakar and the nearby Cape Verde peninsula constituted two zones ravaged by plague in 1914, a third area was the Pout district near Rufisque. Seven villages with a combined population estimated at 1,300, said to have been located on a route frequented by Fuulbe herdsmen, suffered varying degrees of infection from plague. Official documentation only began in August when Dr. Huot arrived in the area.[21] It was determined through oral testimony that the first two isolated cases had occurred after contact with a plague locus in the Rufisque suburb of Mérina. By August, the villages were experiencing the full force of the second wave of plague. Worst off was the village of Keur-Gallo-Isser, some 5 kilometers from Pout, whose widely scattered population of 115 persons endured the death of 76 persons within a twenty day period in August, that is, two-thirds of the village. By contrast, nearby Keur-Masamba-Diop lost only one person to plague. As sanitary agents burned condemned compounds and transported their inhabitants to a single common lazaretto set up near Pout, they were said to have met with "energetic opposition from a part of the population," particularly at Nguer. Still another locus of plague was the small village of Mérina, a small village just east of Rufisque's city limits and separated from the town by a canal. The official death count for Rufisque and region for the entire 1914 epidemic was 144, with a substantial number of deaths occurring in the early phase of the epidemic from May through July.

Radiating out further from Dakar and Rufisque, the plague had reached the *cercles* of Thiès and Bawol in May, though most cases there occurred during the second phase of the epidemic in August and later. Most of the infected villages were located just to the south of the rail line, and included Guélor, Tatène, Ndiaganiao, and Thiomboledj.[22] Guélor, some 18 kilometers from the rail line at Khombole, first came to the attention of officials as early as 22 May, when two villagers who had been working as dockers in Dakar died of plague shortly after reaching home. They had travelled on foot and had managed somehow to break through the *cordon sanitaire* erected at Hann in the Cape Verde peninsula. A day later, a brother of one of the deceased fell sick and died within hours. The homes inhabited by the three deceased were immediately burned as well as their effects. Some forty-two persons living in or beside the compound were isolated in a makeshift lazaretto established at a distance from the village. In their fifth day of isolation, all were compelled to accept vaccination with two cc. of the Haffkine serum. In addition, the entire remainder of the village of Guélor was inoculated with one cc. of the Haffkine vaccine.

This effort to contain the plague failed. The plague locus at Guélor remained active in July, and was said to be responsible for a second outbreak of plague in the village. One of the newly infected villages, Tatène, located 18 kilometers southwest of Thiès, was more ethnically diverse than it may have seemed at first. Lying on the road to Nianing in a region generally inhabited by Sereer farmers, the district in fact consisted of two distinct villages of strangers some 1,500 meters apart, one inhabited by Bambara speakers and the other by Tukolor. Only the Tukolor village of some 300 people was touched by plague, a fact which prompted the health authorities to leap to the conclusion that humans and not rats were involved in the transmission of the disease. Though they had no hard evidence, the medical authorities viewed Tukolor laborers as both victims and carriers of plague. They claimed that "farm labor is often lacking, so each family head is obliged to import or to stop those passing through and hire them as workers. These individuals come from diverse regions, only stay a short time in the villages, and are constantly being replenished. This heavy circulation . . . explains why the Tukolor villages are more frequently struck by epidemics, which they help to spread all over the colony."[23] While such theories based on human propagation were flawed, a greater volume of human traffic did mean more opportunities for plague vectors to be transported, so the incidence of plague could have been linked to Tukolor migration.

The spread of plague to the densely populated Sereer canton of Ndiaganiao in Thiès *cercle*, with some 4,230 people distributed among twenty-two different villages, was also held to have been the result of contamination from Guélor, but perhaps by a different social mechanism. According to French medical reports, the carriers were two Sereer traditional healers who had gone to Guélor to treat plague cases and had brought the infection back with them to their respective villages, Keur-Oussemane-Sy and Coquiane. The large Sereer funerals which were traditionally required found in turn mourners transporting plague back to their villages.[24] Between September 1914 and January 1915, the Ndiaganiao canton suffered some 137 deaths resulting from 198 reported cases.

Two regions only mildly infected by plague in 1914, and where plague did not later become endemic, were the more distant *cercles* of Diourbel and Kaolack. Diourbel recorded seven deaths during the outbreak, while the toll for Kaolack was thirty-six. If the medical report is to be believed, the transmission of plague to Kaolack illustrated the near impossibility of containing plague during a full-fledged epidemic. A woman from Dakar traveling with a sanitary passport as proof that she had received a Haffkine vaccination a few weeks earlier became ill with what was presumed to have been septicemic plague and died in Kaolack in mid August. Before passing away, she distributed her clothes among friends living in various parts of the town. By the time medical authorities were made aware of her death ten days later, a mild epidemic was under way. By early November, when the region was declared plague free, Kaolack, which was then a very small town of 500 inhabitants, was said by officials to have suffered no more than eleven plague deaths.

COSTS OF THE 1914 PLAGUE EPIDEMIC

The social and economic costs of the 1914 bubonic plague outbreak cannot be measured. The death of at least 4,000 people, and perhaps as many as twice that number, was one incalculable cost. So too were the long-term consequences of allowing the plague bacilli to find a permanent reservoir in the countryside, and to create an endo-epidemic situation over the next thirty years. Material losses can be tabulated, although the destruction of goods and property no doubt far exceeded the half million francs paid out as compensation. The record of official expenditures dedicated specifically to the health emergency has survived, but not the 1914 health budget for Senegal, which listed regular health expenses.[25] Still, the 1.1 million francs in emergency funds spent in 1914 represented a sum three times as large as the entire average annual health budgets of Senegal in the years leading up to 1914.[26] Of these emergency funds, the construction of the segregation village cost just under 260,000 francs. A sum of 513,000 francs was spent on compensation claims. this left roughly 327,000 francs to pay for such items as the new lazaretto at Bel-Air, the purchase of extra vaccines, and the temporary hiring of personnel.[27]

The colony of Senegal could not meet these expenses and requested help from the federation. Governor Antonetti asked Governor-General Ponty for a supplementary allocation of 800,000 francs, and Ponty allocated 700,000, obliging the colony to dip into its Caisse de Réserve to provide an additional 410,000 francs.[28]

The governor of Senegal chose not to inform the General Council of Senegal of these expenditures until some time after the fact. When Antonetti got round to presenting these costs in October 1915, François Devès expressed his unhappiness that the council had never been given the opportunity to discuss such expenditures.[29] Councillors had no power to demand such disclosures, but they could express their unhappiness with Antonetti in other ways. They ended the debate by passing unanimously a motion which mildly reprimanded the administration for its dilatory response to the plague emergency. The motion stated that in future epidemics the administration should "not delay in furnishing sanitary authorities with all the means necessary to respond."[30]

An evaluation of the 1914 Senegalese plague epidemic must also assess the performance of French biomedical efforts, in the context of international public health standards of the day. First, political and economic pressures clearly operated on the medical officials charged with protecting public health, as they always do in a medical emergency. The two major conjunctions, a dramatic election in May and the outbreak of First World War in August, certainly heightened tensions and allowed political considerations to trump medical ones at every turn. The political considerations explain, in part, why the health emergency was lifted for several weeks when the epidemic was far from over. Second, it must be recognized that most if not all efforts to control the spread of bubonic plague failed during the third pandemic. One of the striking consequences of this pandemic was to create new rodent reservoirs of *Y. pestis* where none had existed before. Senegal conformed to the typical global pattern. Plague would first break out in an urban port setting, and then spread widely into the countryside, despite the sometimes frenetic efforts of governments, sanitary officials, and medical researchers to prevent this. Third, it would be unfair to criticize health officials both for intervening and for failing to do so. For example, a swifter and better coordinated response might have reduced the magnitude of the epidemic in Dakar, and might even have prevented the endemic and enzootic catastrophe that resulted from the development of a permanent reservoir of *Y. pestis* in the countryside. But, given the political and social climate of Senegal in May 1914, such prompt and decisive action would clearly have generated even stronger African opposition. On the other hand, given the crude, blunt sanitary instruments and techniques then available to health officials, more intervention would surely have produced more blunders and avoidable deaths. It is not easy to resolve this conundrum.

Extenuating circumstances aside, the Senegalese epidemic of 1914 was marked by one blunder after another, as eyewitnesses and even historians sympathetic to the colonial state have acknowledged. The Dakar Laboratory director, André Lafont, admitted that while plague was new to Senegal, it had broken out elsewhere in Africa, and the medical authorities should have been on their guard. Yet, despite Dakar's past and recent experiences with cholera, yellow fever, smallpox, and malaria, when it came to plague, "everything had to be improvised."[31] Bruno Salleras blames the cumbersome three-tiered political system for the inertia and delay displayed by French officials in 1914, but even he argues that previous experiences with yellow fever should have been sufficient for officials not to have been surprised by plague.[32] A much sharper critique comes from Elikia Mbokolo, who argues that an atmosphere of "incoherence and inefficiency" prevailed until July, when actions finally started to match intentions.[33]

When the plague struck, the medical community lacked clear indicators of its seriousness. The physician who monitored death rates reported to the Dakar Health Service only at the start of a new month. Not until early May, therefore, did the Health Service discover that the April death rates had been double those of the previous year; nor, even then, did the doctor in charge see any cause for alarm.[34]

Similarly, the colonial bureaucrats were poorly informed about the urban situations they faced. In June, when Governor Antonetti sought legislation making it compulsory for each of the four communes to issue a weekly report with statistics of morbidity and mortality, and causes of death in the quarters affected, the project had to be abandoned because there were no maps of the communes which delineated the various quarters.[35]

When control measures were at last adopted in May, they were inconsistently applied. The only lazaretto in Dakar lacked sufficient space and could only hold 700 or 800 sick and suspects for a period from five to ten days, instead of the internationally recommended ten.[36] Several individuals who were discharged early from the lazaretto later contracted fatal cases of plague. One observer, Paul Rousseau, claimed that some suspects were released after only three days "in order not to displease the large local commercial houses," who regarded themselves as "veritable states within the state."[37] Indeed, as Lafont observed, some Europeans who owned commercial warehouses had found a number of dead rats but had "had hidden this carefully" from health authorities so that their businesses would not be affected.[38] These same self-serving forces pressured medical officials into granting thousands of daily passes so that business in Dakar could continue as usual.[39] The decision to limit quarantine to the African quarter of Dakar, thus exempting the racially mixed residential area and the port district, was another politically inspired decision. For the first two months of the epidemic, therefore, stevedores, stokers, and outfitters boarded every ship which called. When the entire city was finally declared under quarantine, the ships called at Rufisque instead, which changed nothing because by that time the plague had extended through the entire peninsula.

When it came to cleansing and burning operations, the authorities showed a similar lack of planning. They were quick to destroy African dwellings but slow to provide for relocation, thus contributing to the overcrowding in previously uninfected districts of the city, and raising the danger of plague infection when *Y. pestis* inevitably reached these districts. When officials finally created a new African segregation village, they chose an insalubrious site and paid little attention to sanitary rules about housing construction at the residentially segregated location.

Vaccination therapy and rodent control, newer measures to fight plague, brought with them further problems. The first vaccines from France were delayed until late May because the ship failed to bring them directly.[40] Second, health officials were confused about proper vaccine dosage, despite proven experience with the vaccine elsewhere. Attempts at control of the rodent vectors placed the very lives of men, women, and children at risk when authorities encouraged the handling of rat cadavers, some of which were still flea-infested. The death of Niaki Senn may have been only one of many that resulted from a practice that, admittedly, was common throughout the world at that time.[41] Nevertheless, dangerously high doses of vaccine applied to those incubating the infection served not only to increase the death toll but also to discredit French interventionist measures.

Arguably the single greatest medical disaster was the tragedy which befell the fishing community of Yoff, where the *cordon sanitaire* left the villagers without food or water for so long. The Yoff tragedy represents one extreme, namely, how a blindly enforced and ill-considered public health intervention could make a bad situation worse. Isolation against plague by means of a *cordon sanitaire* was never effective against the almost invisible vectors of infected fleas. In the case of Yoff it caused immense harm by depriving the besieged villagers of the sustenance their bodies needed to fight off virulent infection. Rousseau, the only contemporary observer to draw attention to officials' negligence in the Yoff case, was clearly the strongest critic of the way in which the entire 1914 medical crisis was handled. He pointed to the recurrence of plague in 1917 in the *cercles* of Tivaouane and Louga as the most serious consequence of the Colonial Health Service's mismanagement. "The most manifest incompetence, the greatest incoherence, together with the fear of taking responsibility, and, no doubt, the concern not to compromise promotion (a major factor), prevailed during the entire epidemic. Sanitary measures which were required and which were clearly set down in laws, regulations and international agreements, were never applied; the time delays for quarantine and surveillance [were] never respected."[42]

Rousseau's accusations ranged from mistakes and misdemeanors to capital offenses. They included allowing Muslims to wash bodies ritually, permitting natives to rebuild houses with contaminated material, and allowing bubonic plague to spread from Senegal to France itself.[43] Rousseau, however, lacked evidence for these eccentric charges, which undoubtedly discredited him with many readers. In any event, no official mention of Rousseau or of any of his accusations ever made their way into the established medical journals.

André Marcandier's critique was more reasoned. Although he chose his words carefully, he found medical officials in 1914 wanting, both in their slow response to the initial outbreak and in their vacillation throughout the nine months of its duration. The decision to begin control measures so late, and especially the decision to abandon isolation measures in June, produced a "disaster." By July, when isolation measures were again resumed, it was too late to prevent the plague from spreading throughout the city and into the interior.[44]

EPIDEMIC PLAGUE AND SENEGALESE SOCIETY, 1914–18

For Senegal, bubonic plague was a new disease, arriving as part of the world's third pandemic, but also as part of the medical crisis in Africa attendant upon European conquest and the establishment of colonial rule. As was the case throughout the Third World, such factors as urbanization and changes in diet, work, and living patterns combined with the introduction of new disease organisms to place human and animal immune systems under enormous pressure.

The scourge of bubonic plague exposed the deep gulf separating groups within colonial society in Senegal. Not only had the overwhelming majority of plague victims been African rather than French, but the two communities had perceived the epidemic in profoundly different ways. For the majority of the French, the plague strengthened their racist assumptions about African inferiority. The French believed that Africans' ignorance made them incapable of understanding that sanitary control measures were introduced by Western biomedical practitioners in the public interest. So Africans hid their dead, trafficked in inoculation certificates, and spread the disease. Yet this French paternalist discourse overlooked a basic contradiction. If it were in the public interest to receive anti-plague vaccination, and to accept strict controls on travel, why did these rules not apply to the entire population? To be fair, some French voices sounded a minority note. Dr. Rousseau, perhaps out of bitterness, ruthlessly exposed what he saw as carelessness and outright incompetence in the health sphere, while Dr. Marcandier alone took the trouble to investigate the harmful impact of control measures on the population of Dakar. Yet even these two exceptional voices were very much in agreement with the virtually unanimous call for residential segregation.

The sanitary argument rationalizing residential segregation was very much in evidence during the plague epidemic. The French in Senegal, like Europeans all over Africa at the turn of the century, preferred not to have Africans as their neighbors, and the 1914 health emergency gave them a window of opportunity. Residential segregation arose from prejudice and from an unwillingness to accept culturally different ways of living. The medical theories of the day reinforced these sentiments by arguing that Africans also represented a potential or real hazard to the health of Europeans. To express this sentiment is one thing; to pass formal legislation to bring about residential segregation is another. Recognizing that Africans would legitimately resist such programs, colonial governments had to take the social costs into account, and were therefore reluctant to permit whites to have their way completely on such fundamental issues as urban residence.

For Africans, the bubonic plague ordeal of 1914 was a political and not a medical event. Sanitary controls, far from being humanitarian in inspiration, were to Africans an elaborate smoke screen motivated by a desire, first, to disallow Blaise Diagne's electoral victory, and, second, to camouflage the grabbing of Lebu property and to remove by force all Africans from the Plateau. Some went further, and saw in the vaccination campaign a conspiracy to intimidate, and even to assassinate, Diagne. On the other hand, it must be noted that opinions were not entirely polarized along racial lines. A minority of influential Africans, including Diagne eventually, and also Malik Sy and Ahmad Bamba Mbacké, came round to the position that French medical officials acted from disinterested motives even if land speculators did not.

For the Lebu community of Dakar, the plague had been a political as well as a medical drama. Their own medical traditions probably embraced control measures such as quarantine, but certainly not on the scale imposed by the 1914 *cordons*, and nothing they had known matched this extensive intrusion into their lives. Sanitary controls affected traditional practices such as visits to the sick, attendance at funerals, burial practices, and possibly also traditional medical therapy. These controls deprived the community of valuable weapons used by people everywhere to ease social tensions at times of traumatic illness, death, and mourning. It must have been a tremendous hardship for people not to be able to show respect to the dead during the medical emergency.

Plague not only affected older social practices, it also disrupted new practices. It meant school closures, and the prohibition of both public meet-

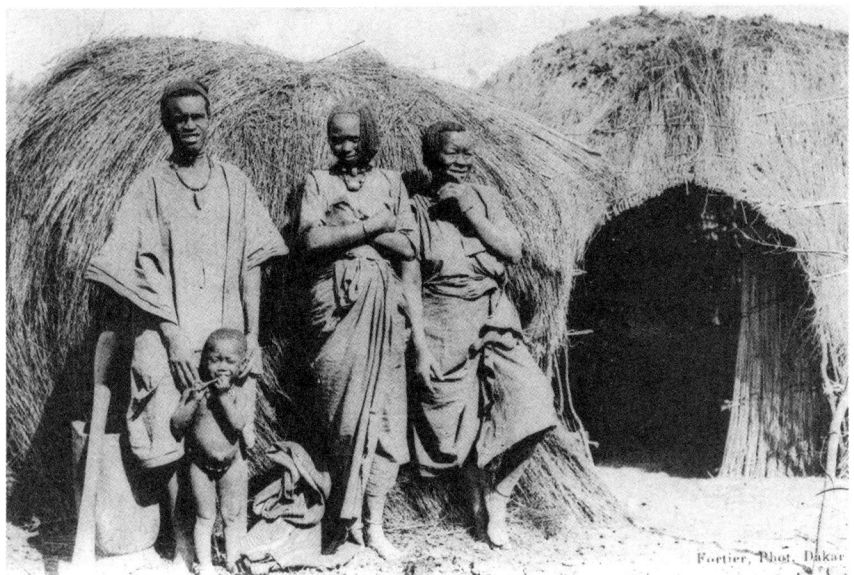

Photo 6.1 Fuulbe Pastoralists in Their Temporary Homes Northeast of Thiès, c. 1912. Some observers believed that their thatched straw dwellings provided harbors for plague-infected rodents. Courtesy of the Archives Nationales du Sénégal. All rights reserved.

ings and the free circulation of trade goods and persons. Before 1914, while French colonialism had brought with it enormous economic and political changes, the pace of social change had been slower. French rule had given Africans space and latitude in their social and cultural affairs. Not only political and economic issues but also this sense of social invasion help explain the depth of the African response to plague control measures in 1914.

While the political protests can be documented from French archival records, much remains unknown about other African responses. Whether new Lebu medical therapies emerged in the wake of the plague, for example, is a major unanswered question. Judging from evidence from rural communities afflicted by plague, one hypothesis may be suggested. Lebu healers, or *saltigis*, would most likely have refused to put their reputations on the line by claiming to be able to cure so implacable a scourge as *Y. pestis*.

Like other epidemics, the plague of 1914 brought out the best and worst in human behavior. Acts of kindness certainly occurred, with people insisting on visiting and tending to the sick, whether or not this placed them at great risk of infection. On the other hand, evidence of fear and inhumanity could also be found, as in the cases of migrant laborers without kin whose bodies were unceremoniously dumped into the street by landlords seeking to avoid having their property condemned. Scapegoating was present in both communities. Both the French and the Lebu of Dakar held strangers and outsiders—for example, Moroccan merchants or Fuulbe pastoralists—responsible for transmitting plague.

None of this should be surprising. The tendency to blame victims is deeply rooted. During the second pandemic of bubonic plague in the fourteenth century, minorities like the Jews, or majorities like the poor, were scapegoated. Dorothy Nelkin and Sander L. Gilman have observed that "in a situation of communal anxiety, locating blame for disease is in effect a strategy of control. . . . Placing blame defines the normal, establishes the boundaries of healthy behaviour . . . and distinguishes the observer from the cause of fear."[45]

Some would argue, as has Frantz Fanon, that Africans' opposition to Western medicine throughout the continent was predetermined because their refusal represented one of the few defensive responses to domination open to the colonized. To a degree, this view seems to be corroborated by events in Dakar during the 1914 epidemic. Yet closer examination shows that the African reaction was rational rather than reflexive and predetermined. If Africans rejected health control measures, they did so because the procedures were ineffective if not injurious. In reality, no scientific case can be made to show that the French health specialists made a serious impact on the course of the plague during the war years. Despite their best intentions, they lacked truly effective biomedical weapons and misused the tools at their disposal that might have made a difference.

Another feature of the plague outbreak was the self-interested behavior of certain groups, and the absence of a wider civic sense that public health was a matter of concern to the entire community. If the French business community had its own agenda, so too did the senior colonial administrators, the Diagnists, and the Lebu urban elite. Significantly, the first victims of forced removal to the new segregation village were those with the least power, namely, the most recent urban migrants. Many among this group were condemned to suffer as plague victims, and perhaps to die, without the presence of families to offer care and comfort.

William Ponty has acquired a reputation as a decisive administrator and a leading architect of French colonial rule in West Africa. His skilful handling of such difficult issues as the abolition of slavery, the acquisition of political rights in the four communes, and military recruitment during the First World War have all been cited in the historical literature.[46] Judged by his handling of the plague epidemic, however, this view requires revision. Ponty vacillated throughout the crisis between support for the medical experts and political expediency. Nor did he show any reluctance to use the stick rather than the carrot. As late as November 1914, Ponty was prepared to use armed force against angry and distraught Lebu civilians. Only when his minister in Paris warned of the dangers of shedding the blood of Senegalese Muslims in particular did Ponty quickly reverse himself. Prepared at one point to follow the heavy-handed advice of Governor Antonetti, a week later Ponty blamed Antonetti for having broken the word of the French administration to the Lebu property holders. Nor did Ponty or any of his successors display much of their vaunted humanitarianism toward those Dakarois forced to inhabit the Médina, which remained an example of urban blight for much of its existence.

Some years later, many in Senegal still took issue with Ponty's handling of the 1914 crisis. The conservative French community felt that Ponty had capitulated to the Lebu. As *L'AOF* bluntly stated in its issue of 3 August 1916, "the demonstrators had made the governor-general tremble."[47] Two years after that, Governor-General Angoulvant took the unusual step of criticizing his deceased predecessor: "he [Ponty] wanted to conciliate all the interests involved when it was necessary to know which ones to sacrifice."[48] Similarly, Inspector of Colonies Revel's report at the end of the war found that "M. Ponty was more concerned to avoid difficulties than to overcome them, more desirous of concealing the reality than of finding a solution; he preferred not to see the danger and refused to recognize its nature."[49]

For quite different reasons, Blaise Diagne was also critical of Ponty. In June 1915, he told a gathering of African residents of the Médina that "the governor-general was wrong to have moved you here under the open sun and not to have concerned himself with your housing."[50] Diagne, in fact, conducted himself with integrity during and after the plague epidemic of 1914. Once he had secured confirmation that his election would not be revoked, he used his considerable skills as a mediator to induce his Lebu constituents to accept reasonable sanitary control measures. Given the patriotism of Ponty and other republicans, Diagne was concerned that, once war broke out, political considerations would trump medical ones. During the war years, Diagne fought tenaciously to make the acquired rights of the *originaires* secure, but he did not ignore land or health issues. He continued to press for a just resolution of Lebu land claims, and for a color-blind application of health measures such as vaccination during the 1918 plague outbreak.

Widespread and high mortality from bubonic plague in 1914 did not lead to health reform, although the war certainly impeded such a development as well.[51] During the war, overcrowding and social inequality persisted in the urban areas of Senegal. The health of the African public did not improve, and it probably deteriorated, in this trying period, though there is no quantitative way to determine this. Many medical features of bubonic plague continued to mystify Western biomedicine. Like their counterparts elsewhere, the French medical authorities could not account for the appearance of bubonic plague in 1914, nor could they explain its temporary retreat in 1915 and its reappearance in 1916. When a major outbreak occurred in Saint-Louis and in the *cercles* running south to Thiès in 1918, it became clear that no empirical, let alone scientific, lessons had been learned from the 1914 experience. The colony remained as vulnerable as before. In short, when it came to plague and perhaps other afflictions as well, the Senegalese population had little reason to believe in the efficacy of Western medicine.

Nevertheless, by the war's end, the politics of accommodation between the French administration and the African political and religious elite had prevented the worst features of a limited and racially focused health policy from developing. A new political equilibrium had been established, one which recognized the electoral power of Africans. The African elite, for example, now had sufficient power to prevent the worst forms of residential segregation, which were emerging in other parts of Africa, from taking hold in Senegal.[52] While it is true that the Médina had become an economic and to some degree a racial ghetto, the European residents of Dakar were forced to acknowledge that complete racial segregation was unattainable. Along with the recognition of French citizenship, Diagne had secured for better-off Africans, *originaires,* and even subjects the right to live in any part of Dakar they could afford.

NOTES

1. The official estimate is found in Collomb, Huot, and Lecomte, "Note sur l'épidémie de peste au Sénégal en 1914," *Annales de Hygiène et de Médecine Coloniales* 19 (1921): 60.

2. André Marcandier, "La peste à Dakar (1914–15)," *Archives de Médecine Navale* 106 (1918): 139.

3. Collomb, Huot, and Lecomte, "Note," 40.

4. Marcandier, "La peste," 143.

5. For a fascinating discussion of diagnosis in the pre- and post-laboratory phases of plague history, see Andrew Cunningham, "Transforming Plague: The Laboratory

and the Identity of Infectious Disease," in *The Laboratory Revolution in Medicine*, edited by Andrew Cunningham and Perry Williams (Cambridge: Cambridge University Press, 1992), 209–44.

6. Collomb, Huot, and Lecomte, "Note," 58.

7. The official report noted that death figures were "recorded as precisely as possible from the information furnished by local authorities." Collomb, Huot, and Lecomte, "Note," 58.

8. Collomb, Huot, and Lecomte, "Note," 60.

9. André Lafont, "Une épidémie de peste humaine à Dakar (avril 1914–février 1915)," *Bulletin de la Société de Pathologie Exotique* 8 (1915): 663.

10. Marcandier, "La peste," 144.

11. Alexandre Kermorgant, "L'épidémie de peste qui a sévi à Dakar et au Sénégal d'avril 1914 à février 1915", *Bulletin de l'Academie de Médecine* 76 (1916): 133.

12. Lafont, "Une épidémie," 661.

13. Kermorgant, "Epidémie," 133. The stricken Syrian was Amin Gaouy, who was described by *L'AOF*, on 16 May 1914, as having had a "mild case of plague." Whether he recovered or not was not reported.

14. Marcandier, "La peste," 143.

15. Kermorgant, "Epidémie," 133.

16. This is not to argue the case for significant human transmission of plague; that would only have been true of pneumonic plague, and victims of this form of plague were usually too ill to travel any distance. But human traffic did provide an opportunity for rodents, their flea vectors, and, of course, *Yersinia pestis*, to seek wider opportunities.

17. Marcandier, "La peste," 136 and 144.

18. Angélique Diop, "Santé et colonisation au Sénégal, 1895–1914" (thèse de troisième cycle, Université de Paris I, Paris, 1982), 291.

19. The portraits are drawn from Marcandier, "La peste," 136–43.

20. Unless otherwise stated, all references to plague in the interior are from Collomb, Huot, and Lecomte, "Note," 46–56.

21. The villages were N'Dara, Khayes, Keur-Moussa-Bougane, Keur-Gallo-Isser, Keur-Masamba-Diop, N'Guer, and Diarrhérat.

22. The Guélor of 1914 was southeast of Khombole, but the newer villages of Guélor Sérère and Guélor Ouolof are to be found a dozen kilometers away, south and west of Khombole. For the most part I have used spellings currently in use in Senegal, such as Ndiaganiao in preference to Diagagniao, and Tatène for Tattène.

23. ANS\H55, Dr. L. Huot, Director of the Health Service of Senegal, "Rapport d'ensemble sur l'épidémie de peste 1914–1915", Dakar, 3 March 1915 (hereafter cited as Huot, "Rapport d'ensemble").

24. The villages listed were Diaye-Diaye, and Guedj in October; and Soussoum, Diarao and Gondj, in early November. Collomb, Huot, and Lecomte, "Note," 56.

25. Acting Governor Antonetti, session of the General Council on 5 November 1914, in *Conseil Général, procès-verbal des délibérations*:sessions of October 1914 (Paris and Saint-Louis: Imprimerie du Gouvernement, 1915), 143.

26. Diop, "Santé," 40, gives early health budgets running to slightly over 200,000 francs per annum at the turn of the century.

In 1914, the French franc was worth slightly more than U.S. $2, so 1.1 million francs was equivalent to roughly $2.3 million.

27. Antonetti to General Council on 5 November 1914, 143.

28. Session of the General Council on 18 October 1915, in *Conseil Général, procès-verbal des déliberations*:sessions of October 1915 (Paris and Saint-Louis: Imprimerie du Gouvernement, 1917), 20.

29. Session of the General Council on 18 October 1915, 21.

30. Session of the General Council on 21 October 1915, 131.

31. Lafont, "Une épidémie," 674.

32. Bruno Salleras, "La peste à Dakar en 1914: Médina, ou les enjeux complexes d'une politique sanitaire" (thèse de troisième cycle, Université de Paris, École des Hautes Études en Sciences Sociales, Paris, 1984), 106.

33. Elikia Mbokolo, "Peste et société urbaine à Dakar: L'épidémie de 1914," *Cahiers d'Études Africaines* 22 (1982): 23, 26. Mbokolo concludes that the forceful control measures, especially large-scale vaccination and systematic deratting, enabled authorities to succeed, "not without brutality," in controlling the epidemic. Such a cause-and-effect assertion cannot be proven. More recent research, in fact, suggests that deratting during an epidemic may have helped spread plague, and that vaccination after an epidemic had begun was far less significant than preventive vaccination a month or two before the plague season began.

34. Mbokolo, "Peste," 19.

35. Mbokolo, "Peste," 24.

36. Huot, "Rapport d'ensemble."

37. Paul Rousseau, "Au sujet de la peste du Sénégal," *Journal des Praticiens* 31 (1917): 743.

38. Lafont, "Une épidémie," 677.

39. Rousseau, "La peste," 743.

40. Mbokolo, "Peste," 23.

41. British colonial authorities, for example, paid such generous and extensive bounties for rat tails during and after an epidemic in Malawi that the premiums paid out actually had an impact on the local economy. The head of the Livingstonia Mission instructed the headmasters of primary schools to accept payment of school fees in the form of rat tails. M. C. Musambachime, "The Bubonic Plague Epidemic in Karonga (Northern Malawi) and the North East Luangwa Valley (Eastern Zambia) between 1916 and 1920," unpublished paper, Department of History, University of Namibia, 1999. In Kampala, Uganda, in 1920, enthusiastic health officers proudly arranged stacks of rat tails to form the word RATS. Megan Vaughan, *Curing Their Ills: Colonial Power and African Illness* (Stanford, Calif.: Stanford University Press, 1991), 41–42.

42. Rousseau, "La peste," 743.

43. Noting that a few cases of plague had been reported in Paris, Rousseau went so far as to suggest that criminal proceedings, including "civil degradation, and fines or imprisonment leading even to forced labor or the death penalty" should be invoked against certain unnamed medical figures for their negligence in Senegal. Rousseau, "La peste," 744.

44. Marcandier, "La peste," 217.

45. Dorothy Nelkin and Sander L. Gilman, "Placing Blame for Devastating Disease," *Social Research* 55 (1988): 362–63.

46. G. Wesley Johnson, "William Ponty and Republican Paternalism in French West Africa, 1866–1915," in *African Proconsuls: European Governors in Africa*, edited by

L. H. Gann and P. Duignan (Stanford, Calif.: Hoover Institution, 1978), 127–56; James F. Searing, "Accommodation and Resistance: Chiefs, Muslim Leaders, and Politicians in Colonial Senegal, 1890–1934" (Ph.D dissertation, Princeton University, Princeton, 1985), 237–39; Martin A. Klein, *Slavery and Colonial Rule in French West Africa* (Cambridge: Cambridge University Press, 1998), 126.

47. *L'AOF*, 3 August 1916.

48. Salleras, "La peste," 170. Salleras excuses Ponty because of the pressures of war and politics but agrees that he took half-measures.

49. Cited in Salleras, "La peste," 170.

50. Cited in *L'AOF*, 22 June 1915.

51. While I regard Elikia Mbokolo's article on the 1914 plague outbreak as an outstanding work of scholarship, I am in disagreement with him on this one point. He suggests that bubonic plague awoke the colonial administration from its torpor and forced it to put urban public health high on its agenda. As will be demonstrated in Part Two, the administration's record with regard to public health in the cities remained dismal until after the Second World War. Mbokolo, "Peste," 44.

52. John Iliffe, *The African Poor, a History* (Cambridge: Cambridge University Press, 1987), 167–68.

PART II

KOOXA DOOMA KA: "ACUTE HEADACHES," 1919–38[1]

Part Two focuses on the environmental, social, and cultural impact of bubonic plague in both rural and urban Senegal between the two world wars. Chapter 7 studies the physical and human ecology of the emerging "plague zone." Chapter 8 shifts attention to the responses of rural Senegalese toward the calamity in their midst. The text draws on African collective memories of the plague years, as voiced by plague survivors and their kin. Chapter 9 examines plague in urban Senegal, together with the role of the French medical establishment in the continuing struggle to control it.

The data in Table A.1 in the appendix show that bubonic plague became virtually an annual visitor to Senegal after 1919, making it endemic to some regions, epidemic in others, and (to use the awkward medical term), endo-epidemic overall. For the Senegalese communities at risk, an important change in attitude was taking shape. Bubonic plague, and the obnoxious control measures accompanying each outbreak, were becoming burdens to be endured even while they were contested. While many continued to resent and oppose the unpopular control measures imposed upon them, others began to cooperate cautiously with French health workers. A minority of Senegalese joined the colonial medical services, albeit in subservient positions, and participated not only in plague control, but also in the gradual extension of public health facilities throughout the colony.

As the years between the wars passed, French medical responses to bubonic plague remained rigid and unchanging. Although it gradually became understood, certainly by the late 1920s, that the rat flea *Xenopsylla cheopis* was the critical plague vector, control measures remained focused on control of the movement of humans, rather than rodents and their fleas. If it could be said by the end of the 1930s that plague was receding or even dying out in Senegal, it was more likely to have been the work of natural forces than calculated human intervention.

If persistence was the hallmark of *Yersinia pestis* and its French medical adversaries during the interwar period, the same term seems appropriate for Senegal's perennial deputy, Blaise Diagne. He consolidated his power in 1919 by winning the first peacetime election against strong French colonial opposition, but soon afterward, he negotiated a pact of accommodation with the powerful French commercial houses of Bordeaux. This pact guaranteed him reelection until his death in 1934. The class-based privileges Diagne secured for the small Senegalese elite during the First World War were never extended to the great majority of the largely rural Senegalese population, who continued to be viewed in French colonial law as "subjects" of an autocratic regime. For the next generation, Senegal would be governed through patronage involving a complex working arrangement among the French colonial administration, Diagne's patronage machine, the Lebu elites, and the Muslim religious leadership.

NOTE

1. The phrase and its translation are from Guedj Faye, interviewed at Ngayokhème, 3 October 1990. He has worked as an interpreter and assistant in various medical projects among the Sereer of Siin, including two of the Siin Sereer villages where Marguerite Dupire and her colleagues conducted fieldwork in the 1960s, and which had been struck by plague around 1920. See Marguerite Dupire, André Lericollais, Bernard Delpech, and Jean-Marc Gastellu, "Résidence, tenure foncière, alliance dans une société bilinéaire (Serer du Sine et du Baol, Sénégal)," *Cahiers d'Études Africaines* 55 (1974): 417–52.

7

"THE PLAGUE LEAPS OUT OF THE GROUND": PLAGUE ECOLOGY IN SENEGAL[1]

This chapter examines the complex environmental changes which occurred in the plague zone of Senegal, and then introduces the plague zone's inhabitants to the reader. Muslim Sereer and Wolof members of the Tijaniyya brotherhood developed a response to endemic plague which was different from the majority of Sereer Ndut. Taking their cue from their leadership, the Muslim community in and around Tivaouane and Thiès came to accept plague as an act of God, and ended their resistance to the interventionist approach of the French medical establishment. Non-Muslim Sereer Ndut, meanwhile, continued to oppose the maladroit and sometimes brutal anti-plague measures.

Changes in the environment have often been a critical factor in the interaction between parasites and their hosts. While the linkage between European conquest, changes in land management, and the spread of sleeping sickness in Central and East Africa is clear, the connections between human actions, environmental change, and the spread of bubonic plague in Senegal are less so.[2] The present study cannot resolve this complex issue, but the preliminary discussion which follows would seem to be merited.

THE PHYSICAL ENVIRONMENT OF THE PLAGUE ZONE

As plague returned to Senegal year after year, it became evident that a relatively small but highly important region was being continually victim-

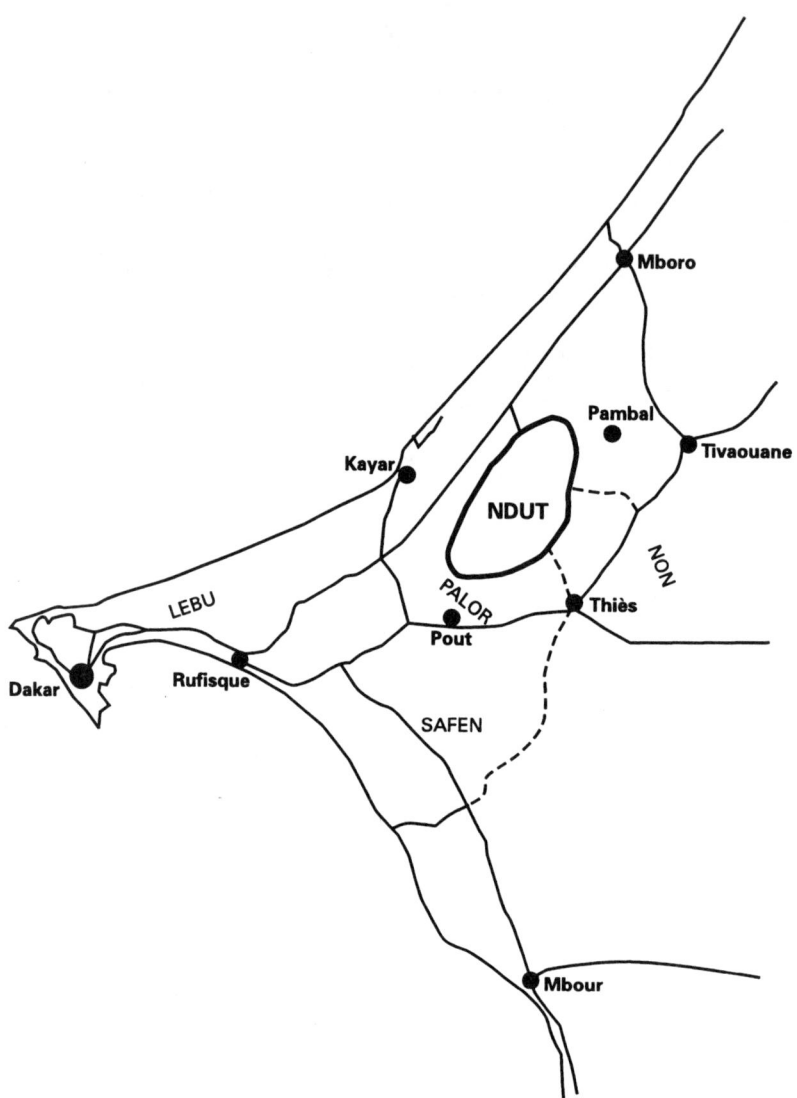

Map 7.1 Sereer Ndut and Their Neighbors. This map has been adapted by the author from Charles Becker, "Les Serer Ndut: Études sur les mutations sociales et réligieuses" (Mémoire de l'École Pratique des Hautes-Études, Paris, 1970), 2.

ized. Labeled the "plague zone" by French public health officials, the region formed a triangle stretching from Dakar through the Cape Verde peninsula to the major inland towns of Thiès, some 50 kilometers east, and

Tivaouane, 80 kilometers to the northeast. Thiès was the railway capital of Senegal and plague infection there presented a constant threat, unrealized as it happened, that the disease would spread deep into the hinterland of French West Africa. Tivaouane, the Senegalese headquarters of the Tijaniyya brotherhood, was a locale frequently visited by the Muslim faithful. In the interwar period, the plague zone included roughly 20 percent of the country's entire population, including the federal capital, port, and rail center, and one of the country's three major religious centers.[3] While most of the population consisted of townspeople, there were three rural, agricultural districts within the zone: the mixed Lebu, Wolof, and Sereer truck farming villages of the Cape Verde peninsula; the Sereer villages known colloquially as "Mont-Roland" on the Thiès escarpment; and the area inhabited by mixed Lebu, Wolof, and Sereer farmers who exploited a tiny, fertile area called the *niayes*, or dunes. A narrow band of land about 7 kilometers wide, and in some places only 4 or 5 kilometers from the sea, never expanding more than 60 kilometers to the east, this micro-region began near Rufisque and ran north throughout the zone until it petered out at a point just south of Gandiol.[4]

Blessed with an attractive environment similar to that of a desert oasis, the *niayes* could retain fresh rainwater, sometimes for an entire year.[5] This tiny microclimate was attractive to a variety of plants and animals, ranging from small rodents to humans; it may have been a propitious environment for microbial parasites as well. An early colonial medical report noted that people inhabiting the *niayes* had been ravaged by sleeping sickness, and spent only the amount of time in the area that was absolutely necessary to maintain their small plots.[6] Despite these risks, few farmers could resist the temptation to exploit the *niayes*. These risk-takers benefited from access to water, date palms, fruit trees, and small but fertile farm plots. In earlier times, Lebu and Wolof fishing villages were located near to the *niayes*, with easy access to both the sea and fresh water. Transhumant Fuulbe also used the *niayes* to water their herds while moving them south from the Senegal Valley. As cities and towns sprang up along the Dakar-Saint-Louis rail line, which ran just to the east of the *niayes*, the oases proved a valuable area in which to practice market gardening. Indeed, a considerable urban population could be found on the line stretching from Dakar through Rufisque to Thiès, and then north via such rail towns as Tivaouane, Meckhé, Kébémer, and Louga. Lying at the very center of the region was Lake Tanma, itself very close to the Sereer Ndut lands. At the same time, the carrying capacity of this area was extremely limited.

While it can be documented that the *niayes* attracted a variety of rodents, in the absence of any studies we can only speculate as to whether the microclimate enabled such microorganisms as *Yersinia pestis* to gain a niche.[7] The arrival of *Xenopsylla cheopis*, the most efficient flea vector of plague, is an equally intriguing puzzle. *X. cheopis* is today found worldwide, especially between latitudes 35 degrees south and north of the equator, but we do not know if its wide distribution is the result of a recent species invasion.[8] No evidence exists to support the speculation that it may have been introduced into Senegal, on the back of a rat perhaps, as a result of the expanded international trade of the late nineteenth century, just in time to be in place when *Y. pestis* reached West Africa. What is clear is that the first scientific survey of flea distribution in Senegal, which began in 1928, found *X. cheopis* to be the most common flea in the area on both sides of the rail lines stretching from Dakar north to Louga and east to Diourbel and encompassing the *niayes*.[9]

The persistence of plague for three decades and its endemicity in the region suggest that plague bacteria did find a wild rodent reservoir in one of the few environments in Senegal that could bring together all of the organisms required to produce both epizootics and epidemics. The *niayes'* microclimate probably also solves two mysteries which baffled French scientists of the day. First, the rodent reservoir would explain why the plague seemed to "leap out of the ground" on an almost annual basis, without benefit of importation via the sea lanes from abroad. Second, the failure of the plague to spread significantly to the east and the north was a function of the drier, hotter temperature there, which was inhospitable to fleas. The window of opportunity in which the bacteria, the rodents, the fleas, and the humans were all in place was closed for a far greater part of the year outside the well-defined plague zone.

THE INHABITANTS OF THE PLAGUE ZONE

The communities inhabiting the plague zone were heterogeneous. In the majority was an autochthonous agricultural population of northwestern Sereer; Wolof farmers were part of a more recent influx; and a small number of Fuulbe pastoralists lived part of every year in the region as a function of their transhumant migrations. Distinct from the numerous Sereer-speaking peoples of the old kingdom of Siin, the northwestern Sereer were stateless segmentary groups divided into five small subgroups named Safen, None, Léhar, Palor, and Ndut.[10] Relatively more is known about the last mentioned, the Sereer Ndut, and they have been chosen as a case study of rural response to endemic plague in the interwar era.[11]

Plague Ecology in Senegal 143

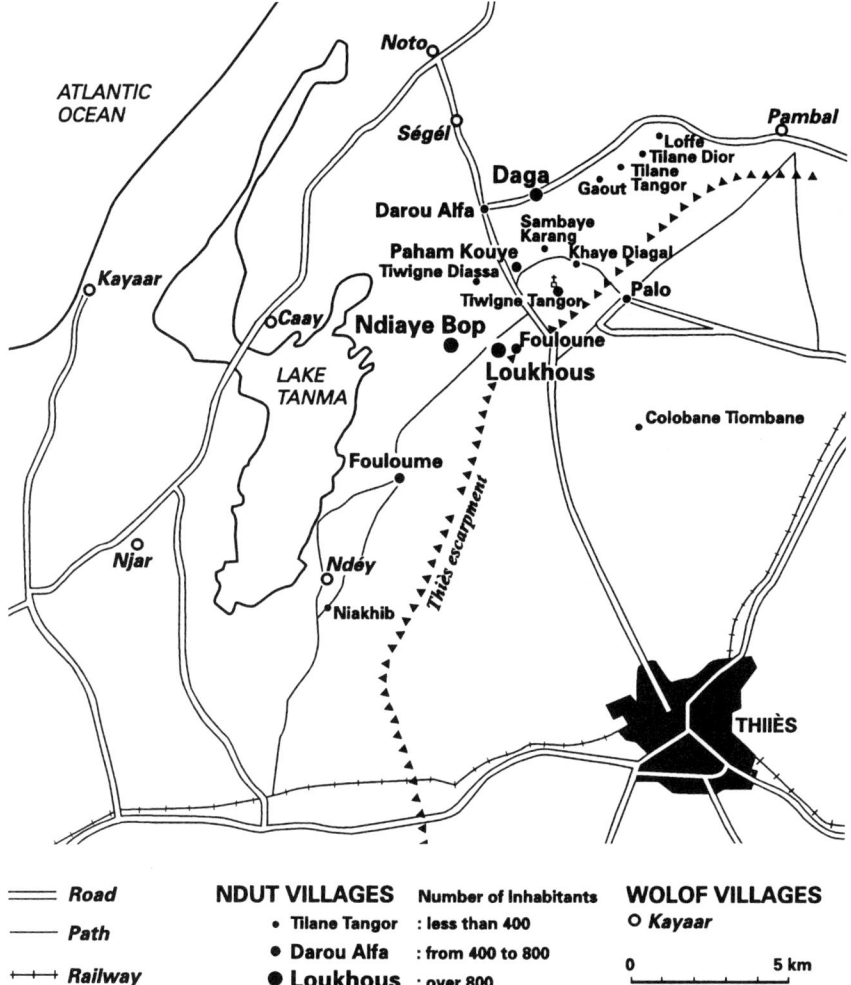

Map 7.2 Sereer Ndut Region. This map has been adapted by the author from Marguerite Dupire, *Sagesse sereer: Essais sur la pensée sereer ndut* (Paris: Karthala, 1994), 6.

The northwest Sereer inhabited the southern frontier region of the Wolof kingdom of Kajoor and the western frontier of Bawol, at the time an area more forested and difficult of access than it would later become under French rule. Subjected to slave raiding by *ceddo* warriors, as well as the vicissitudes of irregular rainfall, periodic drought, and epidemic disease, the northwest Sereer were typical of those classic segmentary societies which were able to preserve their cultural autonomy, but only at considerable social and demographic cost. Among the many Senegalese who were victims of the Atlantic slave trade, the northwest Sereer were despised as "savages" by their Muslim neighbors, and withdrew into their then forested regions.[12] The first French accounts of the Sereer Ndut describe a tiny, enclosed society, hostile to the outside world of more powerful Muslim and Christian forces. A census of 1865, for example, counted only 1,756 people living in a total of thirteen small Ndut villages; no community was larger than 310 and most consisted of about half that number.[13] In comparison, the Sereer region of Siin, while also densely populated, extended over a much larger territory.[14]

Sereer Ndut country is located approximately 100 kilometers to the east and northeast of Dakar, and some 15 kilometers north of Thiès. The region, known colloquially in the twentieth century as "Mont-Roland," and by the Ndut as Tiwigne, forms part of the Thiès escarpment.[15] The Ndut land traces an arc of a circle around a promontory on the escarpment, and is bounded on the south by scrub brush known as "tangor," and on the west by the Lake Tanma depression.[16] All told, the Ndut villages occupy a band of land 25 kilometers in length and varying in width from 1 to 7 kilometers. This valley includes the fertile *niayes*. To the east, a barrier of scrub land separates the Ndut from the Sereer None, whose lands begin at the village of Pambal.

The Ndut are subsistence farmers of millet, maize, and beans, with some export production of peanuts. They also maintain small cattle herds, which are often consigned to Fuulbe pastoralists. Little out-migration occurred among the Ndut until after the Second World War.[17] Like other Sereer, the Ndut had close ties with Lebu fishing communities, which were themselves of mixed origins. One theory held that the Lebu village of Ouakam, for example, was originally founded by migrants from the Sereer Ndut region.[18] Many matrilineal and patrilineal names are the same in both cultures.[19]

Colonial rule began with the construction of forts at Pout and Thiès in 1863. The French completed the annexation of the lands of the northwestern Sereer, and set off a series of dramatic changes, when they defeated the last Wolof ruler of Kajoor, Lat Dior, in 1883.[20] Earlier, camel caravans had brought goods to the Senegal River or to ports at Dakar, Rufisque, and Saint-Louis. But after the 1870s, the rail lines pushed through the heart of the Wolof state of Kajoor, close to the northwestern Sereer, and enabled the cultivation of peanuts to spread.[21]

Administratively, the Sereer Ndut were placed within the French colonial *cercle* of Tivaouane, even though the region would later enjoy easier communication by means of a better road to the closer *cercle* capital of Thiès.

The demographic trends in the plague zone were characteristic of those in western Senegal as a whole under French rule. In the period leading up to the First World War, there was significant urbanization, with the towns of Thiès and Tivaouane benefiting from their strategic location on the rail line. At the same time, overall densities of population in and around the plague zone continued to be among the highest in all of Senegal.[22] Population increased markedly throughout Senegal after 1920, and the plague zone was no exception.[23] At the micro level, data are scanty. The twin Ndut villages of Tiwigne Tangor and Tiwigne Diassa were said to have included only 200 persons between them in 1865. In 1927, they had grown, respectively, to 233 and 899 persons.[24]

THE CHRISTIAN SEREER OF MONT-ROLAND

Somewhat unusually for Senegal, a large minority, perhaps 20 percent, of the Sereer Ndut are Roman Catholics.[25] Their conversion, which began in the 1890s with the establishment of the mission of the Congrégation du Saint-Esprit (Pères Spiritains), accelerated considerably after 1925.[26] There was a rush of conversions in the mission's first decade, a time when Father A. Sebire, the author of an important study of the useful plants of Senegal, was stationed in the Ndut area.[27]

In 1901 Father J. Boutrais began his forty-seven-year mission to the Sereer Ndut at Mont-Roland. Throughout the plague years of the interwar period, the Christian mission among the Ndut was dominated by his presence. A tenacious and stolid man, he persisted despite the failure of the tiny congregation to attract many converts until the 1920s. It might be tempting to speculate that the long ordeal of the Ndut through many plague epidemics accelerated the pace of conversion, except that there is no evidence at all to support such a contention. Charles Becker's more plausible account is that the first wave of converts was composed of adolescents, but that after 1901, Ndut elders opposed conversion.[28] When Father Boutrais returned in 1918 after an absence during the war, he was able to overcome this opposition. Conversions in the 1920s averaged about 60 a year, and over 100 annually in the 1930s. The best single year was 1929, when 132 conversions were recorded.

Although the order's archives at Chevilly-Larue near Paris contain Father Boutrais's correspondence with the mother house, the references to plague, although poignant, are sparse. What is striking is the almost complete absence of a healing dimension. Father Boutrais was, in short, as far from a medical missionary as it was possible to be.[29] His first reference to plague occurred in 1926, when he reported: "Plague still has not disappeared and has killed 22 Christians and catechists. Lots of pagans have been baptized on their deathbeds. Plague since Easter; never lasted this long before, [it] may be due to the fact that the rains were not strong, and did not destroy the fleas."[30]

The following year saw not only plague but yellow fever hit his parishioners:

> When I left Thiès last week, the plague had just made its appearance. Poor Senegal! All the epidemics congregate here. You have no doubt heard that we also have yellow fever. Tivaouane and Mbour were very hard hit. At Tivaouane there were nine deaths; the tenth fled before the quarantine, and died on arrival at Diourbel. The Europeans have evacuated Tivaouane; there is hardly anybody there now. I made seven trips there, but almost always for burials. Only one patient requested a priest. I was able to arrive in time to hear confession, and one hour later, he died. At Thiès, the sanitary situation was good when I left. Let us hope that this continues.
>
>   At Tiwigne, there was one case of plague close to Easter. . . . [E]veryone stayed at home, for fear of contagion.[31]

In 1928, Father Boutrais provided his superior with his most extensive comments yet on the devastating impact of plague in his parish:

> Our work [building the church] has been delayed because we have had plague at Mont-Roland for three months. This year the plague has been more terrible than in previous ones. There are many cases of pulmonary plague. For many weeks, Mont-Roland has been a real battlefront; all the compounds have been hit, villages entirely abandoned and fires everywhere; and death a permanent fixture. Many Christians have died; all have received the last rites; catechists and others were able to be baptized. People fled from each other; they fled from me as well, since I was in contact with many of the sick and I touched them. The poor patients, they were confined to the fields, far from the houses, and relatives had to be satisfied with looking on from a distance. On more than one occasion, I had to be the one to announce their deaths when passing close to the village. Immediately, the women began crying, with more shouts than tears. That was life in Mont-Roland for several months. For the past two weeks there have

not been any deaths. The third Sunday after Pentecost two women died, right next to the mission. The sick from three villages had been consigned to the hill where the statue of the Virgin is located. Among them were three unfortunates who suffered horribly. I went to see them at night because I could hear their moans from my bedroom, and I baptized all three of them. The first, a woman of about 30, said to me: "I have believed in Jesus Christ for a long time, and I would like to be baptized." The second, a grandmother, extended her two hands to me: "I would like to go to heaven," she said. She was the first to die. The third, who was very young and who was nursing her first-born, said to me: "And I, will I not also be baptized?" "Is this your wish?" I asked. "Yes," she replied, "I have often been to Church." The next day, after Mass, I went to see her; they were digging her grave, and her body was stretched out next to a tree. Last week a small boy was stricken, but he recovered. He was a catechist, very gentle. In his suffering he asked only for one thing, a medal. Last Sunday, I went to see him after Mass. An old man still at the lazaretto said to me: "Oh, Yuya is cured; while you were singing at the church during Mass, he started singing as well; he sang the way you people do."[32]

Father Boutrais also reported in 1928 on deathbed baptisms of plague victims in two Sereer None villages he had visited: "Plague has broken out in two Sereer None villages. There are very few Christians there but a few unfortunate pagans were baptized before they died. In one week, nine have died of plague. One mother, ill herself, has lost five of her children in one blow, four young adults and a girl of fifteen."[33] Fortunately for the devastated community, 1929 did not see plague return to Mont-Roland. Instead, the decade of the 1930s would be marked by the steady retreat of plague from both urban and rural Senegal. Father Boutrais reported happily on the successful inauguration of the new church in 1929, attended by 500 Europeans with some ninety automobiles converging on the small parish. Also present were "a huge number" of Africans, including their chiefs and members of the Wolof cavalry.[34]

THE TIJANIYYA MUSLIMS

Although the Sereer Ndut were hostile toward Muslim traders and clerics from outside their region before French rule, Islam was finally able to make some inroads into the community immediately after the First World War. The first Muslim Ndut villages were Keur Daouda Ciss, founded in 1920, and Darou Alfa, established in 1924 and named after its founder, Serigne Alfa Thiombane. Gradually the Muslim Ndut villages took on a Wolof appearance. The early Muslims were converted to the Tijaniyya ritual by Serigne Sangoné Mbaye, originally from Kajoor, and a disciple of Al-Hajj Malik Sy. He was succeeded by Serigne Alfa Tiombane, a native of the village of Daga, in Ndut country.[35]

In the 1920s, conversion to Islam caused tensions as some young people abandoned the Sereer Ndut religion despite the objections of their elders. Coupled with the plague epidemics, these conversions resulted in a further dispersion of the population since they led to the founding of new Muslim villages and neighborhoods set apart from nonbelievers.[36]

While the plague zone on the Thiès escarpment was religiously pluralist, since the zone included the important religious town of Tivaouane within its boundaries, the plague was a matter of great concern to Senegalese Muslims in general, and to members of the Tijaniyya brotherhood in particular. Some background information is in order.

The Tijani order was founded around 1782 by Ahmad at-Tijani, who was originally from Ain-Mahdi near Laghouat in present-day Algeria, but who founded his *zawiya* at Fez, where he died in 1815 and was buried.[37] The success of the Tijani order in West Africa is associated with the rise to prominence of Al-Hajj Umar Tall, holy man, military leader, and state builder.[38] The movement's most important Senegalese leader was Al-Hajj Malik Sy, born in 1855 in the Upper Senegal Valley, in the very same year that the French were conquering the Wolof kingdom of Waalo.

Malik Sy was one of a new generation of Muslim leaders who came into prominence in the Wolof states after the 1860s. Opposed to military expansion in the name of Islam, these men sought to proselytize by peaceful means. Like Ahmadou Bamba Mbacké, founder of the Mourid brotherhood, Malik Sy was an assimilated Wolof from a Tukolor clerical family.[39] He was, moreover, linked to Al-Hajj Umar Tall and the Tijaniyya when, at eighteen years of age, he came under the tutelage of a maternal uncle who had been initiated into the order by Al-Hajj Umar himself.[40] While still a young man, Malik completed his pilgrimage to Mecca in 1889, and set up a school in Saint-Louis upon his return. Between 1895 and 1902 he lived in the village of Ndiarndé, near Pire, in the Thiès region of Kajoor. The locale had been the site of Muslim scholarly activity in the past.[41] From there Malik Sy soon moved to the new and thriving rail town of Tivaouane to found his *zawiya*, or religious center, and to build a new mosque in 1907.[42] Tivaouane would become his permanent home until his death in 1922.

The fortunes of the Tijaniyya rose with the town. Tivaouane had been the site of a French fort since 1869. The first rail lines were laid in 1885, and the next year, as the French occupied the rest of Kajoor, they chose it as the capital of the new *cercle*. Its population grew from 300 in 1895 to 4,300 by 1904, making it by far the largest new town in the interior.[43] Malik Sy was able to attract students and followers across ethnic lines. He also maintained good relations with Mauritanian Tijanis, and with the central *zawiya* in Fez; the chief of the Tijani order in Fez actually paid a visit to Malik in Tivaouane in 1914.[44] Other Senegalese Islamic notables to visit him included Al-Hajj Abdullah Nayas, chief of the Tijani *zawiya* at Kaolack.[45] Saidu Nuru Tall, the influential grandson of Al-Hajj Umar, was actually entrusted to Malik Sy's care as a child.[46]

Malik Sy's followers came mainly from the middle sectors of rural society. By contrast, the Mourids attracted the top and bottom layers of Wolof society: the displaced aristocrats, their retainers like the *ceddo*, other client groups, and slaves. The Tijanis found their greatest support among urban groups such as merchants and clerks working in the French administration.[47] By 1912, Sy's followers had built a *zawiya* near the African market in Dakar. When the French health authorities were displacing Africans during the plague of 1914, they left the Tijani *zawiya* standing. It is now within the commercial heart of the city. Other Tijani congregations affiliated with Malik Sy in those early years were established in towns near and far, ranging from Pire Gourey, Pire, and Rufisque, to Louga, Pal, Dagana, and even Kaolack.[48]

On this substantial base, the Tivaouane Tijaniyya continued to grow. Today, disciples of Malik Sy are found all over Senegal and beyond. In Fatick in southern Senegal, a recent study found that two of the four leading *marabouts* had received their authority from Tivaouane.[49] Despite the fact that the Mourids may be the fastest-growing Sufi order, Tijani adherents remain the most numerous, both in the Sereer Ndut area near Thiès and in the country as a whole.[50] Among the Sereer Ndut, a survey of the religious affiliation of village leaders after the Second World War revealed that 60 percent were Tijani, 7 percent Mourids, 20 percent Roman Catholics, and 12 percent followers of Ndut traditional religion.[51]

Malik Sy maintained excellent relations with the French authorities. In 1912, he issued a circular letter to his followers recommending that they "show confidence in the French as they show confidence in you.... Know that the French have given full assistance to our religion and to our country."[52] During the First World War, he conducted special communal prayers at Tivaouane for the success of the French forces. In the war, he actually lost his eldest son, Ahmet, who died in France in 1916.[53] In return for his support, the French arranged for twenty-two of his theological and linguistic tracts to be published by Bel-Hassan Frères in Tunis at the expense of the Tunisian government in 1914–15.[54]

It took considerable tolerance and courage at that time for a Muslim cleric to adopt a conciliatory position toward the French, who had followed an ambiguous Islamic policy in the early years of their rule in Senegal. Although they were aware that the *Pax Gallica* was helping to spread the Islamic brotherhoods by destroying the power of the Wolof states and dismantling the old social order, the French feared Islam as a potentially unifying anticolonial ideology. In 1903, the colonial administration had attempted to abolish the Muslim courts in Senegal. A strong reaction led to the restoration of the Muslim tribunals in Dakar, Saint-Louis, and Rufisque, though on a restricted basis. In 1903, also, a decree was promulgated prohibiting Qur'anic schools from opening without governmental authorization, and making them subject to examination of the teachers' skills in Arabic. The religious head of each school, moreover, was required to keep a registry of his pupils in French. Even if some teachers might not have passed muster, this legislation was undoubtedly viewed as outrageous interference in a religious matter. In 1911, the colonial state prohibited the collecting of alms by any *marabout* without a physical infirmity. Although these laws remained on the books, they were not enforced because the French came to fear the disruption an alienated *marabout* could cause.[55]

French policy toward the Sufi orders gradually shifted. While the French were cordial toward Malik Sy and the Tijaniyya, they remained somewhat suspicious of Ahmadu Bamba and the Mourids. In the interwar era, however, the French came to accommodate themselves especially well to the second generation of Sufi *shaykhs*.[56] The French acknowledged their new posture toward Islam in both practical and symbolic ways. In 1936, Governor-General J. M. de Coppet began to subsidize the building of mosques, and initiated the state's practice of bringing expensive gifts while attending important Muslim festivals.[57] As the Mourids in particular continued to contribute significantly to the expansion of peanut production, French colonial cooperation grew even greater. In 1946, the Mourids provided labor to unload ships detained in Dakar harbour by a dock workers' strike.[58]

Malik Sy was no itinerant seller of charms. Nor did he seek simply to ingratiate himself with the colonial administration. He was very well trained in Islamic jurisprudence and literature, possessed an extensive library at Tivaouane, and published widely in the fields of law, theology, and Sufism.[59]

One report stated that his library contained over 900 items.[60] He and his disciples stood in marked contrast to the Mourids on matters pertaining to Western medicine as well as to cooperation with the French generally.[61] Even if some were less enthusiastic than others, no members of the Tijani leadership were ever identified with a public stand against the health program either of the French colonial government or of the independent state which replaced it after 1960.[62]

Far from being hostile toward Western medicine, in 1913 Malik Sy underwent successful cataract surgery at the colonial hospital in Saint-Louis.[63] This may have confirmed what he was able to argue philosophically: that modern Western medicine and Islam were not incompatible. His position on this subject has become much clearer thanks to an important discovery by Papa Amadou Gaye, a young Senegalese scholar working in the colonial archives in Dakar.[64] In a letter written originally in Arabic, Malik Sy responded to a series of French overtures. He stated his willingness to accept the French invitation to be the spiritual leader of the new segregation village, and suggested that it be called Médina, rather than village William Ponty, as the French had originally proposed. He offered to lend his support to the application of health measures in Dakar, including plague vaccination; and he nominated his son-in-law, Saidu Nuru Tall, and his son, Babacar Sy, to serve as his intermediaries. Saidu Nuru Tall would later become France's most prized Muslim collaborator on health as well as general matters. Between the two world wars, he urged Africans to accept vaccination programs and to visit the AMI clinics for medical consultations.[65] The French health authorities received a second Muslim endorsement during the plague epidemic of 1914. Cheikh Sidia Baba, head of the Qadiriyya order in Saint-Louis, called on the Dakar population to "follow the health prescriptions put forward by the government."[66] Such endorsements, together with Blaise Diagne's support, were instrumental in gradually producing a tolerance for Western medical intervention in Dakar after 1914, if not during the 1914 epidemic.

Ever the diplomat, when Malik Sy justified his actions by invoking both prophetic experience and Islamic medical scholarship, he was reflecting practices of considerable antiquity in northwest Africa. By giving prominence to the learned as opposed to the prophetic approach, he was attempting to reconcile Islamic practice with the modernist methods of Western biomedicine in much the same manner as did Islamic modernizers such as Muhammad Abduh in Egypt.[67]

The scholarly Islamic approach, like premodern European medicine, was wedded to Galenic principles of medical thought and practice, such as belief in the four cardinal elements and the four humors, to explain disease and health.⁶⁸ The Muslim physician's responsibility was to aid nature in securing relief for the patient; the cure was in the hands of God. Because the same principles applied to drugs and herbs, Islamic scholarship included an extensive botanical literature as well.⁶⁹ Learned medicine began to decline and prophetic medicine to rise after the twelfth century, as Muslim political structures weakened throughout the Middle East and North and West Africa.⁷⁰ By the nineteenth and early twentieth centuries, with few exceptions, West African Muslims relied on the mystical powers of the *shaykhs* and *marabouts* to protect the community from disease and to bring about healing.⁷¹ Their invocation of the healing powers of verses of the *Qur'an* represented an approach remarkably similar to the divination and clairvoyance used by traditional African healers, and were far removed both from Islamic scholarly medicine and from the new French biomedicine.

The location of the main Tijaniyya shrine at Tivaouane, in the center of the plague zone, posed a major problem both for believers and for the French administration during the interwar period. On several occasions in the 1920s, French medical officials declared the plague zone off-limits to travelers who did not have certificates proving they had received the anti-plague vaccination. During the height of the plague season, an outright interdiction on travel was sometimes imposed. Such control measures represented a major hardship for the Tijaniyya faithful. Not only did the disciples of the Tijani *shaykh* wish to visit him on a regular basis, but once a year believers were expected to visit Tivaouane for the annual *gammu*, their most important celebration. This Wolof term, derived from the name of a pre-Islamic festival held shortly before the start of the rainy season, had come to be associated in the Tijaniyya brotherhood with the Muslim feast of Mawlud, the celebration of the Prophet Muhammad's birthday.⁷² Restrictions and outright interdictions on travel to Tivaouane were particularly difficult for the Tijaniyya to accept since their rivals were not being constrained. The Mourid holy city of Touba and, for that matter, the rival Tijani center at Kaolack lay outside the plague zone, and the annual pilgrimages to these centers were not subject to travel controls.⁷³

The gradual accommodation of Muslim leaders to Western biomedicine constituted an important watershed in the history of public health in Senegal. Closely tied to issues of political power in the country as a whole, the decisions of Malik Sy and his successors to accept even such intrusive health measures as those associated with plague control clearly alleviated tensions in rural Senegal between Muslim communities and the Colonial Health Service in the interwar period. Among traditionalist or even Christian Sereer Ndut, on the other hand, where no stratified hierarchy of political authority existed, a very different set of Sereer visions of the plague emerged. To this subject we now turn.

NOTES

1. Marc Sankalé, "La peste au Sénégal (1914–1938): Données épidémiologiques et cliniques" (thèse de Médecine, Université de Montpellier, Montpellier, 1944), 22, states that the expression was used by the "bush doctors."

2. For Central and East Africa, see John Iliffe, *Africans: The History of a Continent* (Cambridge: Cambridge University Press, 1995), 209–10; Maryinez Lyons, *The Colonial Disease: A Social History of Sleeping Sickness in Northern Zaire, 1900–1940* (Cambridge: Cambridge University Press, 1992), and James Giblin, *The Politics of Environmental Control in Northeastern Tanzania, 1840–1940* (Philadelphia, University of Pennsylvania Press, 1992).

3. Population estimated from data in Charles Becker and Mohamed Mbodj, "Dynamiques régionales au XXè siècle," in *La population du Sénégal*, edited by Yves Charbit and Salif Ndiaye (Dakar-Paris: DPS-CERPAA, 1994), 467–86.

4. Nguyen Van Chi, Régine, ed. *Atlas National du Sénégal* (Paris: Institut Géographique National, 1977), 42 and plate 15 illustrating its vegetation. In French the region is described as "Secteur des Niayes (alizés maritimes)."

5. The fresh water in surface pools, combined with moderating sea breezes, made for a humid yet moderate microclimate, certainly when compared to the hotter and drier continental conditions existing immediately to the east, where the very sandy plains of western Kajoor began. While there was variation from one *niaye* to another, with some holding water in depressions for several months after the rainy season compared to only weeks for others, the actual level of the annual rainfall was the key regulator. For example, in 1946, almost all the *niayes* in the Mboro sector went dry; from 1947 to 1949 they held water for six to eight months of the year, and from 1950 to 1955 they held water the entire year, a function of the succession of rainy years in that period. Jean Le Borgne, *La pluviomètrie au Sénégal et en Gambie* (Dakar: ORSTOM, 1988).

6. ANS\2G13\26, Saint-Louis, Dr. Huot, Annual Medical Report for Senegal in 1913, dated 20 September 1914.

7. See, for example, Jean-Marc Duplantier and Laurent Granjon, *Les rongeurs du Sénégal* (Dakar: ORSTOM, 1993).

8. M. Bahmanyar and D. C. Cavanaugh, *Plague Manual* (Geneva: World Health Organization), 46.

9. In contrast, Wassilief found *X. astia*, a less effective vector of *Yersinia pestis*, in only a handful of villages to the east of the plague zone. See the distribution map in Alexandre Wassilief, "Observations sur les puces de la région de Cayor," *Bulletin de la Société de Pathologie Exotique* 23 (1930): 476.

10. Unlike the northwestern Sereer, the Sereer of Siin have received considerable scholarly attention. The classic geographical and sociological study is Paul Pélissier, *Les paysans du Sénégal* (Saint-Yrieix, France: Imprimerie Fabrègue, 1966), chapters 4 and 5. For the history of Sine-Saloum, see Pathé Diagne, "Les royaumes sérères: Les institutions traditionnelles du Sine-Saloum," *Présence Africaine* 54 (1965): 142–72;

and Martin A. Klein, *Islam and Imperialism: Sine Saloum 1847–1914* (Stanford, Calif.: Stanford University Press, 1968).

11. See especially Charles Becker, "Les Serer Ndut: Études sur les mutations sociales et religieuses" (mémoire de L'École Pratique des Hautes-Études, Paris, 1970); and Marguerite Dupire, *Sagesse sereer: Essais sur la pensée sereer ndut* (Paris: Karthala, 1994).

12. James F. Searing, "Accommodation and Resistance: Chiefs, Muslim Leaders, and Politicians in Colonial Senegal, 1890–1934" (Ph.D. dissertation, Princeton University, Princeton, 1985), 13–14; Charles Becker, "La représentation des Sereer du Nord-Ouest dans les sources européennes (XVe–XIXe siècle)," in *Worso, mélanges offerts à Marguerite Dupire, Journal des Africanistes* 55 (1985): 165–85.

13. Becker, "Les Serer Ndut," 148. A century later, the population of the same Ndut villages totalled 9,133 persons. The Cape Verde peninsula was thinly populated as well. A French census of 1876 counted only 191 persons in the Lebu fishing village of Ouakam, and a total population for Dakar of 1,196. Saint-Louis at that time was much larger, with a population of 14,798. Charles Becker, Victor Martin, Jean Schmitz, and Monique Chastanet (with the collaboration of Jean-François Maurel and Saliou Mbaye), *Les premiers recensements au Sénégal et l'évolution démographique. Partie I, Présentation des documents* (Dakar: ORSTOM, 1983), 103, 225.

14. In 1970, 70 inhabitants occupied each square kilometer of Siin, making a total of 500,000 people, 17 percent of the total population of Senegal. In contrast, the Sereer of the northwest numbered only 60,000. Searing, "Accommodation," 14. For more on Siin demographics and migration, see Pélissier, *Les paysans*, 183–299; and Jean-Paul Dubois, "Les Serer et la question des terres neuves au Sénégal," *Cahiers de l'ORSTOM*, sér. Sciences Humaines, 12 (1975): 81–120.

15. Becker, "Les Serer Ndut," 1.

16. Becker, "Les Serer Ndut," 87. He tells us that the name "Mont-Roland" derives from the sponsors of the first Roman Catholic mission to the Ndut, the Collège du Mont-Roland in Dôle (Jura), which had been the school of Monseigneur Magloire Barthet, the apostolic vicar of the Senegambia in the late nineteenth century.

17. By the 1950s, however, a pattern of seasonal and sometimes permanent migration toward the nearby Cape Verde peninsula and Dakar had become established, especially among young Roman Catholics, who were attracted to the city either to continue their education or to find work. Becker, "Les Serer Ndut," 39.

18. Becker, "Les Serer Ndut," 39.

19. Ismaila Ciss, "Les Sereer du Nord-Ouest" (mémoire de maitrise, Université de Dakar, Dakar, 1981–82), 40.

20. Ciss, "Les Sereer," 52.

21. Philip D. Curtin, *Economic Change in Pre-colonial Africa: Senegambia in the Era of the Slave Trade* (Madison: University of Wisconsin Press, 1975), 508.

22. For example, slightly to the south of the rail line, Niakhar in Siin had a density of about 57 persons per square kilometer in 1900, and Pout, on the rail line, a density of 36 per square kilometer. Becker and Mbodj, "Dynamiques régionales."

23. The overall population increased only modestly from roughly 1.1 million in 1900 to 1.2 million in 1920, but then it jumped to 1.8 million in 1940 and to 2.1 million by 1950. In the interwar years, the plague zone maintained a population density of 50 persons or more per square kilometer. After the Second World War, however, the region began to lose people due to migration into the Cape Verde peninsula and to Dakar itself. By 1971, the plague zone's density had dropped to 35 per square kilometer while the Cape Verde peninsula had jumped to densities of 100 and higher, more than double its density in the 1920s. Becker and Mbodj, "Dynamiques régionales," 5.

24. Becker et al., *Les premiers recensements*, 103, 225.

25. Becker, "Les Serer Ndut," 44.

26. Becker, "Les Serer Ndut," 87.

27. A. Sebire, *Les plantes utiles du Sénégal* (Paris: Baillière, 1895).

28. Becker, "Les Serer Ndut," 87.

29. Archives of the Congrégation du Saint-Esprit, "Dossier 262A, Correspondance Sénégambie." Hereafter cited as ACSE\Sénégambie, followed by the appropriate year.

30. ACSE\Sénégambie, 1926; Father J. Boutrais to Monseigneur Louis Le Hunsec, Thiès to Paris, 23 August 1926.

31. ACSE\Sénégambie, 1927; Father Boutrais to Monseigneur Le Hunsec, Poponguine to Paris, 5 July 1927.

32. ACSE\Sénégambie, 1928; Father Boutrais to Monseigneur Le Hunsec, Thiès to Paris, 3 July 1928.

33. ACSE\Sénégambie, 1928; Father Boutrais to Monseigneur Le Hunsec, Thiès to Paris, 25 September 1928.

34. ACSE\Sénégambie, 1929; Father Boutrais to Monseigneur Le Hunsec, Thiès to Paris, 26 April 1929.

35. Becker, "Serer Ndut," 96.

36. Such was the case for Darou Alfa, Darou Loukhouss, Sintiou Mboul Daga, Medina Fouloume, and Keur Daouda Ciss. Becker, "Serer Ndut," 96.

37. Jamil M. Abun-Nasr, *The Tijaniyya: A Sufi Order in the Modern World* (London: Oxford University Press, 1965), 23.

38. David Robinson, *The Holy War of Umar Tal: The Western Sudan in the Mid-Nineteenth Century* (Oxford: Clarendon Press, 1985).

39. On the Mourids, see Donal Cruise O'Brien, *The Mourides of Senegal: The Political and Economic Organization of an Islamic Brotherhood* (Oxford: Clarendon Press, 1971); and Jean Copans, *Les marabouts de l'arachide* (Paris: Le Sycomore, 1980).

40. Paul Marty, *Études sur l'Islam au Sénégal*, vol. 1 (Paris: Ernest Leroux, 1917), 205–9.

41. Ibrahima Marone, "Le Tidjanisme au Sénégal," *Bulletin de l'IFAN* 32, sér.B (1970): 136–215.

42. Marone, "Le Tidjanisme," 149. Marone adds that Malik considered Louga for his center, but decided against it because of the presence there of an older Tijani *marabout*, Serigne Malick Sall. Malik Sy's original mosque still stands, but is overshadowed by a new grand mosque completed in the early 1990s. Eric Ross, "Cités

sacrées du Sénégal: Essai de géographie spirituelle" (mémoire de maitrîse, Université de Québec à Montréal, Montreal, 1989), 134.

43. Paul E. Pheffer, "Railroads and Aspects of Social Change in Senegal, 1878–1933" (Ph.D. dissertation, University of Pennsylvania, Philadelphia, 1975), 178.

44. Marty, *Études*, vol. 1, 205–9.

45. After the death of these two leaders, their heirs quarreled bitterly, and Tijanism in Senegal would never again enjoy a single spiritual head. See Abun-Nasr, *The Tijaniyya*, 145–47, for the split between the Kaolack and Tivaouane factions. During the election campaign of 1956, Tijani succession quarrels between Ababacar and his brother Mansour boiled over into violence known as the "Tivaouane fire" of 6 March 1956, in which two people died, forty-three were wounded, and 373 houses were destroyed. Ross, "Cités sacrées," 129.

46. Leonardo A. Villalon, *Islamic Society and State Power in Senegal: Disciples and Citizens in Fatick* (Cambridge: Cambridge University Press, 1995), 67.

47. Searing, "Accommodation," 64.

48. Ross, "Cités sacrées," 121–22.

49. Villalon, *Islamic Society*, 132.

50. The Mourids were increasing three times faster than the population of Senegal in the 1970s, when Cruise O'Brien reported that they represented roughly one-sixth of the country's population. Their greatest concentration was in the Diourbel region, home of the Touba mosque, where they constituted 30 percent of the population. Cruise O'Brien, *The Mourides*, 76–77.

51. Becker, "Les Serer Ndut," 44. In 1958, Tijanis constituted 45 percent of the entire Senegalese population, compared to the Mourids at 19 percent, and the Qadiris at 13 percent. Lucy C. Behrman, *Muslim Brotherhoods and Politics in Senegal* (Cambridge: Harvard University Press, 1970), 63. In the 1990s, Villalon stated that Tijanis made up almost half of all the Senegalese Muslims who declared any Sufi affiliation. Villalon, *Islamic Society*, 72, 139.

52. Marty, *Études*, vol. 1, 181.

53. Ross, "Cités sacrées," 123.

54. Marty, *Études*, vol. 1, 181.

55. Behrman, *Muslim Brotherhoods*, 35–36, 40–42.

56. Malik Sy was succeeded by his son, Al-Hajj Abababar Sy, (1885–1957), who was *khalifa* until 1957, and then by another son, Abdul Aziz Sy. Behrman, *Muslim Brotherhoods*, 70. As an example of their willingness to cooperate with the new Mourid *khalifa*, Mamadu Mustafa, in 1930 French authorities arrested his defeated rival, Shaikh Anta, on the trivial charge of having visited the Gambia without authorization. He was sent to prison for eight months, then exiled for ten years because he had allegedly been "guilty of manoeuvres which might have destroyed public peace in Senegal." Shaikh Anta was kept in exile until 1934, when he returned to live in Senegal under close surveillance. The quotation is from the governor-general of FWA's decree of 13 October 1930, quoted in Cruise O'Brien, *The Mourides*, 72.

57. Villalon, *Islamic Society*, 205.

58. Cruise O'Brien, *Mourides*, 71.

59. Behrman, *Muslim Brotherhoods*, 63.

60. Papa Amadou Gaye, "La diffusion institutionnelle du discours sur le microbe au Sénégal au cours de la Troisième République française (1870–1940)" (thèse de doctorat, Université de Paris VII, Paris, 1977), 236.

61. Behrman, *Muslim Brotherhoods*, 51, noted that Saidu Nuru Tall would become France's strongest supporter among the Senegalese Muslim clergy. He traveled all over FWA as a mediator, endorsed health and sanitation campaigns, and encouraged tax payment and peanut production. In return, he was given free travel on the railroad and aboard ships, and decorated with many honors.

62. Behrman, *Muslim Brotherhoods*, 145–47, contrasts Tijani and Mourid attitudes toward Western biomedicine. Later, Mourid suspicions would diminish. In 1965, during a yellow fever scare, the Senegalese government was able to persuade the Mourid *khalif*, Falilu Mbacké, shortly before his death, to support the mass vaccination program in the Diourbel region. Mbacké also thanked the government for sending a doctor to live permanently at Touba and for "purifying" the area around Touba of mosquitoes. Nevertheless, close associates said that he did not approve of doctors and preferred his disciples to seek healing through prayer.

The Mourids were also the most marked in their opposition to the French secular education system.

63. Cataract operations were not unknown to Muslim West Africans. Hausa *wanzami* or barber surgeons in Northern Nigeria were known to have performed eye surgery to remove cataracts, but there is no indication that such surgery was carried out in Senegal. Ismail Abdalla, *Islam, Medicine and Practitioners in Northern Nigeria* (Lewiston, NY: Edwin Mellon Press, 1997), 126.

An excellent piece of detective work by Kalala Ngalamulume has brought this significant event to light, as well as the failure of French authorities to capitalize on a golden opportunity to exploit the success of the surgery. No higher authority responded to the insightful note penned by the local *commandant de cercle* at Tivaouane: "As there would be a high interest that it [eye surgery] succeed and that the *marabout* be cared for with a great deal of attention and consideration during his convalescence, I respectfully draw your attention to his case. In my opinion and if it is feasible, it would not be a good idea to let him share the same ward with the other natives and . . . to charge him for the [surgical] operation and subsequent care. *We would do there a good propaganda in favour of our interests* [emphasis added]." Translated by Kalala J. Ngalamulume, "City Growth, Health Problems, and Colonial Government Response: Saint-Louis (Senegal) from Mid-Nineteenth Century to the First World War" (Ph.D. dissertation, Michigan State University, East Lansing, 1996), 252 and note 11, from ANS\H11, Commandant de Cercle of Kajoor (Tivaouane) to Governor of Senegal, 12 May 1913.

64. The file is ANS\H57. Malik Sy's letter is discussed in Gaye, "La diffusion," 231–33.

65. In his letter, Malik Sy justified his willingness to cooperate on health emergency measures by invoking precedents both from two Islamic texts on medical practice, *Tashil al-Manafi*, "Book of Medicine," and *Kounouz al-Sahati*, "Treasures of Health," written by Azraq Ibrahim Abd-al-Rahman, and also from the *hadith*, or traditions associated with the Prophet Muhammad and his immediate successors. While it was true that a believer was expected to accept adversity as the will of Allah, Malik Sy noted that the Prophet Muhammad had instructed the faithful to avoid contagious diseases and to seek remedies for them when he stated, 'flee the leper as you would the lion.'" Gaye, "La diffusion," 236.

66. ANS\H57, Cheikh Sidia Baba to Governor-General Ponty, Dakar, 8 June 1914.

67. Gaye, "La diffusion," 236, notes that an Arabic translation of a medical treatise from Egypt, originally written in French by Clot Bey, was circulating in Africa. For Egypt, see LaVerne Kuhnke, *Lives at Risk: Public Health in Nineteenth Century Egypt* (Berkeley: University of California Press, 1989).

68. For a general overview of Islamic Medicine, see Lawrence I. Conrad, "The Arab-Islamic Medical Tradition," in *The Western Medical Tradition, 800 B.C. to A.D. 1800*, edited by Lawrence I. Conrad et al. (Cambridge: Cambridge University Press, 1995), 93–138. For West African dimensions, see John Hunwick, *Literacy and Scholarship in Muslim West Africa in the Pre-colonial Period*, (Lagos: University of Nigeria Press, 1974); and Ismail H. Abdalla, "Diffusion of Islamic Medicine into Hausaland," in *The Social Basis of Health and Healing in Africa*, edited by Steven Feierman and John M. Janzen (Berkeley: University of California Press, 1992), 177–94.

69. Ibn Sina's *Al -Qanun fi Al-Tibb* was the standard guide for physicians and pharmacists. Abdalla, "Diffusion," 183–84.

70. This major transformation in North and West Africa was noted by the great fourteenth-century historian and sociologist, Ibn Khaldun, who specifically related the decline of the craft of medicine to the weakening of sedentary culture. Connected with the political and social disarray was an intellectual shift, marked by the rejection of innovation or independent judgment, known as the closing of *bab al-Ijtihad* or "the door of independent judgment." It was now argued that the major *Shari'a* law books were complete and final, and no new interpretation was necessary. Designed to protect believers against nonorthodoxy, this position precluded almost all changes and led to a shift toward the compilation of lexicons, encyclopedias, and commentaries rather than the development of new ideas. One such compilation was *Tibb Al-Nabawi*, "Medicine of the Prophet," dealing with medical aspects drawn from the large corpus of *hadith*. Hunwick, *Literacy*, 26–27; Abdalla, "Diffusion," 186–88.

71. One dramatic exception was the Fuulbe ruler and scholar, Muhammad Bello, who headed the Sokoto Caliphate in Northern Nigeria in the early nineteenth century. In addition to roughly sixty-five works on Islamic sciences in general, he wrote ten treatises on various aspects of medicine, hygiene, and related topics. He also devoted himself to the study of medicinal herbs and minerals found in Northern Nigeria. Abdalla, *Islam, Medicine*, 94–99.

72. Villalon, *Islamic Society*, 162–64, and 170–78, for a description of these events at both holy cities, attended by thousands of people. Villalon notes that important *taalibés* of the head of the order enjoy special seating, and that government officials and politicians now attend since it is important to see and be seen. Elaborate preparations using microphones, singers, and the like are involved, with much jostling to find good positions within sight of the *marabouts*. The songs, almost all of which are in Wolof, are of a religious nature, in praise of the order's founder, and, especially, in praise of Malik Sy.

73. Mourid events are called *maggals*, from the Wolof verb meaning "to celebrate," or "exalt." The Grand Maggal at Touba was initiated in 1928 to commemorate the first anniversary of the death of Ahmadu Bamba. Today, many Senegalese Muslims make annual pilgrimages both to Touba and to Tivaouane, regardless of their affiliation, although it is not known how far back this practice dates. Villalon, *Islamic Society*, 162.

8

VISIONS OF THE PLAGUE: THE RURAL IMPACT

This chapter examines the rural memories of the plague years between the two world wars. These visions of the plague are based upon oral testimonies drawn from two groups, the northwestern Sereer Ndut of Mont-Roland, and the Sereer living in the Niakhar district of Siin. These communities experienced the four standard anti-plague measures (isolation, incineration, vaccination, and vector control), but with some modifications in comparison with control measures in the cities. In part, these differences stemmed from the nature of the rural setting; in part they were an indication of colonial priorities and concern to make the cities safe for Europeans, for international commerce, and for the new elite of African urban clerks and workers.

Themes which emerge from the oral narratives reflect the continuing antagonism between the Western biomedical approach and the local African perception of how to respond to infectious disease. The narratives raise political issues touching on the role of leadership and power; on disease etiology and therapy as practiced by African healers; and on a powerful social dimension, including issues related to inheritance, funerals, and burial practices. The chapter ends with the presentation of six formal funeral dirges specific to Sereer Ndut society.

SEREER RELIGION, HEALTH, AND HEALING

Sudden and unexpected death from bubonic plague represented a severe challenge to the Sereer worldview.[1] It had implications for inheritance, for reincarnation, and indeed, for the well-being of the entire community. The Sereer had observed empirically that a "season for death" occurred "when the millet was high" (September–October).[2] Children were warned not to wander alone in the fields lest they fall victim to sorcery. Of course, this was also the time, just before the harvest, when hunger was greatest, resistance lowest, and the weather most oppressive. Plague, striking just before and during the early rains of June through August, did not coincide with the dangerous period, but it could and did sometimes extend into the "season for death."

Sereer disease etiology recognized three categories. The first, *karanta*, meaning "to pass," referred to physical contagion which could affect anyone. This category encompassed diseases contracted in childhood, such as smallpox, whooping cough, measles, and mumps. The Ndut considered plague, or *pisti*, along with cholera and leprosy, as a contagious disease, and classified it as *karanta*.[3]

The second category was *kadow*, or "evil," and referred to magical contagion aimed at a specific individual. Marguerite Dupire labeled this type "contamination," as opposed to contagion.[4] Afflictions characterized by loss of blood (certain venereal diseases) or repeated attacks (asthma), would be considered *kadow*.

The third category, *nimil*, or "defect," embodied the atavistic notion of the return of a physical characteristic, a defect, in certain people. For example, diseases of the skin were seen as anomalies which appeared at birth and were attributed to the mother and her matrilineage, since skin and bones were held to be feminine. Diseases of the blood, in contrast, were afflictions that appeared later in life and were attributed to the father and his matrilineage, blood being masculine. Many diseases could involve two overlapping causal categories; thus, whooping cough was said to derive from both contagion and atavism, while eye disease derived from contagion and contamination.

Each of these three categories had causal agencies. Thus a physical contagion such as bubonic plague was the product of natural forces. Sereer Christians, Muslims, and animists, like their counterparts throughout Africa and beyond, regarded some diseases (including bubonic plague) as a manifestation of the will of God.[5] Like many African peoples, the Sereer Ndut had a creator god called Kope, who remained aloof from the affairs of men, although he is taking on more importance in contemporary life through the influence of Christian and Muslim monotheism.[6] The object of prayers would have been the divine ancestors called *pangol* by the Sereer of Siin, meaning the forces which controlled the universe. *Yaal pangol*, a ritually prepared libation, for example, could be taken as an antidote to certain illnesses.[7] Al Hajj Serigne Malik Thiombane, a Muslim Sereer, saw plague as an expression of God's will,[8] while a Christian, Thérèse Tisa Mbengue, not only agreed but stated that God, not modern medicine, was responsible for plague's retreat from her region.⁹

The agents responsible for magical contagion were evil spirits known as *madaag* in Siin and *nak* in Ndut. The *nak* were believed to be cannibals who devoured the flesh of their victims. They might be the spirits of the deceased, or worse still, the living dead, individuals capable of leaving their bodies to sally forth and do harm.¹⁰ Still another group of evildoers was the sorcerers, living persons capable of causing others to become ill. In precolonial times, it was said that those found to have practiced sorcery were punished by beatings, expulsion, including sale into slavery, and even execution.¹¹

Sereer Siin society sought protection against the powerful forces aligned against it from specialists known as *saltigi*. These were male commoners who had the power of divination by means of clairvoyance. The *saltigi* could also serve as healers. Their powers were said to have been inherited, and could be transferred equally to males or females by the *pangol*. Not every child of a *saltigi* would inherit such important gifts. Women were clairvoyants, especially gifted at detecting sorcery. Male *saltigi*, however, also claimed to be able to exorcise the *nak*. Ngor Laba Diop, a healer who inherited his powers from his father, maintained that because the colonial state and its successor disapproved of the practice of identifying evildoers, he was unable to act for fear of punishment. If permitted, he was confident of his ability to "sort out" the *nak*.¹²

A *saltigi* could also serve as official diviner for several villages. He was sometimes referred to as "God's little brother," and his main function was to forecast rain and events, especially misfortunes. He acted as the officiating priest at the ritual or symbolic hunt, held before the harvest each year, in which the community sought protection against the *gon paf*, the living dead.¹³ The *saltigi*'s knowledge of talismans was supposed to protect villages from illnesses and other dangers caused by sorcerers, demons, forest spirits, and diviners.

Even those who were not specialists in healing could possess special powers which could be invoked in times of epidemic distress. Thus, the uncle of Dié Yat served as her powerful protector not only because he was head of her matrilineage, but also because, as a twin, he exercised magical powers.¹⁴

Healers were also herbalists. The Sereer term for herbal remedies was *padj*.¹⁵ The common form of this treatment involved the lengthy boiling of a mixture of roots and plants in water to produce a liquid medicine, but roots and plants could also be administered directly as salves to wounds on the skin.¹⁶ One informant maintained that Sereer healers also administered a traditional vaccine against smallpox.¹⁷

Treatment for polluting or contaminating diseases usually involved the use of Senegalese redwood. Redwood resin held powerful symbolic value, because it has characteristics similar to blood: it is red and it coagulates. Another remedy involved rosewood, which had the power to remove impurity and prevent its spread.¹⁸

The Sereer pharmacopia, shared by the Lebu and Wolof, drew heavily on plants common to Senegambia. These included *Calotropis procera*, or silkwood (*bodafot* in Sereer), whose roots were used against eruptions of the skin, and whose fruit was fastened on the doors of houses as protection against sorcery. A plant with powerful properties, its latex was used traditionally in Senegambia as the active ingredient in arrow poisons. Used externally in smaller doses, often mixed with milk, the latex was employed both as an antiseptic and as a sedative. Laboratory testing by the French revealed that the latex was toxic, and that the leaves were a powerful insecticide. The plant's roots were commonly found in the Dakar market, where Joseph Kerharo was told they could usefully treat anxiety and mental illness.¹⁹ A second useful plant was *Cocculus bakis*, a climbing vine, called *peys* in the Thiès area and *bakis* elsewhere. The bitter root of this vine was used to treat fevers and as a diuretic.²⁰ Another interesting plant was the papaya, called *papayo* in Sereer and Wolof, originally imported to Africa from Central America and widely cultivated in Sereer villages. Its fruits were boiled while still green as a remedy for jaundice, and its leaves and roots were used as diuretics. Papaya fruit was often cooked with chicken as a strengthening food for the sick.²¹

Remuneration for healers consisted of payment in kind: a chicken, some millet, or a large block of wood. Some healers today actually live entirely on remuneration for their services, but this was rare in previous times.²² Diviners, on the other hand, could sometimes use their gifts of divination to extract payment from beyond the grave. The soul of the deceased was said to have visited the diviner to inform him of the extent of the deceased's wealth, and the portion he wished to leave to the diviner, who would then request it at the funeral ceremony. To refuse a diviner's request meant contradicting the will of the deceased and risking serious offense.²³

Xa kiid axa'n kooxa dooma ka, "the years of the acute headaches," have a distinct place in Sereer medical tradition.²⁴ Plague has been remembered as an *a sella*, that is, a severe epidemic for which the healers were unprepared.²⁵ Those who suffered from plague recalled symptoms such as severe pain in the armpits and groin.[26] The plague in Toukar was remembered as having caused approximately fifty deaths.[27] One observer labeled it a truly horrible disease, cursed by the population.[28]

Like their counterparts elsewhere in Africa, Sereer healers were reluctant to abandon their notions of causation for Western ones.[29] While one healer demonstrated familiarity with germ theory by stating that the disease was transmitted by infected people, and that it was necessary to burn the infected dwellings to break the chain of transmission,[30] another *saltigi* stated wryly that neither vaccinations nor vaccination cards imparted immunity.[31] Empirically, it was true enough that some people contracted the disease both because of and in spite of vaccinations. While Western practitioners attributed these unusual results to stale or contaminated vaccines, Sereer healers explained such results as due to the success of a sorcerer with great powers in breaking through the individual's defences.[32]

Sereer healers appear to have responded to bubonic plague in a variety of ways. Many reflected the wish, almost universal among healers across different medical cultures, to ease their patients' suffering. A few were audacious enough to claim a cure for such a dreaded disease as plague, while others argued that they had the skills to prevent plague from ever entering their community. One pair of Siin informants believed that while the *saltigi* could not cure *pisti*, they could prevent it. Today, however, they continued, plague had disappeared because of modern medicine.[33] Marguerite Dupire was informed of two treatments practiced by the Sereer Ndut against plague, namely, quarantine, and symbolic expulsion from the community during a community ceremony led by a *saltigi*.[34] Faith in the preventive skills of healers was a tacit recognition of the links between healers, political rulers, and the public's health. Wise and skilled healers and rulers could protect their people; less able ones could not. Thus, when asked why plague struck more severely in the Sereer Ndut region than among the Sereer of Siin, Chief Coumba Ndoffène Diouf replied that the *saltigi* and rulers of Siin together deserved credit for maintaining the good health of the province. These wise men could see the future. They anticipated the epidemic and took measures to prevent plague and treat the symptoms. They counseled their clients on which roots to boil and solutions to drink, and on which charms to buy in order to protect the body. Perhaps, it was argued, the healers and elders of Ndut lacked these talents.[35]

An interesting perspective on plague comes from Ngor Laba Diop, who became a *saltigi* in adulthood, after his own personal deliverance from plague when he was approximately seven years old.[36] The plague had been imported into Siin by Wolof herdsmen who carried it from Diourbel. It struck first at Gossas and then in the village of Tokan where he lived at the time. Hundreds died during the two-year-long epidemic. When Ngor became infected with plague, his father, a lion hunter and healer, intervened. Thanks to his father's skills, none in his family's compound died, despite the severity of the epidemic. His father devised *gris-gris* (charms, usually in the form of amulets) for protection, and treated ganglions with a compound made of herbs and boiled roots. In this way, the father's "magic" caused the ganglion on the son's neck to disappear.

Equally audacious in his claims was the *saltigi* Ko Diouf of Toukar. A well-known healer in Siin, both his mother and father were healers; yet he was the only one of his family to inherit the power, which he exercised for over forty years. Too aged to attend meetings of *saltigi*, he now sends his son. In his day he claimed to have recommended the burning of leaves and roots in smudge pots in each compound to ward off contagion, and to have actually cured plague victims by means of ritual baths.[37]

Both of Ko Diouf's practices had resonance in Sereer traditional medicine in times of an *a sella*, or an epidemic. Sereer herbalists favored specific leaves and roots for their smudge pots. One root came from a tree called *seelunq*.[38] Another Sereer practice was the ritual bath or *bukut*. One informant argues that the *bukut* bath was demanded by the Sereer for those individuals released from the Colonial Health Service's lazaretto before they could be accepted back into Sereer society.[39] A similar recollection was related in Siin, where the bath of purification, called *bogyt*, consisted of a solution of roots boiled in water.[40]

These two intriguing treatments merit comment. The smoke from the smudge pots would certainly have helped protect against a variety of diseases in which insects were vectors, including of course, *Yersinia pestis*. The question arises as to whether Sereer healers had discovered more than simply which plants generated the most smoke. Clearly, any green plant would work better than any dry plant. But the healers may also have determined empirically which plants produced odors which were more effective insect repellents. As for the ritual bath, while it could not have cured plague, it may have had the effect of raising the patient's comfort and confidence level. It stands as a fascinating effort to graft African symbolism and purification practice onto the Western control measure which the plague lazaretto represented.

Sereer medical thought and practice was buffeted by many forces of change in the interwar period. Even in the precolonial era, despite their reputation for closing themselves off from their often hostile neighbors, the Sereers' pharmacology strongly resembled that of their Lebu and Wolof neighbors. Under French rule, the rapid expansion of Islam and Christianity opened the Sereer to medical pluralism. Wolof specialists, for example, installed themselves in Ndut villages, where they sold amulets for sums ranging from 100 to 500 francs. When Ndut migrants moved to the city, Islamic magic became important socially and was held to be necessary for migrants to "succeed" there.[41]

Of the medical therapies open to the Sereer, Western biomedicine was perhaps the least attractive. For one thing, it was the most difficult of access, both because the nearest European clinic was at Thiès or Tivaouane, and because it was costly. More fundamentally, however, Western biomedicine represented a dramatic shift in medical thinking. It offered a much narrower definition of healing, based largely on the curative measures of clinical biomedicine rather than on the broader African tradition of seeking the spiritual and social well-being of the larger society.[42] The reductionist tendency of biomedicine to treat the disease rather than the larger context, troubled those African healers and their patients who were used to seeking out first causes.[43]

Sereer healers under French colonialism found that their very existence was called into question. French legislation had been passed making their profession illegal, even if such laws were next to impossible to apply in practice. A similar fate befell healers and herbalists throughout Africa as colonial health systems took away their control over the diagnosis of illness, and often their right to practice. Steven Feierman has shown that the Shambaa healers in northeast Tanzania had a much wider range of control over the social conditions of health in precolonial times than they were ever permitted under colonialism. Formerly, they could isolate individuals such as lepers or those infected with smallpox; they coordinated the cleaning of irrigation ditches and the distribution of water, and exercised other powers which contributed to the "social health" of the society.[44] Meredeth Turshen, in fact, argues that this was more a political than a medical conflict, because colonial administrations sought to replace the authority of the healer with that of their own personnel, sometimes including their appointed chiefs.[45]

A gendered dimension also prevailed. African women were disadvantaged because their health was undermined by increased work under colonialism. To the extent that they had played roles as healers, herbalists, or spirit mediums, their status was undermined as well. This is not to idealize precolonial social formations, where women were also subjected to subordination. Nevertheless, whereas health and healing may previously have been one of the few opportunities for women to maintain or improve their social status, this capacity was seriously eroded under colonial rule.

SEREER MEMORIES OF COLONIAL HEALTH CONTROL MEASURES

We begin with a single personal narrative of plague. This vivid recollection of a plague experience in Siin comes from an eyewitness and a plague survivor, Dié Yat. While her narrative is only one individual's experience, it eloquently expresses bubonic plague's tragic impact:

> I spent two months at the lazaretto. My mother and older brother died there, after contracting the disease by helping out a neighbor. This other victim was an old woman called Dié Kama, a neighbor who had gone to a funeral at Ndimag. Upon her return she soon fell ill, and behaved as if she were mad. No one fed her so my mother felt sorry for her, took her some food, and caught plague in this way. Mother had stayed a few days with Dié Kama. When she returned, after one week she experienced headaches. She went to the granary, returned to do her cooking, and suddenly fainted. I came home and found her on the floor, unconscious and barely breathing. I immediately called my uncle.
>
> All told, we were seven people in the lazaretto. My uncle was the watchman at the lazaretto. He was a powerful man, so strong he could never become infected with plague. He was not a warrior but he was powerful enough to protect us from the plague. Even when both of us were at the lazaretto the plague was not able to attack us. I fed the sick and he buried the dead. It was in the time of Massène Sène. My uncle was a twin and that is why he was invulnerable.
>
> The patients prepared their own food. If they were not able to do so, it was necessary to ask the suspects to help. I was very young, not even ten years old, but I was obliged to cook and to take care of the sick. There were others in the lazaretto, strangers who came with the doctor. In the evenings, the men who were in the lazaretto went out to find millet from the granaries. The women pounded it. People had fled their concessions because of the epidemic. For water we used a stream that was assigned to the lazaretto. It was in *hivernage*. When graves were needed, burial was in three common ditches.
>
> After my release, people were afraid of me. My father had died well before the epidemic so I was now an orphan. They tried to send me to relatives in Bawol, and in another village, Kahone, near Kaolack, but no one wanted to accept me, so I stayed with my uncle until the

epidemic was completely over. Within a month or so, I was again accepted by the villagers here at Toukar, and I never experienced problems in later years. In the epidemic people panicked, and looked after only themselves. I bear no grudges, but I still grieve over my lost loved ones. As I look back on those sad memories, I ask myself why this happened to me. The health service ordered us to bring in rat tails and from this we later deduced that rats brought the disease. But I have to believe that even if this was so, it was all because of God's will. We have to accept it.[46]

In the centralized Sereer polity of Siin, the oral history of the plague epidemic reflects aspects of power and authority, as is clear from the testimony of a descendant of the rulers of Siin, Coumba Ndoffène Diouf.[47] Talking about events which took place before his time, this informant stated first that plague had a very limited impact in Siin because of the skills of the state's medical and political leaders. According to M. Diouf, when a few small epidemics did occur, these visitations were the result of a curse placed on an unpopular and illegitimate ruler, a former noncommissioned officer in the Tirailleurs Sénégalais named Massène Sène. On his retirement from military service, Sène had been illegitimately appointed *chef de canton* over the Sereer, a French practice that was as unpopular as it was common.[48] Not being of royal descent, a *lam diafadj*, as tradition demanded, Massène Sène offended the ancestral spirits and this brought down epidemics upon Siin for the first time. Eventually, the French recognized his incompetence and corruption; he was suspended and fled to Gambia. The population rejoiced when Coumba N'Doffène Diouf's father, Farba Diouf, son of the *bour siin*, was appointed in Sène's place. Thereafter, no further epidemics occurred and there was great improvement in the local economy.

The current chief or *diaraf* of Toukar, Cheikh Dieng, also stressed the political dimensions of the epidemic in his testimony. His version attributed the arbitrary and unpleasant actions of the state not to the Colonial Health Service but to the same Massène Sène. Sène is alleged to have isolated patients in lazarettos and to have banned formal burials.[49] The chief's brother, Ibrahima Dieng, a healer in his own right, praised the skills and power of his fellow *saltigi* as protectors of the community. When the first plague cases in Siin occurred near Toukar, the disease was highly contagious and deadly, killing a person every second day. Far from being at a loss, healers had responded even before the disease reached Siin. They predicted that no more than two cases would occur in the polity, and that is what happened. The victims were a man called Biram Yat and a woman named Dié Kama.[50]

Among the stateless Sereer Ndut, plague was not directly linked to illegitimate political authority. The only connection between plague and local political authority was seen as accidental. Plague in the Thiès escarpment was inadvertently associated with the life of Shaykh Serigne Alfa Thiombane, an important Muslim notable of the region, and the founder of a village that bears his name. One legend has it that he came to the site of Darou Alfa because he was fleeing the plague; this is, however, denied by Dauda Mbengue, who states that Shaykh Thiombane created a new village because he needed to distance himself from non-believers.[51] Another informant recalled that despite his charisma and powers, the *shaykh* could not prevent his first wife from dying of plague.[52]

The French Colonial Health Service was deeply involved in plague control measures at the village level. Indeed, the outbreak of an epidemic often led to a greater state presence than villagers had ever known before. Recollections of this state involvement became deeply embedded at Mont-Roland among the Sereer Ndut, and at Toukar among the Sereer of Siin. In Mont-Roland, memories include the precise location of the lazaretto constructed by the Health Service. It was just outside Daga, in a hamlet called Wangal, near Lake Makka.[53] An area of 5 kilometers long was covered with tents all the way to Nguick.[54]

The staff of the Health Service were remembered as intrusive and largely unpopular agents of the state.[55] Transport most likely was difficult. One informant remembers being the youngest patient in the lazaretto and seeing his first European, a French doctor, who arrived on horseback. The medical workers with him built a large ditch and a palisade separating the lazaretto from the rest of the community.[56] These state employees were supervised by soldiers, Tirailleurs, who all came from Tivaouane; they were remembered as having been under the command of Diawara Sall, the *diaraf* of Tivaouane.[57] In Siin, according to one observer, prisoners under military guard were required to perform some of the difficult tasks at the lazaretto.[58]

The tasks were certainly unpleasant. Whenever a village compound was condemned, guards soaked the houses, together with all the material possessions, in kerosene and burned everything. The loss of irreplaceable material possessions must have taken a heavy emotional toll, especially in the homes of elders where sacred objects were housed.[59] Those who could recall the raids and village burnings that accompanied the French conquest could hardly be blamed for seeing health control as yet another harsh imposition. The Health Service insisted that the clothes of those who had died of plague be included in the incineration.[60] Worse, as two informants independently attested, the health brigades would attach chains to the feet of corpses and drag them through the dust to be buried.[61] Not surprisingly, such actions provoked profound irritation and resistance. But when people protested, the guards struck them. People hated the degradation and the lack of Christian burial.[62] One informant, it should be noted, disagreed with the consensual view, and argued that the health brigades, in doing their difficult job well, were trying to help the local community.[63]

The Health Service legitimately believed that Sereer funerals were a significant means of propagation of plague. During a plague emergency, large funerals, and perhaps small ones, were made difficult if not impossible by the interdiction on travel. For Christians, Muslims, and traditional Sereer alike, this was painful. Perhaps no solution would have proved acceptable. Much later, under an independent government, Senegalese public health officials argued that the funerals of cholera victims were helping propagate the disease more widely, and urged tighter control measures.[64]

Another imposition was the *cordon sanitaire*, which not only prohibited strangers from entering villages, but kept people from visiting their wells and streams. Water was imported by the Health Service, but many people suffered from shortages. Food was also at a premium and people ate manioc; others had to make do with fruits and peanuts during a two-year plague visitation.[65]

Collective memories recalled Sereer experiences with anti-plague vaccinations. One informant graphically described the huge syringe used to administer painful injections to the backside and recalled that some even died after receiving the injections. For a combination of reasons, fear led people to flee the Health Service, not realizing, the informant added, that it was designed to protect them.[66] Vaccination cards were issued to those who had been inoculated. They were remembered as blue with a diagonal red band. No one was permitted to travel outside the Mont-Roland area without one.[67]

Resistance to the Health Service could involve other tactics in addition to flight or avoidance of vaccination. To fool French authorities, some people took to burying their bracelets, rings, and other valuables, to be dug up later in the *hivernage* season, after the epidemic had ended.[68] The fact that health workers burned property but did not compensate people may have led to this activity.[69]

Pest control was an area to which the Health Service devoted a great deal of attention. Marie-Anne Yaayo Diouf recalled how the Health Service, after explaining that rats brought the plague, distributed rat cages to the public.[70] Villages were assigned a quota of rodents to be caught and had no choice but to comply. The cages were placed in the paths

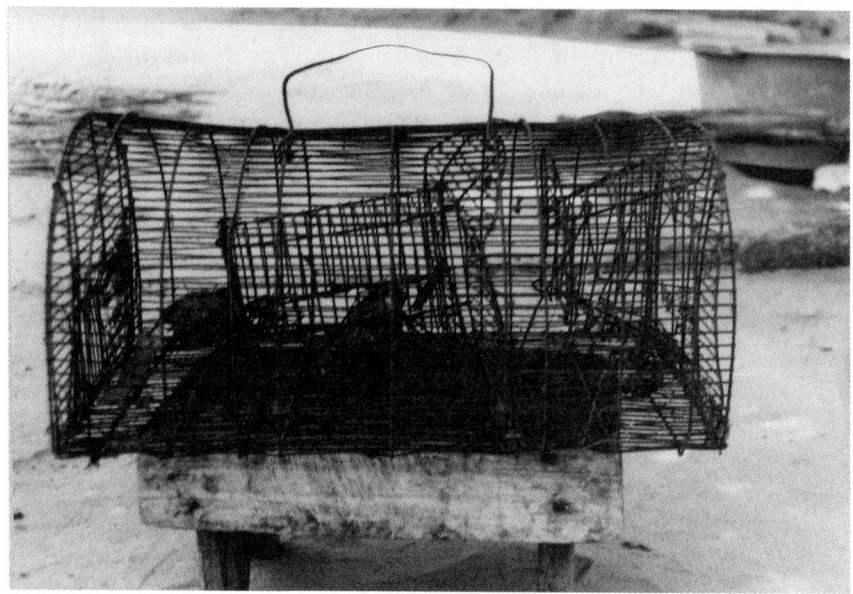

Photo 8.1 Rat Cage Distributed by the Health Service. Rat cages such as this one, the property of Marie-Anne Yaayo Diouf of Tiwigne Diassa, were distributed by the Health Service throughout the plague zone during the 1920s to help villagers meet their quotas of captured rodents. Author's photograph.

frequented by rodents and in the granaries. Cages were baited with pieces of fruit, usually apples. The informant remembered catching as many as twenty rodents a day, whose tails were cut off as proof of success. Fleas, on the other hand, were too numerous to count and tally in any way. Instead, poison immersed in an oily liquid was placed in a dish and set under the bed. A candle was used to illuminate the plate and attract the fleas.[71]

The brothers Adama and Mor Ciss noted that it had once been common among the Sereer to eat wild rodents. The Sereer believed the health authorities insisted on an end to this practice in their campaigns to eradicate rodents. Instead, the young people were obliged to capture rats, burn the carcasses, and turn the tails over to the Health Service.[72]

Sometimes, pest eradication campaigns led to confusion and rumor. In Siin, a story circulated, which the informant did not personally believe, that rats' tails were to be used to prepare a medicine against plague. He regarded this as a device to get people to carry out the unpleasant task of catching rats.[73] Still another informant recalled the rat-killing campaigns but not whether the population was ever told why they had to bring in rat tails.[74]

These preventive campaigns made their mark in various ways. Changes in house construction techniques and in cultivation practice can be linked to rural plague epidemics. The brothers Ciss remembered that at the time of the plague, few houses were built with cement floors, and the prevailing sandy floors permitted far larger numbers of fleas. While the health authorities called for cement floors, few villagers could afford the extra cost.[75]

Plague epidemics affected Sereer farming practices as well. Next to the staple of millet, manioc was a desirable secondary crop, although grown only by those with abundant land. Less manioc was grown in times of plague, perhaps because it involved traveling to distant fields.[76] To keep rodents from sheltering among the large stalks of millet, the Health Service persuaded villagers to cultivate manioc closer to the houses and to confine the millet to fields further away.[77]

Oral tradition in Siin suggests that plague epidemics reduced contacts between communities and could lead to ostracism. Cattle turned over to pastoralists for grazing, for example, could not be recalled if an epidemic had been declared, as all contact with outsiders was interdicted. According to Tekheye Diouf, a person sick with plague and sent to a makeshift lazaretto came in time to be regarded as a social leper, and was not immediately welcomed back even if he had survived the dread disease.[78]

Fifty years later, distress remains evident in Sereer memories of the plague years. On the other hand, the terror of those days, so brilliantly captured in the oral testimony, is rarely observed in the detached, clinical writings of French observers. Exceptionally, in a medical thesis written in 1944, Marc Simond illustrated the horrors of the plague epidemics in Senegal and Madagascar. He described how a "suspect case," someone exposed to a plague patient, could enter a lazaretto in good health only to exit four days later as a cadaver, transported in a truck by masked men to a special "plague" cemetery, where his body would be covered with lime and buried in a common grave with the bodies of other plague victims. Parents and kin would have no rights to visit the patient, to comfort him in his last moments, or to participate in his burial.[79]

THE SOCIAL DIMENSION:
INHERITANCE AND FUNERAL PRACTICES

"The years of acute headaches" placed great stress on the Sereer social system, as oral testimonies make clear. The Sereer of Siin practised a system of double descent. In the inheritance of goods and property, the matrilineage predominated, while the patrilineage was involved in the transmission of status.[80] Among the northwestern Sereer, only the Ndut and Saafen have preserved the matrilineal system, but even here, patrilineage has grown more important with time, partly though the influence of Wolof neighbors, and partly because of the increasing importance of Islam and Christianity.[81]

The matrilineage was required to pay for funeral obligations, and claimed the personal property of the deceased.[82] This included livestock and clothing, but also cooking utensils and jewelry in the case of women.[83] One exception to these customary rules among the Sereer Ndut occurred in the case of a venereal disease unique to women, called *lewre*. When a woman who had been infected with this disease died, as a preventive measure her clothes were washed and sold, rather than being given to the matrilineal relatives.[84] Such deviation from custom was important, because it shows that the Sereer had been able to make empirical changes in their customary rules based on hygienic observations. It suggests that had the Colonial Health Service been more adroit, the service would have been able to persuade the Sereer to make similar changes regarding goods suspected of contamination during bubonic plague epidemics. Unfortunately, the tendency of the colonial system to command compliance in hierarchical fashion precluded the nuanced approaches that would have included social considerations of this sort.

Another Sereer exception to custom involved tobacco utensils. Pipes and snuffboxes were considered to be the most personal objects of an individual. Women smoked pipes, while snuffboxes were the property of men. These items would be inherited by a close friend, rather than the matrilineage.[85]

The Colonial Health Service's fundamental control measures during plague epidemics involved the destruction of contaminated property, and the banning of traditional funerals and wakes. However justified these measures were,[86] they nevertheless constituted a dramatic intrusion into Sereer rites of passage and, naturally, generated bitter resentment.[87] The failure to consult local people, together with the high-handed methods of the medical guards, intensified resistance to measures that constituted a major affront to local custom. No compensation was provided for property;[88] burial in mass graves was carried out by strangers. It was therefore not surprising that the Sereer, like plague-infected communities throughout the world, resisted the Health Service's measures at every opportunity. People refused to declare plague deaths so funerals would not be banned. When plague deaths could not be hidden, they buried the clothing and other valuables of the deceased, inadvertently helping to spread contagion.

In these situations of stress and tension, the best and the worst of human behavior could be discerned. The treatment of plague victims as social outcasts was evident in the funeral dirge recounting the hardships of Yaa el (see below). On the other hand, Dié Yat's account illustrates her mother's compassion in caring for a sick neighbor and contracting plague in the process. Dié Yat also maintained that the social stigma did not last very long in her case and that it was the product of temporary fear. The brothers Adama and Mor Ciss maintain that the common struggle to rid the community of plague actually brought people closer together. The general group interest in getting rid of plague overcame the tendency of some individuals to make personal denunciations of each other.[89]

Funeral practices among the Sereer were particularly intricate, given the complexity of their double descent system. The patrilineage, the weaker group in Sereer society, was able through funerals to assert the rights accorded to it by means of a viri-patrilocal residence pattern.[90] At the same time, funerals had tremendous religious implications. Burials, for example, had to be conducted in a strictly prescribed manner to allow the reincarnation of an individual to occur. Cremation, which French plague control rules frequently ordered in mass burials, was anathema to the Sereer, who believed reincarnation could only occur within a limited time period, before the skeleton decomposed.[91]

The Sereer followed a set of precautions in preparing a corpse for burial. The ears and nose were blocked with cotton to ensure that earth did not enter, as this would cause deafness and nose problems in the reincarnated newborn. The members and fingers were stretched out, and the hands opened to avoid deformities. A baby born with its hands closed was considered to be the reincarnation of a leper. The corpse was wrapped in a mat and placed in the grave, on its left side if male, on its right if female, and covered by pieces of palm trunk and fronds. In the first years following death, matrilineal relatives swept the tomb to ensure it did not cave in, which could damage the corpse and cause the newborn to be a hunchback.[92]

Marguerite Dupire has provided a detailed description of a Sereer funeral ceremony.[93] Since the patrilineage was responsible for assisting the departed soul in its journey to the next world, patrilineal relatives washed corpses ritually and dressed them for burial.[94] After washing, the corpse was covered by one or several woven wraps and the marriage mat. An iron tool was placed on its stomach to keep the soul from "wandering." The corpse was brought to the burial site on a stretcher and placed in the grave. It was covered by the roof of the deceased individual's house; then everything was covered with earth. In the past, and even in the present in the burial of important figures, the entire straw hut and bed would be placed in the grave. These distinctive earthen mounds, three meters or more in height, all surrounded by a circular ditch, marked the continuity of Sereer burial practices stretching back to proto-historic times in Senegambia.[95]

Following the burial, a funeral ceremony was held at the deceased's compound. It could be divided into three phases: condolences and presentation of gifts; preparation of meals and feasting; and dancing and festivities, sometimes ending with copious drinking. Participation in a funeral was the principal occasion on which uterine relatives could express their solidarity. Contributing to the cost of the funeral provided an opportunity for the settling of debts within a matrilineage. At a more lavish ceremony, the patrilineage could also contribute, for example, to paying the musicians (*griots*).

The father's matrilineage of the deceased had a distinct role. A young member of this group washed the corpse and dug the grave. He wrapped the body with a cotton cloth, which served as a shroud. Once the body was lowered into the grave he ripped off a strip of the shroud which was given to the children of the deceased to be worn for a week as a sign of mourning. Following the funeral ceremony, a representative of the deceased's father's matrilineage would send an emissary to request *mbap*. This was compensation due to the matrilineage of an individual who, in his role as father, did not receive from his children as many services and goods as he provided in the payment of bride-price. This was partial compensation for the fact that a father had few rights over his children.

FUNERAL DIRGES OF THE SEREER NDUT

This section is based on a series of six formal funeral laments touching on plague and composed by two women elders among the Ndut Sereer of Mont-Roland. The first five dirges were composed by Marie-Anne Yaayo Diouf of Tiwigne Diassa, and the sixth by Coumba Gaye of Darou Alfa.

Customarily among the Ndut Sereer, certain talented women performed formal functions as singers and poets at the funeral rites of distinguished elders. Coumba Gaye and Marie-Anne Yaayo Diouf were two such remarkable singers. Their stylized dirges are more than praise poems to the deceased. Part of a diversified and specialized tradition of singing among the

Ndut Sereer, these dirges play a central role in the social drama of funerals. Their themes are a mix of the sacred and the profane, ranging from consideration of the vanity of humans to the impotence of man before his destiny, the condition of the humble, and the memory of a dear one taken before her time. The songs express collective feelings such as joy, suffering, and hope. They are rich in codes and language, and have elaborate oral systems of notation, narrating myths, beliefs, social conflicts, and initiation systems.

The songs which follow are those of affliction and sadness, composed in periods of disaster. They are at the same time complaints, cries from the heart, and resigned revolts against the inevitable and the irreparable.

The Five Songs of Marie-Anne Yaayo

First Song: "Bisi, bisi (Wolof, Wolof):[96] the mother of Saliu is angry."
Text in translation:

> Wolof, Wolof, oh the mother of Saliu is angry with the
>   the father of Malik Puy.
> How can a girl be angry with her matrilineage?
> She is angry with her mother, the mother of Njaay Fay.
> How can a girl abandon her matrilineage, father of Mbanik Gey?
>   The Fuulbe of Jama[97] is the vital ingredient in
> her mother's soul.

Interpretation. This dirge alludes to the importance of the matrilineage, and to the inability of even the wealthy to avoid their destiny. Saliu was a wealthy and sophisticated shopkeeper who died of plague. Adopting the voice of the mother of Saliu, the mourner criticizes the maternal uncles for failing to protect her son. By means of haunting melody and lyrics the mother is made to express her deepest feelings for her son, and to worry about how this untimely and awful death will affect his immortal soul, or *coona*.

Second Song: "Baa Njeeme" (Homage to the father of Njeeme).
Text in translation:

> The father of Njeeme, my uncle the elephant, has fallen.
> Oh, an elephant has fallen, a noble Sereer. Oh truly a noble Sereer.
> The father of Njeeme, my uncle, but it is truly an
>   elephant that has fallen.
> Those men there do not remember the days when Njeeme

had harvested his millet at the place called "Gel."
Isn't it then the mother of Samba Baam?
Members of our lineage, know that the noble father of
Njeeme is dead.
The father of Njeeme, my uncle the elephant,
has fallen.
Oh truly an elephant has fallen. Noble Sereer,
oh Sereer king.

Interpretation. Njeeme's father was a prosperous landholder whose fields yielded a large crop of millet the year that plague struck him down. Well regarded by his society, he was a man of stature and dignity, compared in this dirge to an elephant. Using the voice of one of his nieces who is paying him homage, the Sereer text employs Wolof words describing wealth and civility. Implicit in the lament is the point that even the most powerful and successful in Sereer society are not immune from the ravages of plague.

Third Song: "Mi min bini leetar koonoo" ("If I could write a letter").
Text in translation:

If I could write a letter,
I would warn Mbisaan, the father of Tilaan,
that his sister, the descendant of Don Gey,
is currently being confined in the king's prison.
If I could write a letter,
I would warn Amad, the father of Sewru,
that his sister, the descendant of Don Gey,
is currently being confined in the king's prison.
   I am punished, but what is it that I have done,
Timbeey Juuf, Jeey, Anca?
If it were not for those bad marriages
I would not be punished and banished to the bush.

Interpretation. This song describes the hardships of Yaa el (also known as Mélanie Alima Mbengue), a woman afflicted with plague who was shunned by her village, denied food and water, and banished from the community for having brought plague to the village. In her poem, Yaa el attributes this shabby treatment to the absence of her brave older brothers, whom she had lost long before, and who would have protected her from such abuse. The poem therefore interprets practices such as isolation and banishment not as collective acts to ensure public health, but as unjust punishments of marginal members of the group. Once again, the point is made that the consequences of plague penetrate deeply into Sereer Ndut society.

As a footnote to the story, Marie-Anne Yaayo Diouf recounts the role played by the Catholic missionary, Father Boutrais, during the plague epidemics. One Sunday during the time of the plague, he decided to visit the village of Tiwigne Diassa. When he reached the quarter of Ngoh he was intercepted by a woman who suspected plague in a sick woman. She asked the priest to visit the sick woman. When the priest determined that it was plague, without telling any one, he informed the Health Service, which came that same Sunday night and burned all the homes after evacuating the entire quarter. It was this event which the village blamed on Yaa el, holding her responsible for their misfortunes.

Fourth Song: "Mi na looy koowi yaal" ("I grieve over my misfortune").
Text in translation:

> I mourn the brother of Baa Ngeeni Njoon
> because something happened to me.
> Every one is talking about the sister of Baa Tilaan
> Mbisaan.
> And yet my brother is very much feared,
> because with one finger he could knock down men.
> Bull of my matrilineage, come to my aid, descendant of
> Don Gey;
> observe the misfortune which strikes me now.
> See how a giant has struck the sister of Baa Tilaan of Yaa Muse.
> Another giant also came to strike the sister of Baa Tilaan
> of Yaa Muse.
> But something happened to these people at the compound of
> Pena Puy.
> Bull of my matrilineage, come to my aid, descendant of Don
> Gey;
> observe the misfortune which strikes your sister now.

Interpretation. This song continues the previous one, describing the misfortune of Yaa el. Not content to deprive her of food and water, before banishing her the villagers sent two men to beat her. She again deplores the absence of her father, Tilaan Mbisaan, and hopes that her matrilineage may yet come to rescue her reputation. She maintains that this isolation and marginality, which resulted from her contracting plague, ruined her life. It led her to enter into a poor marriage, and cast a permanent stigma over her.

Fifth Song: "Wuna Farba Duum: The Niece of Farba Duum"
Text in translation:

> Inhabitants of Diassa, I ask every one of you to come
> and see what has happened. A bullet of an epidemic has
> just struck down the beautiful one, the beautiful one
> of Farba Duum.
> And yet she told me that she spent the night at the
> funeral rites of Baa Ti Gey Sam and that she did not
> tarry long there.
> Ngoy Duum, with what shall your aunt warm herself now?

Interpretation. This song calls on the inhabitants of Diassa to hear the sad story of Farba Duum. Only one of her children, a daughter, lived to adulthood, and that daughter had only one child, a beautiful baby girl. When she grew older, the child represented her grandmother at the funeral of a relative who had died of plague in another village. Alas, when she returned, she too succumbed to plague, leaving her bereaved grandmother to ask, "who will gather firewood for me in my old age?" Thus the song metaphorically refers to the spiritual and material poverty of those deprived of kin as a result of the plague.

The Song composed by Coumba Gaye: "Yaa Maan-ce kud-te" ("The punishment of Yaa Maan-ce")
Text in translation:

> Yaa Maan-ce has brought unhappiness to the home of Baa
> Mbeet. She has not been spared since she was brought
> down at Ba'jataa where she was buried. Being taken to
> the lazaretto is better than contracting plague.

Interpretation. This lament indicates that succumbing to plague is a punishment for violating Sereer codes of conduct. Yaa Maan-ce was held responsible for having infected her quarter (Faam Baa Mbeet) with plague. She traveled to a neighboring quarter, Ngiik, and was offered manioc. She brought some back and shared it with a pregnant woman named Paana Mbay. The next morning Paana developed a severe headache and ganglions, symptoms of plague. She died soon afterward, and a few days later, so did Yaa Maan-ce. Yaa violated Sereer practice which prohibited a pregnant woman from eating special foods not immediately available to her, such as would have probably been the case with manioc. Violation of this taboo was said to produce stigmata on the newborn.

The important place assigned to Sereer women in the mourning process helped empower them in their society.[98] Comparative studies of oral literature in a variety of cultures in Africa and elsewhere suggests that women have usually expressed grief differently from men.[99] The specialized art of lamentation, however, has deeper and wider dimensions. Laments as a genre used in mourning are linked not only to death, but to the passing of a way of life. In societies as far apart as Celtic Britain and ancient Greece, laments became an art form of women. They may have been expressed through possession, in which the dead were seen to address the living, either to bring solace or to call for the redress of real or imaginary grievances. Because social tensions could be exacerbated by strong rhetoric inciting men to take revenge, funeral laments were actually banned for a time in Athens and other Greek city states.[100] Although there is no evidence that Sereer women went as far as this, clearly they used laments as an opportunity to state their sometimes angry views about the unfolding of events in their community, and vent their grievances.

NOTES

1. Sereer belief systems in their complex variety have been treated at length in Marguerite Dupire, *Sagesse sereer: Essais sur la pensée sereer ndut* (Paris: Karthala, 1994). Also valuable are Charles Becker, "Les Serer Ndut: Études sur les mutations sociales et réligieuses" (mémoire de l'École Pratique des Hautes-Etudes, Paris, 1970), 120–40; and Ismaila Ciss, "Les Sereer du Nord-Ouest" (mémoire de maitrîse, Université de Dakar, Dakar, 1981–82). For the more elaborate but similar healing cults and practices of the Lebu, see Georges Balandier, *Afrique ambigüe* (Paris: Plon, 1957), chapter 3.

2. Becker, "Les Serer Ndut," 120.

3. Dupire, *Sagesse sereer*, 48.

4. Dupire, *Sagesse sereer*, 50.

5. See Steven Feierman, *Peasant Intellectuals: Anthropology and History in Tanzania* (Madison: University of Wisconsin Press, 1990), 253–56, for very similar distinctions drawn in Tanzania between diseases "of God" and those caused by human malice or breach of custom. The first type simply happened, with no human causation. Treatment might consist of rest, herbal remedies, devoted nursing, and occasionally isolation.

6. Becker, "Les Serer Ndut," 127–28. For comparisons, see E. B. Idowu, *Olodumare: God in Yoruba Belief* (London: Longmans, 1962).

7. Interview with Guedj Faye.

8. Interview with Al Hajj Serigne Malik Thiombane.

9. Interview with Thérèse Tisa Mbengue.

10. Interview with Guedj Faye.

11. Interview with Marie-Anne Yaayo Diouf.

12. Interview with Ngor Laba (called "Goudi") Diop.

13. Marguerite Dupire, "Chasse rituelle, divination et reconduction de l'ordre sociopolitique chez les Serer du Sine (Sénégal)," *L'Homme* 16 (1976): 5–32.

14. Interview with Dié Yat.

15. Interview with Guedj Faye.

16. Interview with Goudi Diop.

17. Interview with Goudi Diop.

18. Dupire, *Sagesse sereer*, 52–53.

19. Joseph Kerharo, *La pharmacopée sénégalaise traditionnelle. Plantes médicinales et toxiques* (Paris: Éditions Vigot frères, 1974), 211–14; and A. Sebire, *Les plantes utiles du Sénégal* (Paris: Baillière, 1895), 228.

20. Sebire, *Les plantes*, 8.

21. Kerharo, *La pharmacopée*, 323–24; Sebire, *Les plantes*, 20–21.

22. Interview with Guedj Faye.

23. Marguerite Dupire, "Funérailles et relations entre lignages dans une société bilinéaire: Les Serer (Sénégal)," *Anthropos* 72 (1977): 376–400.

24. Interview with Guedj Faye.

25. Interview with Guedj Faye.

26. Interview with Coumba Gaye.

27. Interview with Ko Diouf. This informant was renowned throughout Siin as a powerful healer or *saltigi*.

28. Interview with Al Hajj Serigne Malik Thiombane.

29. Maureen Malowany, "Medical Pluralism: Disease, Health, and Healing on the Coast of Kenya, 1840–1940" (Ph.D. dissertation, McGill University, Montreal, 1997).

30. Interview with Chiekh Dieng, Ibrahima Dieng, and Mandione Dieng.

31. Interview with Goudi Diop. He observed that plague was imported into Siin by Wolof herdsmen traveling south from Diourbel.

32. Interview with Aissatou Gaye.

33. Interview with Sitor and Amad Diouf.

34. Dupire, *Sagesse sereer*, 48.

35. Interview with Coumba Ndoffène Diouf.

36. Interview with Goudi Diop.

37. Interview with Ko Diouf.

38. Interview with Guedj Faye.

39. Interview with Marie-Anne Yaayo Diouf.

40. Interview with Étienne Faye, together with Dièn Dione.

41. Becker, "Les Serer Ndut," 123. Maureen Malowany has suggested that, on the Swahili coast of Kenya, there were four therapies from which to choose: African, unani, ayurvedic, and Western. Malowany, "Medical Pluralism."

42. "Introduction," in *The Social Basis of Health and Healing in Africa*, edited by Steven Feierman and John M. Janzen (Berkeley: University of California Press, 1992), 19.

43. For example, a healer in Ufipa expressed his contempt for the Western practice of attempting to cure a deeply rooted illness without first determining its hidden cause. Roy Willis, "Magic and 'Medicine' in Ufipa," in *Culture and Curing: Anthropological Perspectives on Traditional Medical Beliefs and Practices*, edited by Peter Morley and Roy Willis (London: Peter Owen, 1978), 142–43.

44. For details see Feierman, *Peasant Intellectuals*, chapter 4.

45. Meredeth Turshen, *The Political Ecology of Disease in Tanzania* (New Brunswick, N.J.: Rutgers University Press, 1984), 148.

46. Interview with Dié Yat.

47. Interview with Coumba Ndoffène Diouf. He bears the name of his grandfather, the *buur siin*, who was the titular head of Siin until his death in 1923. Martin A. Klein, *Islam and Imperialism: Sine Saloum 1847–1914* (Stanford, Calif.: Stanford University Press, 1968), 204.

48. James F. Searing, "Accommodation and Resistance: Chiefs, Muslim Leaders, and Politicians in Colonial Senegal, 1890–1934" (Ph.D. dissertation, Princeton University, Princeton, 1985), 322–23.

49. Interview with Diaraf Cheikh Dieng, together with Ibrahima Dieng, younger brother, a healer or *saltigi*, and Mandione Dieng, wife. M. Dieng was said to be between ninety-five and one hundred years old, while his wife Manione was described as being roughly eighty years of age. Had the interview focused on politics, it is highly unlikely that M. Dieng would have invited his wife to participate. But since the subject of health and disease is so strongly gendered, the *diaraf* felt obliged to call on his wife's expertise. This pattern was to be repeated throughout the Sereer interviews.

50. Interview with Ibrahima Dieng.

51. Interview with Dauda Mbengue.

52. Interview with Al Hajj Serigne Malik Thiombane.

53. Interview with Coumba Gaye. As a young girl, she was a plague patient there. Another informant, Thérèse Tisa Mbengue (interview, Tiwigne-Tangor), was sent to Wangal as a suspect on no less than on three occasions over several years.

54. Interview with Gaye Faye.

55. Megan Vaughan has noted a similar aversion in colonial Nyasaland (Malawi) to what the local population called the "smallpox police," squads organized to carry out military-style vaccination campaigns. Megan Vaughan, *Curing Their Ills: Colonial Power and African Illness* (Palo Alto, Calif.: Stanford University Press, 1991), 43.

56. Interview with Dauda Mbengue.

57. Interview with Thérèse Tisa Mbengue.

58. Interview with Goudi Diop.

59. Charles Becker, *Vestiges historiques, témoins matériels du passé dans les pays sereer* (Dakar: ORSTOM, 1993), 8.

60. Interview with Adama and Mor Ciss. Like virtually all the informants, they testify that the lazaretto was located at Wangal, near Lake Makka.

61. Interview with Marie-Anne Yaayo Diouf; and interview with Coumba Gaye.

62. Interview with Marie-Anne Yaayo Diouf.

63. Interview with Gaye Faye.

64. I am grateful to Charles Becker for this reference; he graciously afforded me access to his correspondence with a team of physicians and researchers investigating a cholera outbreak in the 1980s. The team consisted of Olivier Fontaine, Bernard Maire, Michel Garenne, René Collignon, and D. Schneider. There were about twenty-five, possibly twenty-nine, cholera deaths in the Niakhar region.

65. Interview with Goudi Diop.

66. Interview with Marie-Anne Yaayo Diouf. She compares the plague vaccination to the one against smallpox, which required only a single injection, and which had very

mild if any side effects. Coumba Gaye (interview at Darou Alfa) agreed, and recalled having contracted plague despite having been vaccinated twice before on earlier occasions. She adds that people did not refuse vaccinations but were ambivalent about their effectiveness.

67. Interview with Dauda Mbengue.
68. Interview with Marie-Anne Yaayo Diouf.
69. Interview with Goudi Diop, Ndiambour; and interview with Dauda Mbengue.
70. Interview with Marie-Anne Yaayo Diouf. Another informant, Aissatou Gaye, recalls that powder was used in houses to kill rats and mice.
71. Interview with Marie-Anne Yaayo Diouf.
72. Interview with Adama and Mor Ciss.
73. Interview with Goudi Diop.
74. Interview with Sitor Diouf.
75. Interview with Adama and Mor Ciss.
76. Interview with Adama and Mor Ciss.
77. Interview with Marie-Anne Yaayo Diouf; and interview with Adama and Mor Ciss.
78. Tekheye Diouf, interviewed by René Collignon, Niakhar, 17 June 1989. I am grateful to René Collignon for affording me access to his interview notes. The informant was too young to remember the plague years, but as a medical assistant and translator, he took a keen interest in the history of health and disease among the Sereer of Siin. He had been told that plague was so devastating that it had been known to kill as many as ten villagers in a single day.
79. Marc Simond, "Le dépistage de l'infection pesteuse en pratique coloniale" (thèse de Médicine, Université de Montpellier, Montpellier, 1944), 14.
80. Dupire, "Funérailles," 376–400.
81. Marguerite Dupire, "L'ambiguité structurale du fosterage dans une société matrivirilocale (Sereer Ndut, Sénégal)," *Anthropologie et Sociétés* 12 (1988): 7–24.
82. Marguerite Dupire et al., "Résidence, tenure foncière, alliance dans une société bilinéaire (Serer du Sine et du Baol, Sénégal)," *Cahiers dÉtudes Africaines* 55 (1974): 417–52.
83. Interview with Marie-Anne Yaayo Diouf; and interview with Adama and Mor Ciss.
84. Dupire, *Sagesse sereer*, 50.
85. Marguerite Dupire, "La tabatière et les réseaux de l'amitié chez les Sereer: Extrait d'objets et mondes," *Revue du Musée de l'Homme* 23 (1983): 143–54.
86. Interview with Dié Yat. She recalls how plague came to her village after a neighbor traveled to a funeral in another village.
87. Interview with Sitor Diouf; and interview with Gaye Faye, who deeply regretted not having been permitted to attend the funeral of a relative who had died of bubonic plague.
88. Interview with Dauda Mbengue.
89. Interview with Adama and Mor Ciss.
90. Dupire, "Funérailles," 376–400.
91. Dupire, *Sagesse sereer*, 32–36. Coincidentally, the Merina of Madagascar were another group profoundly affected by endemic plague, and also strongly resentful of intrusive colonial health control measures. There too, interference with their elaborate

burial practice was particularly galling. For example, their *famadihana* ceremony required the exhumation of a corpse after a period of several months, followed by reburial in a new, permanent tomb. Cremation, or even the hasty mass burials practiced by health officials during plague epidemics, made such ceremonies, designed to permit rebirth, impossible. The classic account of Merina funeral practice is Maurice Bloch, *Placing the Dead: Tombs, Ancestral Villages, and Kinship Organization in Madagascar* (London: Seminar Press, 1971).

92. Dupire, *Sagesse sereer*, 35.

93. Marguerite Dupire, "Les 'tombes de chiens': Mythologies de la mort en pays Serer (Sénégal)," *Journal of Religion in Africa* 15 (1985): 201–15; and Dupire, "Funérailles," 376–400. The point is made by Becker and Martin that the twentieth-century impact of Islam and Christianity has brought considerable changes to Sereer funeral practices. See Charles Becker and Victor Martin, "Rites de sépulture préislamiques au Sénégal et vestiges protohistoriques," *Archives Suisses d'Anthropologie Générale*, Génève, 46 (1982): 272.

94. Interview with Tekheye Diouf. He reported how plague struck at Diakhao and Diambane, and how traditional healers were at a loss to cure the victims.

95. Becker and Martin, "Rites de sépulture," 261–93; and Ismaila Ciss, "Les Sereer du Nord-Ouest" (mémoire de maitrîse, Université de Dakar, Dakar, 1981–82), 33.

96. "Wolof" in this Sereer usage connotes affluence and civility.

97. Fuulbe (speakers of Halpularen) are regarded by the Sereer as beautiful; hence the term here is synonymous with "beauty."

98. The empowerment provided to women through funeral lamentations thus deserves consideration alongside similar exercises in other African cultures. A generation ago, I. M. Lewis drew our attention to the power of women's possession cults such as those known as *sar* (*zar*) in Ethiopia, Somalia, the Muslim Sudan, and Egypt, and as *bori* in Hausa society in West Africa. These cults were often linked to situations in which women did not otherwise receive deference and respect. I. M. Lewis, *Ecstatic Religion: An Anthropologic Study of Spirit Possession and Shamanism* (Harmondsworth, England: Penguin Books, 1971), 31, 76–79.

99. For a pioneering comparative study, see P. C. Rosenblatt, R. Walsh, and A. Jackson, *Grief and Mourning in Cross-Cultural Perspective* (New Haven, Conn: Human Relations Area File Press, 1974). For Greece, see Gail Holst-Warhaft, *Dangerous Voices: Women's Laments and Greek Literature* (London: Routledge, 1992); Margaret Alexiou, *The Ritual Lament in Greek Tradition* (Cambridge: Cambridge University Press, 1974); and Loring Danforth, *The Death Rituals of Greece* (Princeton, N.J.: Princeton University Press, 1982). Elizabeth Schmidt has shown how Shona women in Zimbabwe used songs as a tool of empowerment. Elizabeth Schmidt, *Peasants, Traders and Wives: Shona Women in the History of Zimbabwe, 1870–1939* (Portsmouth, N.H.: Heinemann, 1992), 20.

100. For an intriguing discussion, see Holst-Warhaft, *Dangerous Voices*.

9

PLAGUE IN THE CITY: EPIDEMICS IN DAKAR, RUFISQUE, AND SAINT-LOUIS

Urban living conditions continued to present a challenge to public health authorities throughout the interwar period. As Dakar and the rail towns grew rapidly, overcrowding increased, and with it the threat of a more serious epidemic impact from bubonic plague or yellow fever, as well as a rising incidence of chronic diseases such as tuberculosis. This chapter focuses on bubonic plague outbreaks in the cities of Dakar, Rufisque, and Saint-Louis, and examines the efforts of the French medical research community as it struggled to contain bubonic plague between the two wars. Although Africans in small numbers began to take part in colonial medical efforts, the continuing reluctance of French medical authorities to consult with the Senegalese community contributed to their failure to gain acceptance of biomedical interventions.

PLAGUE IN DAKAR

Plague-free since its last case in January 1915, the city of Dakar was struck for a second time in the first days of June 1919. Before it subsided in the fall, bubonic plague killed at least 712 Dakarois, half the fatalities of 1914 but representing the third worst outbreak in the city's unhappy twentieth-century struggle with *Yersinia pestis*.[1] To the consternation of the authorities, who were wont to blame plague outbreaks on the insanitary practices of Africans, the first cases appeared on Boulevard Pinet-Laprade, in the heart of the European city, in the presumably pristine premises of the Convent of the Sisters of the Immaculate Conception. The convent was located next door to the warehouse of the Compagnie Française, where stores of peanuts and grain attracted a plentiful number of rats. Two European nuns and two Creole girls in their charge came down with what was quickly confirmed by the Bacteriological Institute to be bubonic plague.[2] The rest of the inhabitants of the convent were sent to the European lazaretto at Cape Manuel where five new cases soon materialized. It took the European sisters several months of convalescence, but they survived their ordeal. Two of their students, one described as Creole and the other as Wolof, were not so fortunate. For almost six weeks there were no other signs of plague in the city. Then, on the French national holiday of 14 July, an African child was found on the quay writhing in great pain. Rushed to the Native Hospital, he died soon afterward of septicemic plague. Before long, *Y. pestis* appeared in the Médina and in the western part of Dakar, fanning out along streets such as Malenfant, de Thiong, and Raffenel, where shacks and straw huts were numerous, and threatening to move down to streets such as Victor-Hugo, Félix-Faure, and Jules-Ferry, and the Boulevard de la République in the city core.

Despite the experience of 1914, authorities were once again slow to respond. The first meeting of the Municipal Hygiene Committee of Dakar to deal with the new outbreak did not take place until 31 July, when Chief Medical Officer Heckenroth outlined a plan of action. He called for the usual methods: the isolation of suspects at the Cape Manuel lazaretto for Europeans and "favored" Africans, and at the segregation camp of Bel-Air for Africans; and cleansing, burning, and compulsory Haffkine vaccination for all noncitizens. On 2 August, the governor of Senegal instituted a limited quarantine over the African sections of the city. Heckenroth had also requested that the port be placed under quarantine but neither the military nor the merchants supported him.[3]

Because the port was declared to be plague-free, port physicians continued to issue clean bills of health to ships provided that all Syrian, Moroccan, and "native" passengers had sanitary passports indicating they had received full vaccinations against plague. Navy physician A. Esquier was critical of ships' captains, who, he claimed, did not comply fully with rat prevention measures on their ships nor conduct adequate surveillance of their native crews and the dock workers.[4]

African resistance continued against the sanitary measures and the men charged with enforcement. Cases went unreported, bodies were buried clandestinely, and health agents were attacked when attempting to perform their duties. Vaccination centers were deserted as "intense propaganda" was mounted against the sanitary measures by Lebu elders.⁵ Areas of infection spread from the western side of Blanchot Street to the east, closer to the European neighborhoods. Numerous cases broke out in the city core around Félix-Faure, Victor-Hugo, Jules-Ferry, and the Boulevard de la République.

In a scene reminiscent of their public resistance in November 1914, a large demonstration of Lebu residents gathered on 29 September 1919, to express in public their refusal to evacuate three Lebu compounds, as ordered by the Health Service.⁶ The next day the governor's delegate, M. Henry, suspended the orders to "avoid serious disturbances." During the next two weeks, frequent meetings took place between the heads of government and the health service and the Lebu leaders. Governor Lévecque, who had traveled to Dakar from Saint-Louis, granted three major concessions to the angry residents, over the objections of Heckenroth. Lévecque made the anti-plague vaccination voluntary; he reduced the quarantine confinement at Bel-Air from ten days to five for all those who had been vaccinated twice within the previous six months; and he allowed residents to isolate their sick themselves if they chose not to use the lazaretto at Bel-Air at all.⁷

Although Lévecque returned to his capital in late September optimistic that the concessions he had granted would result in cooperation, he was to be disappointed. His delegate in Dakar, M. Henry, wrote Lévecque to say that in the face of "implacable hostility from the totality of the natives," he could not ask civilian officers to risk their lives in trying to enforce health measures. People were now so angry they refused even to help destroy mosquito larvae. Either the public health measures had to be abandoned completely or the state would have to resort to force.⁸ Lévecque wrote to Governor-General Merlin, stating that the *chefs de quartier* were in fact willing to cooperate but could not get their people to follow them. He suggested that as a good-will gesture Merlin should suspend some of the legal steps being taken by the police against a number of violations of the health code.⁹

Merlin and Lévecque still remained unable to decide whether to confront the population with force. On 5 November, Merlin told Lévecque that he had informally called in all the notables in town, European and African, to consult on a course of action.¹⁰ Angry European commercial interests, such as the Union Coloniale, urged the Government to take "rapid and energetic measures" to end their "policy of hesitation and procrastination."¹¹ Fortunately for Merlin, nature provided a temporary solution to his dilemma. The cooling breezes, which were late in coming in 1919, finally arrived in mid November, and with them, a respite from plague. By December, the scourge had diminished, even if a handful of cases continued to be recorded until mid February 1920, when the city's quarantine could finally be lifted.

Throughout the medical emergency, Governor-General Merlin insinuated that African resistance had been politically inspired. Without mentioning names, he clearly suggested that Blaise Diagne was behind "the harmful propaganda in the light of the coming electoral period," arguing that "certain personalities, anxious to preserve their popularity, were not giving us the cooperation we had a right to expect from them."[12] Later, Merlin would complain to the Minister of Colonies in Paris that the "same elements of the population of Dakar which opposed us in 1914 were doing so now."[13]

The medical authorities, as they had five years earlier, preferred to continue to blame African victims and lack of political will for the persisting medical crisis. Esquier described Dakar as a filthy city and Africans as undisciplined and ignorant of hygiene. His predictable conclusion was that strict segregation should be imposed until education brought Africans to a higher level of understanding:

> It must be admitted . . . that Dakar is a dirty city. Latrines do not exist and the natives are not embarrassed about relieving themselves in broad daylight, and on the prettiest avenues, actions that would result in stiff fines in the neighboring British colony [Gambia]. We know with what promiscuity and dirt the Black lives. As long as his sanitary education is not addressed—and there is no effort now to do so—segregation, the absolute separation of native and European quarters, will remain an absolute necessity.[14]

PLAGUE IN RUFISQUE

In contrast to Dakar, colonial health statistics and accounts of plague in Rufisque and Saint-Louis are much more sparse. What evidence exists suggests that control measures in the smaller towns were less elaborate than in Dakar, but more extensive than in rural areas. As the statistics in chapter 1 indicate, Rufisque, lying in the heart of the plague zone, experienced four major outbreaks and recorded 1,383 deaths during the entire endo-epidemic period.

The 1919 epidemic in Rufisque, which killed at least 437 residents, was typical and repeated the Dakar experience.[15] Despite a *cordon sanitaire* established in June, separating the European section of town from the neighboring African villages, the plague swept over this barrier and engulfed the entire town. Caught unprepared, local health officials felt obliged to isolate 180 plague suspects in a makeshift lazaretto set up at the old military arsenal, which had a capacity for only twenty beds. The majority of suspects were therefore forced to sleep in the open, without mats, and had good reason to complain of the appalling conditions they were forced to endure. Heckenroth reported that the toilets were in terrible condition and the showers in need of repair; no soap had been distributed; and the military physician in charge, Dr. Collomb, was simply overwhelmed by the situation. Two health department guards looked after security, but they did not conduct surveillance at night, making escape relatively easy.

It is little wonder that the townspeople of Rufisque were as opposed to control measures as their counterparts in Dakar. They too refused to report cases, failed to declare their burials at the two native cemeteries, and avoided vaccinations when they could. Compared with the residents of Dakar, however, they were under far less scrutiny from municipal authorities. The Rufisque Municipal Council was entirely absent during the 1919 epidemic, save for one councillor, Moumar Sène, described by Heckenroth as a man of goodwill but both illiterate and ineffectual.[16]

When plague struck again the following year, Rufisque found itself only slightly better prepared. A health inspector, M. Alexis, found six newly erected dwellings at Dr. Collomb's temporary lazaretto, able to hold some 600 suspects.[17] The construction had been carried out in two days by the Tirailleur Sénégalais battalion of Rufisque. The real purpose of Alexis' visit was to study the possibility of the construction of a permanent lazaretto built with cement, not straw. He also discovered that two of the sanitary guards had died of plague, and asked the General Council to provide modest compensation for their widows. Councillor Galandou Diouf, whose constituency was Rufisque, supported the request, noting that the guards were badly paid for the terrible risks they ran, and that the primitive conditions at the lazaretto during the rainy season were very hard on the people.[18]

A common and justified cause of resentment was the obligation of the populace to contribute their labor to the building of health facilities, and to the implementation of such unpopular tasks as vector control. In August 1924, residents of Bargny, a suburb of Rufisque, protested that, as citizens of a commune, they could not be compelled to help build the lazaretto or comply with other aspects of the public health legislation. A senior colonial official was called in to calm them down. A similar popular protest had occurred a month earlier in the nearby African quarter of Thiès-Bambara, where a large crowd of local residents refused to participate in rat hunts unless citizens of the four communes were made to do the same thing. Order was restored and the rat hunt was held only after a senior official from Dakar arrived and promised to hear the people of Thiès-Bambara's grievances against the local *commandant de cercle*.[19]

PLAGUE IN SAINT-LOUIS

The Senegalese colonial capital of Saint-Louis lay to the north of the plague zone, and visitations from plague were less frequent than within the zone. Nevertheless, five major outbreaks between 1917 and 1929 resulted in a minimum of 1,923 deaths, and caused much suffering and hardship. Saint-Louis had a larger population of European officials, private citizens, and African government clerks than Rufisque. Control measures were therefore more extensive and commentary from the General Council, which met in the city, more frequent.

The failure of the state to provide adequate compensation for destroyed property was one issue which resonated in the General Council. At its session of 14 December 1918, as the plague epidemic of that year was winding down, Councillor François Devès expressed his anger that the entire district of Guet Ndar was condemned to be burned, that the people of Guet Ndar had been ordered to build new homes of wood, and that they were being poorly compensated. The administration spokesman replied that had people cooperated with authorities during the epidemic it might not have been necessary to burn everything. He pointed out that compensation had been calculated according to the old price of lumber, 2 francs a meter, not the newly inflated price of 12.5 francs. Devès also expressed his fear that there were plans to build a segregated native town in Saint-Louis along the lines of the Médina of Dakar, a plan supported by the French councillor, G. Dupit.[20]

The council also discussed plague issues on 25 December 1920, when Diagnist councillors spoke critically of the practices of the colonial health officials. Duguay-Clédor described the "deplorable state" of the lazaretto in Saint-Louis, which was particularly dangerous to its patient population because of its proximity to the sea and its cold breezes. Jules Sergent objected that, despite the Diagnists' numerous requests for changes, people were still obliged to sleep on cement floors, were exposed to the elements during the rainy season, and required to eat "detestable food." The council adopted a resolution expressing the wish that the lazarettos be improved as much as possible to "assure the security of their patients," but it appears that the administration was unwilling to spend the money necessary to provide even a minimum standard of comfort.[21]

The 1929 plague outbreak at Saint-Louis, which resulted in 314 declared deaths out of 502 cases, sheds some light on who was at greatest risk during an urban outbreak.[22] The first cases of plague appeared just after the prayers celebrating the festival of Tabaski in late May. *Marabouts* and their *taalibés* were believed to have imported plague as a result of their travels and studies within the plague zone to the south in the *cercles* of Tivaouane and Thiès.[23] Whether this was true in 1929 is unclear, but Muslim teachers and their students frequently appear to have been victims of plague. Professional health workers, of course, were also more often exposed to the plague bacillus than the general population.[24] So too were prisoners. During the Saint Louis epidemic of 1929, some 24 out of the prison population of 108 were assigned as *corvée* laborers to the Saint-Louis Health Service for the duration of the epidemic. Most worked as boatmen conveying corpses to the cemeteries located on the small islets scattered around the town, but some also labored at the lazaretto and in the disinfection of contaminated houses. From this group, no less than seven prisoners contracted plague; they were infected despite taking such precautions as changing their clothing in a special room and soaking their clothing in a creosote solution, according to Dr. Lefrou, a military physician who was present during the epidemic.[25]

Conditions at the lazaretto, located at Pointe aux Chameaux, continued to be far from ideal.[26] A delegation from the General Council consisting of two councillors, Abdou Salam Kane and Khayar Mbengue, reported that conditions which violated cultural norms had been corrected, but that the food needed improving; in particular, more meat needed to be added to the ration. They also requested that trousers no longer be issued to women after disinfection. It appeared that, previously, men, women, and children were all placed in the same room to be disinfected, suggesting a violation of proper modesty. The governor's representative replied and promised improvements along these lines.[27]

URBAN LIVING CONDITIONS IN THE INTERWAR ERA

In the aftermath of the 1919 Dakar plague outbreak, the French medical authorities attempted to take stock of the sanitary situation. Ferdinand Heckenroth, by this time chief medical officer for Dakar, and a research physician with a solid grasp of the importance of demography and epidemiology, was commissioned to study sanitation in Dakar. His report of over 400 pages has not survived in its entirety, but what remains gives a sobering picture of the sanitary problems which continued to confront Dakar at this time.[28] Using the census data from 1918 and earlier, Heckenroth demonstrated that Dakar was a very unhealthy place for the African population, which in 1920 endured a mortality rate of 41.6 per

1,000, more than double the overall rate of 20 per 1,000 in France at the time.

Refreshingly, in comparison to his peers, Heckenroth chose not to blame the victims. He instead attributed the high African mortality rates to the rapid growth of the city and the failure of Dakar to develop housing and food reserves sufficient to accommodate this growth. Africans came from the countryside to stay for several months at a time as workers, traders, and artisans. A certain number chose to stay and found a family. But these immigrants were poorly fed, lived in miserable dwellings, and were easy prey for disease.

Heckenroth's report was sharply critical of each and every one of the four standard plague control procedures: racially segregated quarantine and isolation; disinfection and burning; vaccination; and vector control. The African lazaretto at Bel-Air remained as unattractive and insalubrious as when it first opened in haste during the plague emergency of 1914, resembling a prison much more than a medical facility. It consisted of three long wooden barracks, five isolation courts, a small four-room lodge to house the security guard and the medical assistant, and two sets of showers, one for each sex.[29] Some 300 meters away was a rudimentary hospital for those infected with bubonic plague. The entire compound was surrounded by a double barbed-wire fence. The site was swampy and mosquito-ridden, which was not surprisingly one of the main complaints of the people who had been forced to spend time there. No wonder, Heckenroth concluded, that Africans tried to avoid confinement in the lazaretto at all costs and continued to hide from the sanitary brigades, the physicians, and the state.

The second major control measure consisted, as in the past, of disinfection and burning. Heckenroth noted that the only control measure readily accepted by the Dakar population was the disinfection of their homes. Clearly, Africans recognized the benefit of ridding of their dwellings of vermin and insects. Unfortunately, short-staffed health squads, rather than taking the time and trouble to disinfect, preferred the quicker and more destructive option of burning infected native houses in their entirety.

Another problem concerned the difficulty health authorities faced in locating the precise sources of infection. Street numbers in Dakar often designated compounds rather than individual dwellings, and health teams were often not convinced they had the right house. During epidemics, moreover, some people threw the clothing and bedding of the sick or deceased into the street to avoid detection of houses. Health guards were under strict orders to destroy such apparel, but they did not always reach the goods before the poor, who appropriated the clothing either to sell or to wear.[30]

Vaccination, the third main control measure, no longer enjoyed the uncritical support of Heckenroth or other medical specialists by 1920. Africans submitted to vaccination only when they were obliged to travel and needed to have official proof that they had received an anti-plague injection. Cheating and traffic in such documents was rampant, and control therefore illusory. For example, in an effort to clamp down on abuses, health officials obtained government permission to board trains outside Dakar in 1920. They not only discovered Africans by the dozen without adequate health papers, but actually found people dying of plague aboard cars and in stations. In sum, Heckenroth observed that by 1920, physicians' confidence in the anti-plague vaccine "had diminished each day . . . to the point where it could no longer be considered a functioning sanitary measure."

The fourth major anti-plague measure was vector control. Despite the primary role of fleas in transmission, however, the medical focus continued to be on rodents. A commission appointed by the governor-general of FWA recommended that in the cities, personnel should be trained by teams of ratters imported from France. In the countryside, the local people were to be used, and the BLFWA should assign a scientist to study the problem of vector control more closely. Heckenroth was pleased that in 1921, his report resulted in action when the federal government signed a contract with a professional ratter, recruited from Paris, who would bring two rat-catching dogs with him to Dakar, and train local dogs and agents of the Health Service in the latest techniques.

More practically, Heckenroth had also recommended preventive approaches which hinted at an awareness of the structural problems underlying public health issues in urban French West Africa. Housing and public buildings should be constructed so that rats were unable to find shelter, and the question of their food supply should also be addressed. Empty lots in Dakar should be fenced off to prevent garbage from being dumped there. Permanent grain depots should be distanced from the city center. Dakar should develop a separate section of its port for grain. In villages, millet granaries should be built at some remove from dwellings. Such reforms cost money which the colonial administration was not prepared to spend, although the importation of ratters from Paris had no doubt not come cheap. Had reformist approaches been followed, they might very well have yielded far better results than the antiquated and futile policy of species eradication.

Heckenroth concluded his lengthy investigation of sanitary conditions in Dakar with judgments aimed more at official slackness than at alleged African backwardness. The state itself set a bad example in its own public buildings. The Dakar prison dumped its soiled water in the street. Very few schools had drinking water for their pupils. The École de Médina lay beyond the area served by the city water supply and was obliged to rely on an uncovered well for its water. Lastly, practitioners of Western medicine needed to do more to win the confidence of Africans. One way to do this was to bring medicine to the people. Dividing the Médina into five zones in 1920, each with a physician responsible for the sector, the French hoped, would lead each doctor to seek out the sick, treat patients in their homes, and record births and deaths. The reality, however, was far from this ideal. Physicians in the Médina took long and frequent holidays and were not immediately replaced, so that doctors did not build up a personal clientele. The diagnosis of death was always arrived at by observation of the corpse, or from hearsay information, since families refused bacteriological examination of the body. In short, Africans continued to distrust Western medicine, would not willingly allow Western physicians into their homes, and would only try Western medicine as a last resort. Heckenroth predicted it would be many years before public confidence would be achieved.

SCIENCE IN THE PERIPHERY:
THE PASTEUR INSTITUTE AND PLAGUE IN SENEGAL

For most of the thirty years in which Senegal struggled against endoepidemic plague, the Pasteur Institute of Dakar (PID) stood in the vanguard of the energetic but unsuccessful efforts of the colonial research community to deal with the disease. The expansion of the Pasteur Institute overseas reflected the close ties between French science and imperialism, "strongly flavoured with French chauvinism."[31] While its roots in Senegal can be traced back to the old Bacteriological Laboratory of FWA (BLFWA), which had been established in Saint-Louis at the turn of the century, the Dakar institution became formally affiliated with the Pasteur Institute of Paris in 1924, under the directorship of Marcel Léger.

Under Léger and his successors, the PID's research record was undistinguished. Unlike branches of the Pasteur Institute in North Africa or Indochina, which contributed significantly to the development of science, and also concentrated on applied, practical research of particular use to the colonial economy, the PID seems to have struggled from epidemic to epidemic. The Pasteur Institute in Tunisia, for example, under the inspired direction of Charles Nicolle, stood in marked contrast to the institute in Dakar.[32]

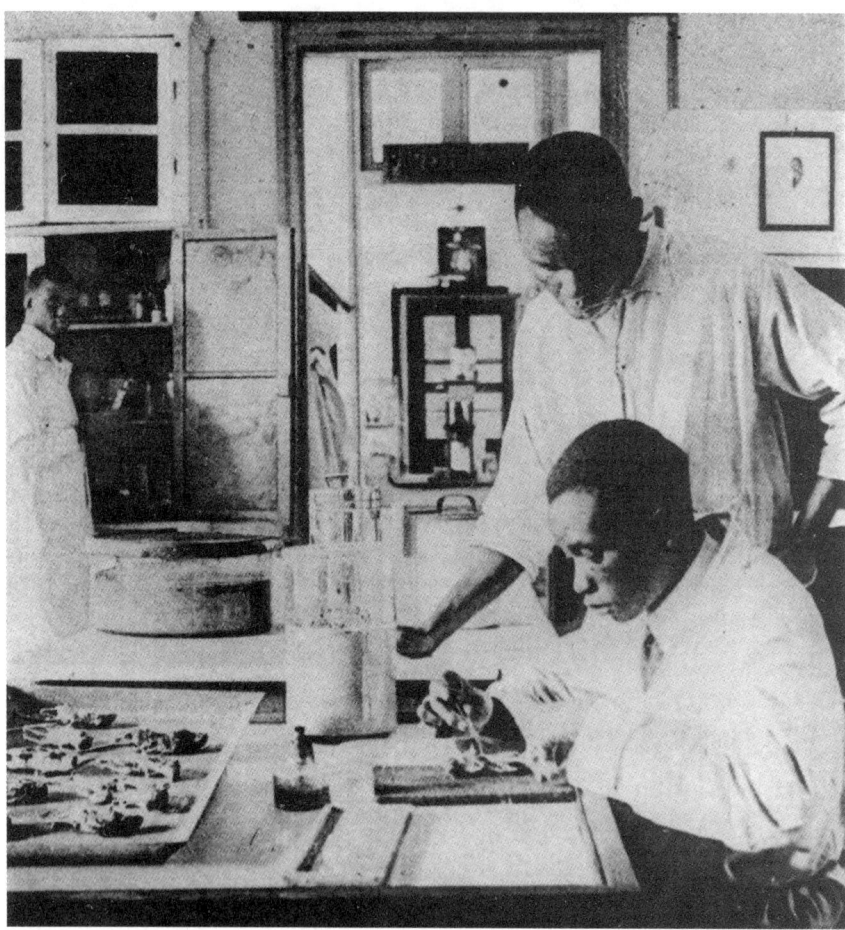

Photo 9.1 African Laboratory Workers at the Pasteur Institute of Dakar (PID) Dissecting Rat Cadavers for Signs of Plague, 1920s. With the singular exception of the deputy's son, Adolphe Diagne, Africans at the PID did not rise above low-level technical positions. From Constant Mathis, *L'oeuvre des Pastoriens en Afrique noire, Afrique occidentale française* (Paris: Presses Universitaires de France, 1946). Courtesy of Presses Universitaires de France. All rights reserved.

Nor can it be said that the PID did much to train a new generation of researchers among the colonial population of Senegal. While a long parade of directors and assistants kept coming from the metropole, the only local name associated with the PID before 1945 was that of Adolphe Diagne, son of Deputy Blaise Diagne, who remained a junior researcher until after the Second World War.[33]

From time to time, particularly when the city of Dakar was spared an annual visitation from plague, French medical authorities would argue that their plague control measures were working.[34] In fact, however, nothing seemed to alter except the irregular rhythm of illness and death. One significant reason for failure was the wrongheadedness of Marcel Léger during the early 1920s, when he directed PID's research in Senegal.

Born in Guadaloupe, Marcel Léger spent most of his career in the colonial laboratories of Indochina.[35] He was an extremely active researcher. In the three short years he spent as director of research in Dakar, over seventy publications appeared under his name. No less than thirteen of these (authored or co-authored by Léger) were on plague. The titles of several of these publications on plague reveal Léger's controversial research positions.[36]

While the volume of his work was certainly impressive, there is much doubt about the quality of Léger's science. In *L'oeuvre des Pastoriens,* a publication devoted to praising the achievements of colonial medicine in general and the African Pasteur Institutes in particular, it is rare to find criticism. Yet, Constant Mathis, the author, and Léger's successor, felt compelled to write that several of Léger's ideas about bubonic plague were questionable, especially the argument that humans could serve as a reservoir for bubonic plague.[37] In his discussion of plague in Senegal later in his book, Mathis's criticism was more explicit and more devastating. Indeed, Mathis organized his entire section on plague around four of Léger's major propositions, each of which Mathis proceeded to demolish.[38] These were (1) bubonic plague in Senegal occasionally occurred independently of any epizootic, which might occasionally follow, but did not necessarily precede, an epidemic; (2) in the absence of rodent infection, inter-human transmission played a primary role in endemicity, which can only be explained by the existence of healthy (and dangerous because undetected) carriers who could even serve as reservoirs of plague;[39] (3) rates of cure of bubonic plague were higher in Senegal than elsewhere; (4) plague, even in its pulmonary form, could sometimes result in a cure, and, thus, the research community had exaggerated the danger of contagion. Mathis and his associate, Marcel Advier, attributed these fallacies to gross misdiagnosis, and concluded that plague in Senegal and in West Africa was no different from anywhere else in the world.[40]

While Mathis's critique of Léger was devastating, his argument did not begin to appear in print until the early 1930s. This allowed erroneous or misleading hypotheses about plague in Senegal to circulate, at least within the French scientific community, well after Léger's departure in 1924. Usually, Léger's influential pen was at work. For example, in 1926 Léger published a lengthy overview of plague in Senegal in which twenty-nine pages, two-thirds of the article, were devoted to his human plague transmission theory.[41] In a 1929 text on tropical medicine, Léger's collaborators, Jules Guiart and Charles Garin, wrote the entry on plague and made a point of presenting the Léger theory about healthy ambulatory human carriers as if it were an established truth, despite the absence of any new evidence to support it.[42]

Clearly, the PID proved very slow to dispense with incorrect hypotheses, reluctant to get out of the laboratory and into the field,[43] and weak in its understanding of plague research and breakthroughs in other parts of the world. It might be argued that language and colonial barriers could have prevented Pastorian scientists in Senegal from following the work, for example, of the India Plague Commission and its successors.[44] But what is extraordinary about the contemporary scientific literature emanating from Senegal is the almost complete absence of references to other researchers' publications, even those of researchers working at other Pasteur Institutes such as the important center in Madagascar, where endo-epidemic plague was also a continuing threat to public health. Tananarive-based researchers like G. Girard, J. Robic, and their colleagues, who published in French in the same journals that the Dakar personnel used and presumably read, not only managed to keep abreast of international plague research but also were able to make significant contributions.[45]

The question arises as to whether a better scientific grasp of the medical and ecological dimensions of plague was indeed possible in Africa between the two world wars. Girard and his team in Madagascar provide one example of what could be accomplished. Another interesting example comes from the British colony of Kenya in the same period. There, R. N. Hunter, an obscure British physician assigned to plague control in the Kenya Health Service in the 1920s, published a short but insightful article containing a sophisticated evaluation of standard international plague control measures. Although it focused on Kenya only, Hunter's critique could easily have applied to Senegal as well. Hunter argued succinctly that the most effective control measures were those which separated rats from humans by improving both rural and urban housing.[46]

Seen in a different light, however, the spotty track record of the PID in plague research may not have been the real issue. What probably mattered more was the symbolic authority of the PID and its close connection to the colonial state. While its limitations should be acknowledged, Michel Foucault's concept of power-knowledge sheds light on this question.[47] The PID and its directors were the leading custodians of Western biomedicine, a body of knowledge upon which French claims to power and control, in part, rested. For powerful researchers like Marcel Léger to admit error risked calling into question part of the foundation of colonial rule.

AFRICAN RESPONSES

African voices were muted in response to the harsh urban living conditions many were forced to endure in the interwar period. One potential source of criticism might have been the new class of petit bourgeois government clerks, schoolteachers, technicians in the health sector, and professional politicians at the municipal and state levels. But this group, able to afford improved living conditions within the racially mixed Plateau district of Dakar, for the most part made conscious choices not to criticize the insanitary conditions endured by their less privileged countrymen living in the squalid Médina. The leading voice of protest on behalf of Africans during the during the 1914 epidemic, Blaise Diagne, joined the camp of Dakar boosters willing to overlook the city's insalubrity. African health workers and schoolteachers, coopted into the colonial civil service at junior levels, risked their careers by speaking out. Nevertheless, a few insights into working-class living conditions can be gleaned from interviews conducted by the François Manchuelle ten years later. The remarkable response of a Dakar school prinicipal named Abdoulaye Yaré Fall is especially noteworthy, and is discussed below.

Until his death in 1934, Blaise Diagne held sway over Senegalese politics, but his decisive reversal, which he termed a "commercial marriage" between the capital of the Bordeaux business community and Diagne's majority control of the Senegalese electorate, occurred in 1923.[48] Diagne had been victorious in the elections of November 1919, capturing 85 percent of the vote, soundly thrashing his sole opponent, François Carpot, and signaling the end of Creole influence in the colony.[49] The campaign had been vicious, with the administration as well as French commercial interests showing hostility to the African deputy. Diagne was chastised for having created discord between the two races, and even for being a Bolshevik revolutionary. A French physician writing in *L'AOF* even blamed Diagne personally for half the deaths during the 1914 plague epidemic because his refusal to help health authorities explain the need for basic control measures had allowed the plague to spread.[50] Diagne's newspaper, which changed its name from *La Démocratie* to *L'Ouest Africain Français*, stoutly rebutted these unreasonable charges, painting Diagne as a patriot and war hero.

The French postwar colonial administration, far from inclining toward further reform, had become much more conservative. The new governor-general, Martial Merlin, who presided in Dakar from 1919 to 1923, would usher in a policy called *association* in place of the now discredited *assimilation*.[51] Merlin's successor, Jules Carde, continued with this newer line until the end of his term in 1930. These new proconsuls of empire argued that the older policy of privileging a small urban elite and trying to replace African culture with French culture had not worked well, and should be replaced by a policy which was kinder to the older West African social and political organizations and the chiefs who were the "natural" leaders.

Much of this ideology was a coded declaration of opposition to what the French called "Diagnism." Fearing that Diagne's demands would spread to other parts of the federation, the administration responded quickly to Diagne's 1919 victory.[52] The next year, the administration restructured the General Council to allow an equal number of elected urban representatives and chiefs. Since the governor of Senegal appointed the chiefs, this change effectively thwarted Diagne.[53]

In response to this newer and harsher colonial reality, Blaise Diagne found himself forced to make a momentous decision. He could continue to champion the cause of the colonial underdog in the face of increased hostility from his opponents, or he could compromise. Forced to choose between France and Africa, Diagne chose France. Ever pragmatic, and by now accustomed to an elegant and expensive lifestyle in France, where he spent most of his time, Diagne approached the French business community in Bordeaux in the summer of 1923 with his proposition. Known as the Bordeaux Pact, his agreement with some forty-seven large and small French import-export houses marked the "greatest victory of the colonial system in Senegal," and the end of Blaise Diagne's reform period.[54] He would become French colonialism's most dutiful supporter until his death in 1934. Senegalese politics now took on the flavor of French machine politics or ward patronage, where access to municipal services depended upon the mayor and the municipal councils. Diagne's Dakar machine, although controlled overall by French commercial interests, used patronage to continue to attract numerous African political allies and supporters. Diagne's successor after 1934, Galandou Diouf, maintained the same system until the coming of the Second World War.

In his new role as defender of the colonial order, Diagne allowed his newspaper to laud Dakar's progress and ignore its shortcomings. A 1924 article in *L'Ouest-Africain Français* boasted that Dakar had become the "showpiece city of French West Africa," with more dispensaries and clinics per capita than Lille.[55]

Meanwhile, evidence grew of continued epidemics and the rise of new endemic diseases in the "other" Dakar. Tuberculosis, for example, was on the rise. One physician observed that the rate of positive skin tests among Dakar school children rose from 38.5 percent in 1922 to 43.3 in 1927. He was convinced that overcrowding in the Dakar slums, where up to eight persons shared a room measuring 4.6 by 3 meters, was the primary cause.[56] One of Diagne's opponents in the election campaign of 1932, Georges Barthélémy, had the temerity to raise public health reform in Dakar as a campaign issue. Promising Dakar voters sewers, water pipes, modernization of housing, and a campaign against mosquitoes during the winter season, Barthélémy painted an ugly picture of the city. He noted that once a visitor left behind the grand boulevards and the splendid homes of the federal capital and penetrated inside the interior courtyards of the streets inside the town, he observed simple straw huts, dozens of people living in open courtyards, without running water or sewers, and garbage and debris piled up in filthy mounds.[57] Of course, others avoided structural causation and continued to blame the usual victims, the new Bambara, Tukolor, and Soninke immigrants, who led a "nomadic" life and, it was argued, were unable to acclimatize themselves to the city.[58]

Soninke migrants to Dakar told a different story. According to their narrative, they were able to maintain their culture and social discipline in the overcrowded urban conditions in which they found themselves. Soninke urban workers lived in what they called *chambres*, or *kompe xoore*, that is, "great rooms."[59] A typical example was the *chambre* located on Thiers Street in the old center of Dakar, inhabited by men from the royal Soninke village of Tiyaabu in the Senegal Valley. Few of the *chambres* were located in the Médina; the majority were to be found in the heart of Dakar on streets such as Raffenel, Escarfait, Félix-Faure, and Thiers.[60] These were, of course, streets where overcrowding placed residents at repeated risk from plague. Each *chambre* was under the authority of the oldest man of the chiefly family present in the migratory group; he would be assisted by a member of an artisan family, his client. The *chambre* had a budget, made up of contributions from migrant villagers, to pay for rent and food in the initial stages of a migration. Modeled after the village youth associations back home on the river, the *chambre* would impose fines to maintain discipline within the unit.[61]

Schoolteachers constituted a large part of the new Senegalese elite.[62] While few of their comments on public health issues have survived, one exception is the remarkable exchange of views between the director of the Dakar Health Service and a person he described as a "diligent"

Senegalese school principal named Abdoulaye Yaré Fall.[63] Born in 1888 at Saint-Louis and educated there, Fall had received his *certificat d'études primaires* in 1906 and his teaching certificate three years later. He taught in small towns and had worked his way up to the post of principal of the elementary school in Bakel in 1916, when he was mobilized for military service. As a citizen, he served in the metropolitan army with the rank of corporal, saw action in France, and was demobilized in 1919. Upon his return to Senegal, he was named principal of the École de Médina, a school with almost 300 students.[64]

In 1922, Fall conscientiously submitted an eleven-page handwritten letter to the Dakar Medical Service to accompany the results of a questionnaire the Medical Service was circulating to school teachers on issues related to bubonic plague. He pointed out that the inability of Africans to implement control measures was a function not of indifference but of the expense involved. People were willing and indeed keen to be rid of fleas, for example, but found that the various pesticides such as creosote or tobacco powder were too costly. Fleas proved a terrible nuisance as soon as the hotter months came, beginning in April, and peaking in late July, just before the first rains. The fleas could be found everywhere, in bedding, beds, and linen, in homes and in schools. Some individuals were particularly sensitive to bites and found them painful, even preventing sleep at night. He noted that during the 1919 plague epidemic in Dakar, pharmacies dispensed creosote without cost to the inhabitants, and it was used widely. But once the epidemic ended, the creosote was no longer given out free and people stopped requesting it. Fall ended his comments on fleas by stating modestly that in his view, fleas played the same role in plague as did mosquitoes in malaria and yellow fever, and that, perhaps, free distribution of pesticides should be considered.

Fall also gave his views on rodent control. In response to the question as to whether children could be encouraged to take small steps in the home to guard against rodents, Fall commented that children were receiving the small bounties paid out by the Health Service for deratting, but noted politely that only three or four children out of ten in Médina and the Dakar suburbs could afford to attend school, and that in any event there were only places for this number. He urged the Health Service to confine rat catching to specially hired teams of specialists. Fall gave the same answer in response to the question as to whether rat catching drives were feasible in his neighborhood. People misunderstood the purpose and resented the burden in monetary cost and time.

No personal reply to Fall's letter appears in the colonial archive. There is only a letter of commendation from the director of the Dakar Health

Service to the inspector-general of education of FWA. In it, the director applauded Fall and his pupils for their "magnificent results" during the rat catching campaign in the first quarter of 1922, when they captured 1,482 rodents. Such an achievement "was due entirely to the tireless efforts of the principal . . . an outstanding and disinterested educator" whom the department of education should recognize and compensate accordingly.[65]

Clearly, French authorities entirely missed the subtlety of Fall's response. In a polite and cautious manner, as befitting a grade school principal in the colonial hierarchy, Fall had made the point that rodent and flea control were serious undertakings better left to specialists than to schoolchildren, and that Senegal had a difficult scientific problem on its hands which required the attention of specialists. Implicit also was the argument that structural changes, which would result from greater investment in education, would be the wisest way of improving living conditions in the Médina.

It would be incorrect to assume that the French had no plans for public health reform after 1918, even if economic priorities remained paramount. Under Governors-General Merlin and Carde, the colonial administration included health reform among its postwar initiatives.[66] Perhaps the most significant change in colonial public health between the wars was the exponential growth of a cadre of African health workers, products of the Dakar Applied School of Medicine (L'École pratique de médecine), which opened its doors on 9 June 1918, "in recognition of the services rendered by the African population to save the mother country."[67] In addition to training African "auxiliary doctors" (médecins auxiliaires indigènes, or ADs), the school also had sections for midwives, for pharmacists' assistants, and for veterinarians.[68]

In the early years, recruitment to the medical school was restricted to secondary school graduates of the École Faidherbe on Gorée.[69] Upon entry, students faced four years of study before graduating as ADs. The long course of study and the demanding curriculum deterred many. The first graduating group, or *promotion*, of 1922, was a small cohort of eight. Over the next twenty-four years, until 1945, the school produced a total of 380 ADs, an annual average of roughly sixteen. Overrepresented among these graduates were Christians from Dahomey and Upper Volta, the presumption being that religious reservations detracted young Muslims from a career so closely tied to Western biomedicine.[70]

Life in the bush was not easy for the young ADs. They found themselves having to travel sometimes enormous distances in their *cercles*, on horseback, camel, donkey, bicycle, and even on foot. The local population mistrusted their ignorance of the local language and their youth, since healing was often regarded as a profession of the mature. African healers looked at the ADs askance, possibly because they were in competition, but mainly because they had become bearers of a foreign therapy. Vaccinations, for example, were one of their major responsibilities, yet resistance to the needle, and to the often coercive methods of the health guards who accompanied the ADs, made their work very difficult.[71] One AD recalled that individuals would offer a chicken in an attempt to bribe him not to vaccinate them; others would attempt to substitute relatives.[72] Older African medical assistants, nurses, and medical aides also resented the better-paid newcomers. Finally, the ADs, like their counterparts in other colonial regimes in Africa, had to endure the paternalism and often the outright racism of their European medical superiors.[73]

To summarize, Part Two of this study has shown that while the impact of the plague on the city of Dakar was dramatic, and put lives and the economy of a busy port at risk, the progress of the disease in the immediate hinterland was equally devastating. The conditions for the emergence of a plague zone were both human and environmental, and within a few years, plague had become endemic. The plague zone proved to be a propitious micro-environment for the propagation of plague.

In the Senegalese littoral, while the plague zone shifted somewhat in this period, plague in the Mont-Roland and Tivaouane areas remained endemic, and populations in this region were subject to persistent interference in their daily lives. Although death rates fell off considerably after 1930, the maintenance of strict quarantine and travel control regulations, together with the realization that plague could strike dramatically and without warning, combined to exacerbate tensions between colonized populations and the Colonial Health Service.

One of the most fascinating aspects of the Sereer response to endo-epidemic plague was its gendered nature. Women were empowered by their exclusive right to compose and recite public obituaries. On the other hand, while the impact of the plague on Sereer women may have reinforced their importance in the grieving process, it certainly added to their societal burdens. Oral testimonies stress that women and not men were expected to feed and care for the patients in the lazarettos and isolation huts. In their role as caregivers, women were thus more exposed to contagion, even if those males who worked as health guards were also at risk. Not coincidentally, in every Sereer village in which I conducted interviews, women were far better informed about the events of the plague years than were men.

During the interwar period, French medical authorities in Senegal did not distinguish themselves in their response to bubonic plague. They continued to blame the Senegalese victims and to force preventive measures upon the population while they themselves displayed timidity and downright incompetence in understanding the scientific nature of their problem. When compared to the major contributions of the Pasteur Institutes in Tunisia, Algeria, and Madagascar, the overall performance of the Pasteur Institute in Dakar proved sadly mediocre.

NOTES

1. See chapter 6 and the Appendix for full statistical comparisons. The only published source for the 1919 outbreak was authored by a navy physician who was present at the time. See A. Esquier, "La deuxième épidémie de peste à Dakar," *Archives de Médecine et de Pharmacie Navales* 110 (1920): 187–213. In terms of documentation, the initial 1914 outbreak was covered in greatest detail. Thereafter, especially once plague became an annual event, the yearly medical reports tended to report on events routinely, and increasingly briefly.

2. Esquier, "La deuxième épidémie," 187.

3. Commercial interests were obviously reluctant to see the port quarantined, while the army wished to continue with the demobilization of thousands of African soldiers. ANS\H57, Minutes of the Meeting of the Maritime Council, Dakar, 16 October 1919.

4. Esquier, "La deuxième épidémie," 189.

5. ANS\H57, Dr. Heckenroth, "Brief Summary of the Plague's Progress from 6 June to 10 October 1919," dated 10 October 1919.

6. ANS\H57, Dr. Heckenroth, "6th Report on the Plague Epidemic," 5 November 1919. Heckenroth reported that the most militant Lebu were those living in the rue Grammont, rue Sandiniery, rue Paul Holle, rue de Valmy, and Avenue de la Liberté.

7. Heckenroth argued in vain that plague could flare up at any time and his service would be unable to control it. Given the service's previous lack of success, it is not surprising that the governor opted for the political concessions. ANS\H57, Dr. Heckenroth, "6th Report on the Plague Epidemic," 5 November 1919. See also Esquier, "La deuxième épidémie," 189.

8. ANS\H57, 15 October 1919, Henry to Governor Lévecque.

9. ANS\H57, Lévecque to Merlin, 31 October 1919. There is mixed evidence as to whether such leniency was applied. A procurator's report in 1920 indicated that the Police Tribunal during the period from late October to mid November did drop three charges of obstructing anti-plague measures while it convicted three other people of the same charge and sentenced them to terms of up to two weeks in prison, with a fine of 50 francs, reduced from 500 francs. Three men were sentenced to six days in jail and a fine of 50 francs for using a vaccination passport that was not their own. From mid November to the end of January, 1920, however, once the plague danger was over and resistance abated, sentences were again heavy. Of the twenty cases brought for-

ward for the two offenses noted above, one individual had the charges dropped, three or four were exempted from the prison sentence, but the rest had to pay the full fine and serve the entire two weeks. ANS\H57, Report by the Procurator of the Republic, Rozé, 20 April 1920.

10. ANS\H57, Merlin to Lévecque, 5 November 1919.

11. ANS\H57, Copy on file of M. Chailley to Minister of Colonies, Paris, 19 November 1919.

12. ANS\H57, Governor-General Merlin to Minister of Colonies, Dakar to Paris, 20 October 1919.

13. ANS\H57, Merlin to Minister of Colonies, 22 December 1919.

14. Esquier, "La deuxième épidémie," 203.

15. The source for this outbreak is ANS\H14. Dr. Heckenroth, Mobile Health Inspector for FWA, "Account of an Inspection Mission to Rufisque on 12 August 1919," dated 13 August 1919.

16. ANS\H14, Dr. Heckenroth, Mobile Health Inspector for FWA, "Account of an Inspection Mission to Rufisque on 12 August 1919," dated 13 August 1919.

17. Session of the General Council on 15 December 1920, in *Conseil Général procès-verbal des délibérations:* sessions of December 1920 (Paris and Saint-Louis: Imprimerie du Gouvernement, 1921), 104–5.

18. Session of the General Council on 15 December 1920, 104–5.

19. ANS\2G24\14, Senegal, Annual Political Report for 1924, Saint-Louis, n.d. For continuing tensions within the municipality of Rufisque, see Ndiouga Adrien Benga, "Du modèle dégradé au contre-modéle, la question municipale: Rufisque (Sénégal, 1926–1960)," in *La ville européene outre-mer: Un modèle conquérant? (XVe–XXe siècles)*, edited by Catherine Coquery-Vidrovitch and Odile Goerg (Paris: L'Harmattan, 1996), 261–79.

20. Session of the General Council on 14 December 1918, in *Conseil Général procès-verbal des délibérations:* sessions of December 1918 (Paris and Saint-Louis: Imprimerie du Gouvernement, 1919), 87–88.

21. Session of the General Council on 25 December 1920, 214–15.

22. See the article by the military physician, G. Lefrou, "L'épidémie de peste de 1929 à Saint-Louis du Sénégal," *Annales de Médecine et de Pharmacie Coloniales* 30 (1932): 599–602. The other source is ANS\2G29\25, Annual Medical Report for Senegal, prepared by Dr. Fulconis, Saint-Louis, 23 April 1930. The Fulconis Report was typical of all the annual reports written in the interwar period. It remarked that the epidemic was more severe than in the previous year, having reached farther north into Louga and Saint-Louis than was usual.

23. Lefrou, "L'épidémie à Saint-Louis," 598.

24. Although it was not the case in Saint-Louis, the risk to dock workers from plague could also be very high. In Dakar during an outbreak in 1923, forty workers at the Port of Dakar were among the ninety victims of plague that year. Marc Sankalé, "La peste au Sénégal (1914–1938): Données épidémiologiques et cliniques" (thèse de Médecine, Université de Montpellier, Montpellier, 1944), 55.

25. Lefrou, "L'épidémie à Saint-Louis," 601–2.

26. N. Moreau, "Note sur le service médical du lazaret de Saint-Louis (Sénégal) pendant l'épidémie de peste de 1929," *Annales de Médecine et de Pharmacie Coloniales* 28 (1930): 219.

27. Session of the General Council on 7 June 1929, in *Conseil Général, procès-verbal des délibérations:* sessions of June 1929 (Paris and Saint-Louis: Imprimerie du Gouvernement, 1930), 163.

28. ANS\H22, Ferdinand Heckenroth, "Le problème de la salubrité publique à Dakar," Dakar, Government of FWA, 1921), 436 pp. duplicated report (hereafter cited as Heckenroth, "Le problème"). As the archivist notes at the beginning of the document, pages 123–269 are missing from the report. Unless stated otherwise, all references in this section are to this source.

29. Heckenroth, "Le problème," 296. Each barrack was 73.5 by 4.4 meters; the overall capacity of the lazaretto was 336 beds.

30. Heckenroth, "Le problème," 305. No doubt health officials the world over ran up against these acts of petty defiance, which cumulatively represented a serious threat to public health. Like insurance adjusters, it must have been difficult for them to preserve any confidence in the public. The unfortunate thing was, in their own societies, they attributed such flaws to human nature while in a colonial situation they saw race or ethnicity as the causal factor.

31. Anne-Marie Moulin, "Patriarchal Science: The Network of the Overseas Pasteur Institutes," in *Science and Empires: Historical Studies about Scientific Development and European Expansion,* edited by Patrick Petitjean, Catherine Jami, and Anne-Marie Moulin (Dordrecht, Holland: Kluwer, 1992), 307. The literature linking medical science to imperialism is substantial. A sampling includes: Lewis Pyenson, *Civilizing Mission: Exact Science and French Overseas Expansion, 1830–1940* (Baltimore: Johns Hopkins Press, 1993); Daniel R. Headrick, *Tools of Empire: Technology and European Imperialism in the Nineteenth Century* (Oxford: Oxford University Press, 1981); and Michael Worboys, "The Emergence of Tropical Medicine: A Study in the Establishment of a Scientific Specialty," in *Perspectives on the Emergence of Scientific Disciplines,* edited by Gérard Lemaine et al. (The Hague: Mouton, 1976), 75–98.

32. First assigned to Tunis in 1909, Nicolle made major contributions to the understanding of leishmania, typhus, and recurrent fever, and was rewarded with the Nobel Prize for Medicine in 1928. His reputation attracted researchers from Russia and Eastern Europe to visit Tunis, and he was able to direct what was probably the largest overseas Pasteur Institute, with a staff ranging from twenty-five to forty between 1925 and 1950. Marie-Paule Laberge, "Les Instituts Pasteur du Maghreb: La recherche scientifique médicale dans le cadre de la politique coloniale," *Revue Française d'Histoire d'Outre-Mer* 74 (1987): 33–34.

33. Adolphe Diagne's name appears as junior author with Marcel Advier in the following publication: "Observations épidémiologiques sur la peste à Dakar (Décembre 1932)," *Bulletin de la Société de Pathologie Exotique* 26 (1933): 388–89. In 1952, his name appears as senior author of two short papers on rodenticides. See A. Diagne, L. Michel, P. Koite, and D. Veyret, "Note préliminaire sur l'emploi du dicoumarol comme raticide en A.O.F.," *Bulletin Médical de l'AOF* 8 (1952): 185–87; and the same authors in the same journal, "Sur l'emploi des dérivés de la coumarine comme raticide à Dakar," 9 (1952): 273–300.

34. F.P.J. Sorel and M. Armstrong, "La lutte préventive contre la peste dans la circonscription de Dakar et dépendances durant l'année 1928", *Annales de Médecine et de Pharmacie Coloniales* 27 (1929): 64–72.

35. Constant Mathis, *L'oeuvre des Pastoriens en Afrique noire, Afrique occidentale française* (Paris: Presses Universitaires Françaises, 1946), 66.

36. See, for example, Marcel Léger, "Considérations sur l'épidémiologie de la peste. L'homme peut, comme le rat, être réservoir de virus," *Revue de Médecine et d'Hygiène Tropicales* 15 (1923): 209–10; Léger, "Rôle non exclusif des rats réservoirs de la peste," *Bulletin de la Société de Pathologie Exotique* 23 (1930): 564–68; Léger, "Souche pesteuse isolée des porteurs sains humains et sa virulence comparée," *Bulletin de la Société de Pathologie Exotique* 16 (1923): 54–57; and Léger with A. Baury, "Porteurs sains de bacilles pesteux," *Compte-Rendu de l'Académie des Sciences* 175 (1922): 734–36.

37. Mathis, *Pastoriens*, 69. Mathis wrote: "It must be said that research conducted by others who succeeded him at Dakar has not confirmed the results obtained by M. Léger. Personally, I cannot subscribe to the points of view of our departed friend, and I regret the fact that he was never able to resume his research."

38. Mathis, *Pastoriens*, 285–93. The earliest rebuttal appeared in 1932. See Constant Mathis and Marcel Advier, "Considérations épidémiques sur la peste au Sénégal," *Bulletin de la Société de Pathologie Exotique*, 25 (1932), 941–44.

39. Léger and Baury, "Porteurs sains," 734–36. It was not clear whether Léger was extrapolating for plague what had proven to be the case, for example, with typhoid, or whether he was influenced by the general theories of Charles Nicolle, director of the Pasteur Institute in Tunisia, concerning healthy carriers. Personal communication from Kim Pelis, Department of Medical History, Uniformed Services University, Bethesda, Md.

40. Marcel Advier, "Sur l'épidémie de la peste au Sénégal," *Bulletin de la Société de Pathologie Exotique* 26 (1933): 465–74.

41. Marcel Léger, "La peste au Sénégal de 1914 à 1924," *Annales de Médecine et de Pharmacie Coloniales* 24 (1926): 289–318.

42. Jules Guiart, Charles Garin, and Marcel Léger, *Précis de médecine coloniale. Maladies des pays chauds* (Paris: J. B. Baillère, 1929), 215.

43. For example, it was not until 1929 that a field trip to Kajoor was organized to focus specifically on the role of rodents and fleas. One resulting publication came to the far from startling proposition that fleas as well as rodents could be reservoirs of plague. See Franck Cazanove, "Recherches sur les causes de la persistence de la peste au Sénégal," *Bulletin d'OIHP* 22 (1930): 2103–7. Cazanove's focus on rodents was reflected in two of his other publications: "Le problème du rat dans le territoire de Dakar et dépendances" (Extraits du Rapport à la 2e conférence internationale du rat et de la peste. Paris, 7–12 octobre 1931), *Annales de Médecine et de Pharmacie Coloniales* 30 (1932): 108–44; and "Le rat de ville et le rat de champs à Dakar," *Outre-Mer* 5 (1933): 64–76.

44. It is, perhaps, unfair to compare either the PID or the French Colonial Health Service to the Indian Medical Service. As Mark Harrison has shown, the Indian Medical Service was not subordinate to any London-based oganization, and generated its own knowledge and discourse. Mark Harrison, *Public Health in British India: Anglo-Indian Preventive Medicine 1859–1914* (Cambridge: Cambridge University Press, 1994).

45. Girard, beginning in 1917, spent almost his entire research career in Madagascar. He started working with Robic on an attenuated, live anti-plague vaccine in the

1920s. In 1926 Girard and Robic were able to develop their E.V. strain from a human case of plague. They continued to improve their vaccine so that, between 1935 and 1938, 2 million Malagasy received the Girard-Robic anti-plague vaccination. In the later stages of the Dakar plague epidemic of 1944, Girard was despatched from the Pasteur Institute in Paris to Dakar to lend his assistance. As will be seen in Part Three, Girard would write a scathing report on the shoddy performance of the research community in Senegal, including the PID.

Fabian Hirst considered Girard the foremost French expert on plague. Fabian L. Hirst, *The Conquest of Plague: A Study of the Evolution of Epidemiology* (Oxford: Clarendon Press, 1953), 442–44; see also Pierre Pluchon, ed., *Histoire des médecins et pharmaciens de marine et des colonies* (Paris: Editions Privat, 1985), 388. One journal in particular, published by the Pasteur Institute in Paris, made it clear from its title that it was to be an organ of the Institute branches in Africa. It began publication in 1908 and its full title was the *Bulletin de la Société de Pathologie Exotique et de ses Filiales de l'Ouest-Africain et de Madagascar.*

46. R. N. Hunter, "Plague in Kenya," *Kenya Medical Journal* 2 (1925–26): 75–85. Contemporary French researchers would have had little opportunity to learn of Hunter's views. The point, rather, is that what Hunter grasped from his experience in Kenya could be grasped by others from the evidence of their own situations.

47. Foucault has alerted scholars to the need to look not only at the way in which the state exercises power, but how micro-networks of power work, including those associated with the academic and especially the medical disciplines. On the other hand, in Foucault's work there is no theory of how power actually works, and human agency and time are either diminished or removed from history. Several of Foucault's studies have focused on the "medicalization of power." See *The Birth of the Clinic: An Archaeology of Medical Perception*, translated by A. M. Sheridan Smith (New York: Pantheon, 1973; original edition, Paris: Presses Universitaires de France, 1963); *Madness and Civilization: A History of Insanity in the Age of Reason*, translated by Richard Howard (Toronto: New American Library of Canada, 1965; original edition, Paris: Plon, 1961); and *The History of Sexuality*, vol. 1, *An Introduction*, translated by Robert Hurley (New York: Pantheon, 1978; original edition, Paris: Gallimard, Gallimard, 1976).

48. Iba Der Thiam, "L'évolution politique et syndicale du Sénégal colonial de 1840 à 1936," nine volumes (thèse d'état, Université de Paris I, Paris, 1982–83), vol. 7, 2574.

49. For details of this campaign, see G. Wesley Johnson, *The Emergence of Black Politics in Senegal: The Struggle for Power in the Four Communes, 1900–1920* (Stanford, Calif.: Stanford University Press, 1971), 196–212; and James F. Searing, "Accommodation and Resistance: Chiefs, Muslim Leaders, and Politicians in Colonial Senegal, 1890–1934" (Ph.D. dissertation, Princeton University, Princeton, 1985), 462–63.

50. *L'AOF*, 22 November 1919, ran an article by one Dr. André Thierry, who worked for the AMI, entitled, "Diagne and the Plague." Alluding in wordplay to "these two words, and these two evils," he argued that "Diagne and the plague were perfect partners. They both appeared in Senegal at the same time, they were each very tenacious," 3.

51. Raymond F. Betts, *Assimilation and Association in French Colonial Theory, 1890–1914* (New York: Columbia University Press, 1961); Alice L. Conklin, *A Mission*

to Civilize: The Republican Idea of Empire in France and West Africa, 1895–1930 (Stanford, Calif.: Stanford University Press, 1997), 174–75.

52. For a thorough discussion of the political protests in Dahomey, see Patrick Manning, *Slavery, Colonialism and Economic Growth in Dahomey, 1640–1960* (Cambridge: Cambridge University Press, 1982).

53. Diagne did have some chiefs on his side, notably Mbakhane Diop, son of Lat Dior; Coumba Ndoffène Diouf, the *buur sine*; and Meissa Mbaye Sall, descendant of the *ceddo* lineage of royal retainers in Kajoor. On the side of the French, however, was the powerful Bouna Ndiaye, the *burba jolof*, who rallied most of the chiefs to his side. Searing, "Accommodation," 489–507.

54. Thiam, "L'évolution politique," vol. 7, 2578. See also G. Wesley Johnson, "The Impact of the Senegalese Elite upon the French, 1900–1940," in *Double Impact: France and Africa in the Age of Imperialism*, edited by G. Wesley Johnson (Westport, Conn.: Greenwood Press, 1985), 164–66.

55. Dr. Huchard, "L'essor d'assistance médicale à Dakar," *L'Ouest-Africain Français*, 18 October 1924. Huchard, who had formerly practiced in Lille for five years, had become director of Municipal Dispensary Number One in the Médina.

56. L. Couvy, "La tuberculose à Dakar," *Bulletin de la Société de Pathologie Exotique*, 20 (1927): 229.

57. Cited in Thiam, "L'évolution politique," vol. 9, 3655. Although the Dakar electorate must have shared Barthélémy's disgust with sanitary conditions, they did not vote for him. He ran a poor third behind Diagne and Galandou Diouf in the 1932 elections.

58. Couvy, "La tuberculose," 230.

59. François Manchuelle, *Willing Migrants: Soninke Labor Diasporas, 1848–1960* (Athens, Ohio: Ohio University Press, 1997), 124, and note 25. The term may have originated in Provence in the first half of the nineteenth century, being used for a room rented collectively by migrant laborers.

60. Manchuelle, *Willing Migrants*, 191 n. Overcrowded dwellings in these streets placed residents at repeated risk of contracting plague.

61. Manchuelle notes that Soninke labor migration underwent a major change in the 1930s, ceasing to be seasonal and becoming what he calls "pluriannual." The principal reason for the shift was that urban wages had doubled to roughly 4,000 francs yearly since the 1920s, and were now higher than those paid to agricultural migrants. Manchuelle, *Willing Migrants*, 125, 179, 187.

62. See Peggy Sabatier, "Did Africans Really Learn to Be French? The Francophone Elite of the Ecole William Ponty," in *Double Impact: France and Africa in the Age of Imperialism*, edited by G. Wesley Johnson (Westport, Conn.: Greenwood Press, 1985), 179–87; and Prosser Gifford and Timothy Weiskel, "African Education in a Colonial Context: French and British Styles," in *France and Britain in Africa: Imperial Rivalry and Colonial Rule*, edited by Prosser Gifford and William Roger Louis (New Haven, Conn.: Yale University Press, 1971), 663–711.

63. ANS\1H15\1, Marginal comments by the Director of the Dakar Health Service on a letter written by Fall, dated Médina, 30 March 1922.

64. He was to serve there for sixteen years, until he was transferred to his native Saint-Louis as principal of the École de Ndar Toute. He retired in 1947 at the age of sixty, by which time he was described by school inspectors as a loyal but old-fashioned

teacher with out-dated methods, and "disastrous" results. ANS\1C\10931, Personnel Files for Abdoulaye Yaré Fall.

65. ANS\1H15\1, Director, Dakar Health Service, to Inspector General of Education in FWA, Dakar, 26 April 1922.

66. Conklin, *Mission*, 221.

67. Papa Ibrahima Seck, *La stratégie culturelle de la France en Afrique: L'enseignement colonial (1817–1960)* (Paris: L'Harmattan, 1993), 149.

68. In 1924, the veterinary section was transferred to Bamako, and in 1925 it became the École de Médecine Vétérinaire Autonome. The École des Sages-Femmes Africaines de Dakar officially opened in 1920, and closed in 1957 when it was annexed to the Faculty of Medicine of the Université de Dakar. Marc Sankalé, *Médecins et action sanitaire en Afrique Noire* (Paris: Présence Africaine, 1969), 40.

69. This account of the medical school comes from Aimée Grimaud (née Houémavo) "Les médecins africains en A.O.F.: Étude socio-historique sur la formation d'une élite coloniale" (mémoire de maitrîse, Université de Dakar, Dakar, 1979), 71–113.

70. Among the graduates who would go on to political prominence were Félix Houphouët-Boigny from Côte d'Ivoire, one of thirteen in the class of 1925; Émile Zinzou (Dahomey), one of eighteen in 1940, Justin Ahomadegbé (Dahomey), one of eighteen in 1941, and Joseph Conombo (Upper Volta), one of twenty in 1942. Grimaud, "Les médecins africains," 74.

71. These same obstacles applied to colonial health workers of various categories. One nurse who found himself a sometimes unwilling agent of the colonial administration recalled the difficulties experienced as a member of of the mobile teams organized to fight sleeping sickness: "The population of certain regions of Upper Volta rarely bothered to distinguish between [health] agents and other administration corps. That explains why some of our colleagues found themselves subjected to a barrage of arrows in the exercise of their duties. For what reason? Often an act of vengeance against the colonial administration. That explains the difficulty the nursing metier faced." Étienne-Goama Rouamba, "La vie d'un infirmier du services des grandes endémies," in *La Haute-Volta coloniale: Témoignages, recherches, regards,* edited by G. Massa and Y. G. Madiéga (Paris: Karthala, 1995), 391.

72. Grimaud, "Les médecins africains," 96.

73. For various other types of African medical auxiliaries in Belgian and British Africa, see John Iliffe, *East African Doctors* (Cambridge: Cambridge University Press, 1998), 35–38, and 78–79; Maryinez Lyons, "The Power to Heal: African Medical Auxiliaries in Colonial Belgian Congo and Uganda," in *Contesting Colonial Hegemony: State and Society in Africa and India*, edited by Dagmar Engels and Shula Marks (London: British Academic Press, 1994), 202–23; and Adell Patton, Jr., *Physicians, Colonial Racism, and Diaspora in West Africa* (Gainsville: University Press of Florida, 1996), 187–88.

PART III

"MERELY A DISEASE OF NATIVES": PLAGUE, WAR, AND POLITICS, 1939–45

The concluding part of this work deals with the final episode in Senegal's long ordeal with bubonic plague. It includes one chapter on the 1944 Dakar outbreak and another on the plague's retreat after 1945. In April 1944, on the unremarked thirtieth anniversary of its first appearance in Dakar, *Yersinia pestis* made what was to be its final visit. The major Dakar outbreaks of 1914 and 1944 serve as bookends for this study, and they require comparisons and contrasts to be drawn.

Dakar had changed dramatically by 1944. Its estimated population was now 165,000 and growing daily, making it six times larger than the small colonial town that had first experienced bubonic plague in 1914. If anything, the old urban problems of housing shortage, overcrowding, and bad sanitation had grown worse with the passage of time. Another important change was political. Electoral politics had been suspended after the defeat and collapse of the French Third Republic in 1940, and neither the Vichy regime nor the Gaullists who took charge of French West Africa in late 1942 had been willing to draft a new constitution and restore voting rights.

As in 1914, a conjunction of war and plague would help determine the political construction of the epidemic. A new element this time was the presence of some 5,000 American military and civilian personnel. The American medical intervention against bubonic plague in 1944 was dramatic. Armed with DDT and sulfa drugs, American medics were prepared to entirely transform plague control and therapy, providing they could overcome the bureaucratic and political obstacles placed in their way.

As will be seen, American medical technology was arguably responsible for the subsequent disappearance of bubonic plague from

Senegal, but it did not save lives during the outbreak among those who contracted the lethal disease. Official statistics for the Dakar plague epidemic of 1944 recorded 512 deaths among 570 patients, a 90 percent case mortality rate, but the overall mortality rate from plague, based on an estimated population of 165,000, was 3 deaths per 1,000. In 1914, on the other hand, 1,439 plague deaths among an estimated 26,000 people represented a mortality rate of 55 per 1,000.[1]

While the American presence was clearly an important new variable making the 1944 experience different from 1914, even more dramatic was the lack of resistance to plague control measures this time round. While chapter 10 attempts the perilous and perhaps dubious historical exercise of explaining why an event failed to occur, its main aim is to demonstrate that the 1944 plague epidemic was a watershed in the history of public health in Senegal.

NOTE

1. See Table 6.1 and discussion above, and Table 10.1. The pattern of higher mortality rates for the earlier plague outbreaks was entirely consistent with experiences in other cities, and was, in part, the result of some immunity built up among plague survivors (see chapter 2). See plague statistics for Bombay and Hong Kong in David Arnold, *Colonizing the Body: State Medicine and Epidemic Disease in Nineteenth Century India* (Berkeley: University of California Press, 1993), 201; and Carol Benedict, *Bubonic Plague in Nineteenth-Century China* (Stanford, Calif.: Stanford University Press, 1996), 177.

10

THE DAKAR PLAGUE EPIDEMIC OF 1944

THE AMERICAN MILITARY PRESENCE

After the fall of France in June 1940, a Vichy-controlled administration ruled French West Africa from Dakar through its high commissioner for FWA, Pierre Boisson.[1] Under Vichy, the hard-won electoral power exercised by Africans through the deputyship and in the Colonial Council disappeared as authoritarian colonial officials rolled the clock back to an earlier period of colonialism. Throughout its period of control, Vichy FWA was subject to constant Allied military threats. The British and the Gaullists actually launched an unsuccessful attack on 23 September 1940, in the Battle of Dakar.[2]

Vichy rule in West Africa would endure for the next twenty-nine months, until the Allied landings in Morocco in November 1942. The French military forces in Africa lost little time in ending their association with Vichy. On 7 December 1942, the Boisson-Darlan-Eisenhower Accord was signed, officially bringing FWA into the Allied camp. A few days later, the first high-ranking American officer, Rear Admiral William O. Glassford, arrived in Dakar. His orders were to implement the accord by installing American naval and air facilities in FWA. Having completed his mission by mid February 1943, Glassford returned to Washington.[3]

For several months during 1943, the Allies discussed the fate of Dakar. Although they eventually consented to allow de Gaulle to exercise French civil authority there, the American military presence in Senegal remained independent of French authority throughout the war. According to Glassford, at one stage the Allied plan required the Free French to move their federal administrative capital to Saint-Louis, while Dakar itself "should be taken over eventually by the United Nations to be administered by the United States, as a delegate of the United Nations."[4] During the course of a White House conference on 27 March 1943, with Anthony Eden, Churchill's foreign secretary, Roosevelt had raised the issue of Dakar's sovereignty.[5] The two agreed that Dakar, like Bizerte and Formosa, was a strategic point which should be occupied by Allied forces.[6] Although in the end Roosevelt accepted a compromise, perhaps as a result of British urging that the French should not be humiliated any further, he never abandoned his notion that Dakar was "a continental outpost for the Americans which would start on the Coast of West Africa."[7] Clearly, French suspicions that the Americans sought to take over the French colonies in Africa were far from groundless. It is not surprising that French relations with the Americans in Senegal would remain strained during the last three years of the war.

On at least one occasion, the Americans went so far as to contact potential agents within the Senegalese political community. In one report to Washington, Glassford stated that he had sounded out African opinion regarding required changes and that Lamine Guèye for one had implied that the present French administration was incapable of reform. Glassford leaped to the conclusion from his talks with Guèye "that the French West African native apparently desires to place himself under the direct protection and guidance of the U.S.A. as the delegate of the United Nations."[8] While Glassford was probably misreading the intentions of so loyal a French assimilationist as the lawyer from Saint-Louis, it is equally possible that Guèye had been deliberately ambiguous with Roosevelt's representative. In either case, the French had some reason to be worried about American intentions.[9]

Political and diplomatic wrangling aside, the American military presence in French West Africa was substantial after November 1942. The Americans organized their West African Service Command as part of the North African theater of operations, and by 1944, had close to 5,000 American military and civilian personnel stationed in Dakar. The Americans enlarged the French airport at Ouakam, maintained a seaplane base at Hann beach, and upgraded the small airfield at Bargny, near Rufisque, some 29 kilometers from Dakar. Later, in January 1944, the airfield had to be moved from Bargny to a new site at Yoff, as the original site was found to be swampy and mosquito infested and contributed to an excessively high malaria rate.[10] The American base headquarters and billet for officers was in a government building in the exclusively European quarter south of the Avenue de la République. In addition to the American military personnel who were stationed in Dakar, American civilians were attached to the Consulate General, the Foreign Economic Administration, the Army and Navy Petroleum Office, and various government contract agencies, all of which were located in the Plateau area. This large American contingent, like the rest of the population of Dakar, faced the threat of bubonic plague in the summer of 1944.

OUTBREAK AND SCALE

As had been the case so often previously, the return of *Yersinia pestis* in 1944 caught the Dakar health authorities off guard. By the mid 1930s, plague had retreated in both urban and rural Senegal, and many had come to believe that epidemic plague was a thing of the past. As can be seen from Table A.1 on plague deaths in the appendix, fewer than 50 deaths were recorded in the entire country between 1936 and 1942. On the other hand, plague's reappearance in 1943 should have provided a warning since it took 226 lives in the plague zone and another 26 in two villages, Yembeul and Malika, on the Cape Verde peninsula close to Dakar.[11]

It will be recalled that in the Dakar epidemic of 1914, plague's first victims were the families of African clerks, and in 1919, nuns and their pupils. This time, the first cases broke out among personnel at the Navy Arsenal around 20 April 1944, demonstrating once again that proximity to infected rodents was a more important factor than either the sanitary conditions of buildings or the ethnicity of the victims.[12] The first confirmed case was reported at the Hôpital Principal on 21 April following an autopsy performed on an African *laptot* who had been occupying a guard hut adjacent to the crowded harbor area.[13] While April and May saw only a handful of cases, deaths mounted dramatically in early June, prompting health officials to announce an official declaration of a plague emergency in Dakar on 4 June 1944.[14] Two days later, of course, Allied soldiers were on the beaches of Normandy. The long anticipated news of D-Day reached Dakar at 10:30 A.M. on that fateful day, the same day that the American military command in West Africa declared Dakar off-limits to American personnel because of the plague epidemic.[15]

In the beginning, the plague was confined to the vicinity of the arsenal. The first five victims were African employees living in the Navy yards.[16] In the first ten days of June, however, ten cases and seven deaths occurred at the Dakar-Niger railway station and in its vicinity; the first week in June also saw the first cases break out in the Médina.[17] On 4 June, the same day that officials finally declared a medical emergency, the European station master at the Dakar railroad station was stricken. That same day, an African railroad station employee died at his home in the Plateau area about a mile away. Over the next three days, railroad employees died in their homes in widely separated parts of the Médina.[18] The American consul, Maynard B.

Barnes, reported that a third European, an inspector at Maurel et Prom, had died, as had a railroad worker and his wife together with some of their neighbors.[19] If the medical authorities needed any further convincing, the discovery of plague-infected rats inside a railroad warehouse close to the station on 26 May would have provided further proof that an epizootic was in progress.

By 1 June, then, it can be said that a full-blown epidemic was underway in the very heart of Dakar, at the arsenal area of the port, and in the rail yards and central station a block or so away. For the rest of that month, plague rampaged through most of Dakar. The only exception was the elegant and thinly populated district encompassing the French administrative and directors' residences south of the Avenue de la République.[20] Not all of the well-off were free from danger. In mid June, a second European fatality occurred in the person of the director of a French mercantile company. Rats had been found a few days earlier in a warehouse in which his office was situated. As the Americans put it: "Now the French began to take a serious view of the situation and increased their efforts to control rats, especially in the European sectors of town wherever plague was found."[21]

Nevertheless, as has been the case everywhere in the world, the Dakar plague took a higher toll of the poor. One official reported that 96 percent of the plague cases came from the poor African quarters of town: Abattoir, Ngaraff, Santiaba, Gendarmerie, Colobane, and of course the Médina, where 298 cases were reported.[22] Not all Africans were exposed to the same risks. Along the Boulevard de la Gueule-Tapée, which formed the western boundary of the Médina, and where the first urban project aimed at Africans had resulted in the construction of cement houses, the epidemic claimed only three victims.[23]

Among the groups only lightly touched by plague were the large numbers of French, American, and African military personnel stationed in Dakar in 1944. Of the few cases which developed in this large community, one involved a Tirailleur Sénégalais who had recently returned from leave in the interior of Senegal, where he was said to have "escaped from the discipline of military life." A second case involved a young medical auxiliary student, who was the victim of a professional accident at the Hôpital Indigène, where he was infected by a dirty needle.[24]

Although plague spread to the countryside from Dakar in 1944, its impact was less severe than the previous year. Whereas in 1943, some thirty-six villages had been infected, leaving a total of 226 recorded deaths, in 1944 $Y.\ pestis$ spread mainly along the rail lines and the death toll was limited to 60.[25] More than in other years, the 1944 epidemic was closely tied to human and presumably rodent traffic along the rail lines. One of the

Table 10.1 1944 Plague Epidemic in Dakar

Month	Cases	Deaths	Case Death Rate (%)
April	5	5	100%
May	2	2	100
June	35	29	83
July	93	85	91
August	163	152	93
September	162	139	86
October	80	73	91
November	30	27	90
Totals:	570	512	90

Sources: Annual Report on Health for 1944, Dr. Jardon, ANS\2G44\11, for cases; Paul M. Lewis, Milton H. Buehler, and T. Roy Young, "Report on Plague in Dakar, Senegal, F.W.A., 1944, " U.S. Army Military History Institute, Professional Papers, Box no. 68, for deaths.

early cases involved a young girl living in the quarter immediately behind the train station in Thiès.[26] Subsequently, on 2 July, a medical assistant in the train station of Bambey inspecting the arrival of travelers was told of a "madman" on the train. The individual was found to have had a bleeding thigh and an inguinal bubo. After his death a few hours later at the Bambey dispensary, the train was disinfected, and all the passengers quarantined at the Diourbel isolation camp.

Another region linked to the rail line where plague appeared in 1944 was Kébémer. There, in mid August, a Mauritanian child of ten, the servant of a Moorish merchant who had a stand in the main market, fell into a coma and expired, after having run a high fever for three days. Three days later, in the Bambara quarter, a twelve-year-old child, also the servant of a Moorish family, died of plague. His mother sold goods in a stall facing the shop where the first victim had worked. As the summer continued, a half dozen plague cases occurred in the vicinity of the major provincial town of Diourbel. More serious were the outbreaks in the rail center of Thiès in September, where some twenty-eight cases were reported, most of them fatal, in several quarters of the town: Diakhao, Bambara, Takhikao, and especially the quarter behind the rail depot, where half the cases occurred.

One of the dead was a worker in the Health Brigade; another was an "elderly and important marabout."[27]

As we have seen in the case of earlier outbreaks, detailed statistical analysis of the 1944 epidemic is problematic. Table 10.1 gives the monthly breakdown. Of the 570 plague cases, 144, or 25 percent, were detected in time for hospitalization, in contrast to 1914, when only a handful of cases were treated in hospital.[28] Commenting on the high mortality rate, Dr. Girard argued with considerable validity not only that the 1944 epidemic was virulent, but also that little or no therapy was provided.[29]

LIVING CONDITIONS IN WARTIME DAKAR

When *Y. pestis* made a return appearance in Dakar in 1944, it would have discovered important continuities among many changes. Once again, rapid population expansion was at work. As Table 10.2 shows, Dakar almost doubled in population between 1936 and 1945, with most of the growth occurring after 1942.[30] Once more, in-migration was the main motor of growth, fueled again by a combination of labor demand in the city and poor harvests and drought in the countryside.[31] Significant portions of rural Senegal endured a disastrous drought in 1941, a visitation of locusts in 1943, and bad harvests generally leading up to 1944.[32] Paradoxically, the malnutrition and hardship which the food shortage had brought may have contributed to the years of relatively low plague endemicity, since the near-empty granaries left less food for rats.

A census of Dakar taken in 1941 revealed that while Dakar was primarily a city of male immigrants, both African and European, no longer did it consist primarily of a "floating population" of temporary sojourners, as French officials put it (see Table 10.3). As a knowledgeable contemporary American geographer, Derwent Whittlesey, observed, Dakar contained a "percentage of women and children . . . far higher than in any other place in West Africa."[33]

Housing shortages and overcrowding were the predictable results of Dakar's dramatic growth. Colonial urban planning, in its infancy when war broke out, could not cope, burdened both by lack of funding and a lack of will.[34] Like other colonial powers, the French had vainly attempted to prevent or limit African immigration to their cities, and had directed housing efforts to accommodate the growing numbers of European civil servants, not Africans.[35] One important exception was a government project during the Popular Front period called Gueule Tapée, consisting of three small housing developments, with fifty units in all,

Table 10.2 Population Growth of Dakar, 1936–45

Year	Africans	Non-Africans	Total	Increase per Annum (%)
1936 a.			93,000	
1941 b.	93,000	10,000	103,000	1.8
1942 c.	103,000	14,000	117,000	14
1943 d.	120,000	[16,000?]	136,000	16
1944 e.	145,000	20,000	165,000	41
1945 f.			175,000	6

Sources: a. Assane Seck, Dakar, métropole ouest-africaine (Dakar: IFAN, 1970), 211; b. Annual report of the Dakar Health Service for 1941, ANS\2G41; c. Annual report of the Dakar Health Service for 1942, Dr. Jardon, ANS\2G43\6; d. Frederick Cooper, Decolonization and African Society: The Labor Question in French and British Africa (Cambridge: Cambridge University Press, 1996), 164; e. Denise Bouche, "Dakar pendant la Seconde Guerre mondiale. Problèmes de surpeuplement," in Le sol, la parole et l'écrit: Mélanges en hommage à Raymond Mauny, vol. 2 (Paris: SFHOM et L'Harmattan, 1981), 962, based on ration cards issued; f. Seck, Dakar, 211.

offered in lease-sale to Africans, with ownership to be acquired after twenty-five years.[36]

In 1944, Dakar consisted of three distinctive residential neighborhoods. The first was a very small, exclusively European quarter south of the cathedral reserved for Dakar's high society, the senior bureaucrats, the company directors, and the diplomatic community. At the other extreme was the exclusively African Médina, characterized mainly by thatched huts, wooden cabins with tiled roofs, and a few masonry dwellings. The third sector was an integrated city core where French, Lebanese, Senegalese, and other Africans lived in the same three sorts of housing, but probably in reverse order. It was this integrated sector, with approximately 20,000 African inhabitants, which caused the experienced American observer, Derwent Whittlesey, to remark that, much to his surprise, the French colonial capital was the most integrated city he had seen in West Africa, one where income and historical circumstance rather than race dictated where people lived.[37] Whittlesey, who favoured "sanitary segregation" in Africa, hastened to add that while the city hospitals

Table 10.3 Population of Dakar in 1941

	Men	Women	Children (to age 15)	Total
African	45,600	30,731	16,472	92,803
French	4,347	2,185	1,970	8,502
Foreign	739	329	697	1,765
Totals:	50,686	33,245	19,139	103,070

Source: Annual report of the Dakar Health Service for 1941, ANS\2G41.

were segregated, the "commingling" in Dakar was not a matter for rejoicing because the Africans' "careless attitude towards sanitation" made them a menace to their European neighbors.[38]

Insufficient and inadequate housing affected both Africans and Europeans during the Second World War. In fact, housing shortages for Europeans had been a problem for years. In 1924, an anonymous health official had complained that many Europeans were obliged to seek accommodation in "the native town."[39] Now, with the war on, the director of the Dakar Health Service could only regret that many European families were confined to a single room, and that bachelors lived in corridors transformed into bedrooms. The French vernacular described such accommodations as "stalags," or even worse, "concentration camps," perhaps not realizing the wide gulf that separated them from the reality in Europe.[40] Finally, in 1944, the French authorities took the only measure open to them when they informed their military personnel assigned to Dakar that they could not bring dependents with them.[41] Disingenuously, the health director maintained that it was disastrous for the prestige of Europeans to see many of them more poorly housed than the "natives." What would "native" servants employed in such European slums make of "our civilizing mission"?[42] Yet the health director was no doubt well aware that very few Africans were decently housed. The most wretched of the poor, recent arrivals from the countryside without work, or beggars, lived in thatched huts, twenty or even thirty people to a single room.[43] American reports of African housing were similar, but they stressed the importance of the type of flooring, and whether it was hospitable to fleas. "Furnishings are scant and sleeping huddled together on the sand floor of the hut or on the ground within the compound is the rule. In some sections, sleeping is done in shifts, as high as fifty persons using a 20' by 20' room in one 24 hour period."[44]

If overcrowding and poor housing were two major threats to the public health of Dakar during the Second World War, wartime shortages of medical personnel constituted a third element. By 1943, the Dakar Health Service had lost over half of its staff of nineteen with the departure of one of its four physicians, three of its five sanitary policemen, six of its nine health agents, and its only nurse. Yet the staff's duties had actually increased to include overseeing the new facilities at the mixed prison at Dakar, the penal camp at Hann, and the workers' camp at Yoff.[45] Personnel more directly related to plague control were also affected. Eight of the thirteen rat catchers who worked on monthly salary for the Health Service had quit, lured away by better jobs.

Not surprisingly, both qualitative and some quantitative evidence suggests that Dakar was a very unhealthy place to live in during the Second World War. The Dakar Health Service Report for 1941 provided some statistical evidence of a decline in the general health of the African population. While the city had seen a population increase from 1936 to 1941 of 7.7 percent, general mortality per 1,000 was up 20 percent; malaria deaths rose by 21 percent and tuberculosis deaths by a third in the same period.[46] The report concluded that while the African population "did not always grasp the goal of measures taken on its behalf," the real culprits were the public authorities who were indulgent of violations of the public health codes.[47]

To be fair, the French health officials were overwhelmed by the magnitude of their task during the war. In addition to the three "major" infectious diseases (plague, yellow fever, and smallpox), health authorities were now expected to monitor "endo-epidemiological" diseases such as malaria, bilharzia, and sleeping sickness; diseases common to both the metropole and the colony, such as pneumonia, influenza, tuberculosis, meningitis, and typhoid; and the children's diseases of Europe—diphtheria, measles, and chicken pox. A fourth category included "social diseases" such as venereal disease, leprosy, cancer, and alcoholism. Fifth, an entirely new category of medical reporting covered "maternal and infant protection" measures.[48]

Sexually transmitted diseases received detailed discussion in the Dakar Annual Medical Report of 1942, when they were linked to the Health Service's surveillance of prostitution.[49] The report described how a French navy physician was assigned to inspect brothels, and how attempts were also made to examine "free public prostitutes" as well as clandestine ones. Five brothels were listed by name: Bar Lily Cernay; the Excelsior

Bar; Aux Parisiennes; the American Bar; and the Alhambra. Each was estimated to house from twenty-five to thirty prostitutes, mostly Europeans and North Africans. The women were examined twice a week, and given blood tests every two months. Although the volume of the sex trade was very heavy, with some women allegedly recording fifty daily encounters, and as many as eighty on pay-days and Sundays, few of the women were found to have been infected.[50] The Health Service attributed the low incidence of venereal disease not only to their own control techniques but also to the work of a photographer in the U.S. Army, who provided them with a set of photographs for each of the prostitutes in the five registered houses.

Such tight controls were not possible for the West African and "Portuguese" (that is, Cape Verdian) women who sold sexual services outside the brothels. In conjunction with disturbances of the peace, Dakar police had rounded up sixty-two prostitutes in 1943. After examination, thirty-two were hospitalized and ten were found to have been infected with syphilis. Considering that twice this number of prostitutes were arrested by police during 1942 (though the report is silent on their health), it is likely that sexually transmitted disease was a larger problem than the medical authorities acknowledged.

Dakar's chronic health problems were made worse by environmental misfortune as well as overcrowding. The widespread rural drought of 1941 seriously affected the capital city as well, with only 18 days of rain, compared with 32 the previous year, and 49 in 1939. Total precipitation plummeted from 677 millimeters in 1940 to 343 millimeters in 1941. The authorities stopped the watering of public gardens, imposed water rationing, and kept these controls in place throughout the war.[51] The water ration of some 50 liters a day per person was half what was deemed necessary for a large city in a tropical climate.[52] Water was only available for certain hours each day, and water pressure was insufficient to reach the top of multistory buildings. Meanwhile, inadequate garbage and waste disposal continued to threaten the public health of Dakar. In the core of the city, the sewers overflowed because the conduits were too small in diameter to handle the increased volume of usage. The only concrete improvement in infrastructure was the acquisition by the municipality of garbage trucks in 1944.[53]

The sanitary situation was still worse in the Médina. It had too few sewers, and drainage of any sort was made difficult because the terrain was flat and originally marshy, magnifying the original error of selecting such an inappropriate site.[54] Ground pollution was now said to be making the water obtained from the wells of the Médina unfit for consumption.[55] Women with calabashes and jerry cans could be seen queuing for long hours in front of the few fountains and hydrants; frequently, quarrels broke out.[56]

The Second World War proved to be an economic as well as a political watershed in Senegal and all over the African continent. Although in the long run the changes had positive aspects, the war itself led to hardship for both urban and rural Senegalese.[57] In the city, shortages, irregular employment, and rampant inflation were the rule, while in the countryside, peasants endured an extremely uncertain market in terms both of prices and of export demand.[58] Both exports and imports declined dramatically at the beginning of 1940 and did not begin to recover until 1944. Taking 1936 as an index of 100, imports and exports did not return to this level until 1950.[59]

The cost of shelter, food, and essential goods made Dakar an extremely expensive city. Shelter, estimated to cost roughly 50 percent of salaries, was the biggest contributor to the spiraling cost of living in wartime Dakar. A single room in a wooden shack could cost between 200 and 250 francs a month; poorer workers paid from 150 to 200 francs rent for a traditional straw hut.[60] The presence of the military would have made Dakar an expensive town even without the crisis caused by overpopulation and wartime shortages. Such a heavy concentration of military personnel meant a sharp increase in demand for imports, regardless of the cost of living, because the cost was being absorbed both by the colonial state and the Allies. Prohibitively costly for most were such American imports as rice, maize, and wheat. Despite French efforts at control such as the issuance of ration books and surveillance by an "economic police" force, a thriving black market flourished in the city.[61] Other French efforts involved encouraging the consumption of French West African-grown millet and maize after the authorities had cut the official rice ration by a half. Hunger spread, nevertheless, as the overall food supply for Dakar declined by at least 25 percent while the population was increasing.[62] Without the assistance of the Americans, who were the principal suppliers and paymasters for the city of Dakar and its hinterland in 1944, the French colonial government would not have been able to meet Senegal's food needs.[63]

PLAGUE CONTROL MEASURES

Overcrowded housing and wartime hardships added to the burden of the beleaguered French health authorities in 1944 when they were confronted with yet another outbreak of bubonic plague. Their response was to combine a mixture of old and new plague control techniques. From the official beginning of the emergency on 4 June until its official ending on 7 December, they imposed quarantine in lazarettos and a *cordon sanitaire* for Dakar and the Cape Verde peninsula.[64] Segregation continued to be the rule at the Cap Manuel lazaretto, to which only Europeans and *originaires* were admitted, and at a new lazaretto for African subjects, opened in July 1944, at the Front de Terre.[65] The Cape Manuel lazaretto was hardly a desirable address by 1944, but at least it was not overcrowded. In the interwar period it had been employed to lodge tuberculosis patients, lepers, and the mentally ill. During the course of the 1944 epidemic, Cap Manuel admitted only seventeen contacts, one European, one Syrian, and fifteen *originaires*. In contrast, admissions of Africans to the Rufisque and Front de Terre lazarettos totalled 3,738.

Controls on population movement continued with the issuance of vaccination cards as proof of anti-plague inoculation, which all noncitizens were obliged to show in order to pass through the *cordon sanitaire* separating Dakar from the interior. No less than 24,372 such passports were issued during the emergency. Each document indicated the time and place of the inoculation, and the traveler was required to give the destination, address, and duration of the visit.[66] A measure not introduced in earlier epidemics was the banning of assemblies and the closing of cafés and cinemas during the emergency.[67] Another innovation involved issuing new ration books only to those who could produce a valid anti-plague vaccination card.[68]

The second traditional control measure, cleansing by disinfection and burning, continued to be practiced. In 1944, the Health Service organized Dakar into seven sectors in an effort to clean up unsanitary pockets. Each sector was assigned a European chief with three or four teams made up of two African sanitary guards each to inspect all lands and buildings. Some 186 summonses were issued and the same number of slum sites destroyed during the 1944 epidemic.[69] Resettlement in the Médina was resurrected as a solution to the housing of displaced persons, and the allotments known as Mbopp came into being as a result. The chief medical officer claimed that Africans cooperated this time because the administration dismantled the original dwellings carefully and transported materials and other goods to the Médina, where a lot and title were issued to each owner.[70]

Burial of plague corpses continued to be tightly controlled, but officials did permit the immediate family of the deceased to accompany the body to the cemetery.[71] Wartime shortages contributed a macabre element to plague burials. Muslims preferred percale as a burial shroud for the deceased, but its scarcity caused the Muslim cemetery to be raided and corpses disinterred to obtain the precious percale. When any percale in the market showed signs that it had been in the earth, the authorities were able to apprehend and jail the offenders.[72]

The French medical authorities launched a vaccination campaign as soon as the first cases appeared. They used a live E.V. vaccine prepared by the Pasteur Institute of Dakar from a sample from Madagascar of the vaccine which had been used in 1943 during the small-scale epidemic there.[73] Undoubtedly a vast improvement over the older anti-plague vaccine, this Girard-Robic vaccine had the backing of the French medical community. In contrast to 1914, the French expatriate community participated actively in the immunization campaign, even if vaccination remained voluntary for them, and even if old fears died hard. As one European physician remarked to Maurice Maillat, a French railroad employee, "I have no problems with the yellow fever vaccine. I risk absolutely nothing, but I would not take the anti-plague [vaccine], not for all the world."[74]

Still, medical officials estimated that 90 percent of the total Dakar population of 167,946 (153,078 Africans and 14,868 Europeans) did receive the Girard-Robic vaccination.[75] The PID noted that only one case of plague developed among 149 people who had been vaccinated at least three weeks before coming in contact with plague, giving a case rate of 1.05 per 1,000. In contrast, among the non-vaccinated population and those injected less than three weeks earlier, an estimated population of 15,000, there were 403 cases, or 27 cases per 1,000. The PID concluded triumphantly that the Girard-Robic vaccine offered 25 times more protection than the older vaccine. Clearly the new vaccine did seem to offer considerable benefits, but this was not a scientific trial. R. N. Hunter in Kenya years earlier had made the important point that plague vaccinations which were given after an epidemic manifested itself, when it was already on a natural downswing, were not a true indicator of protection.[76]

Not surprisingly, since they rarely agreed with the French on medical procedures against plague, the Americans did not have confidence in the French vaccine.[77] As early as June 1943, because Senegal was known to be a region of endemic plague, all American military personnel, without exception, were vaccinated before arrival, not with the Girard-Robic preparation but with their own U.S. Army plague vaccine.[78] The Americans found that the French vaccine had significant side effects: pain, swelling, redness at the site, and fever as high as 104 degrees Fahrenheit. Reactions to the U.S. vaccine were said to have been much milder.[79]

If vaccination was deemed a controversial but necessary control measure, what distinguished the 1944 Dakar epidemic from all previous ones was the application of new biochemical products both for plague therapy and for vector control. Once again, French and American opinions varied. In 1944, French physicians chose to treat plague cases with a combination of old and new drug therapies. At the Cap Manuel lazaretto, they employed an anti-plague serum dosage of 200 to 450 cc. per patient. When the serum supply began to run short, the physicians switched partially or totally to two sulfa drugs, Sulfathiazole and Sulfadiazine.[80] Of the 133 cases (with 86 deaths) of Africans treated at the Hôpital Indigène, only 12 received the serum because it was in such short supply; the rest were given bacteriophage and sulfa drugs in combination.[81] French health officials in Dakar lamented their lack of supplies, especially of anti-plague serum, only a small quantity of which they were able to borrow from the Pasteur Institute of Morocco. They hoped in the future to experiment with penicillin, which had been ordered by the Americans, but which, they alleged, had proved to have had little effect on *Y. pestis*.[82]

American sources were silent on the use of penicillin for African plague patients, and it seems safe to assume that antibiotics were not used as part of plague therapy in Senegal in 1944.[83] Perhaps the new wonder drugs did not arrive in time. Perhaps they were not yet recognized as the wonder drugs they would soon become against most bacterial infections, including *Y. pestis*.[84] Instead, the Americans in Dakar in 1944 believed that sulfa therapy was the best therapy available, provided that their high-dose therapy, and not the combined sulfa-bacteriophage regime favored by the French, was prescribed.[85]

During the interwar period, vector control against rodents had evolved considerably in all parts of the world, and Dakar was no exception. Port officials there had tightened regulations, and required a gap of one meter between ship and dock, the raising of all gangplanks, and the use of rat shields on all hawsers. The press of wartime shipping, however, led to a relaxation of these regulations.[86] After the plague outbreak of 1934, French control measures against rats were stepped up. The rats were caught in traps, gassed with sulphur dioxide in burrows, and poisoned with chloropicrin in large sewers. Such measures continued until 1938, by which time the plague had not recurred. Arguing that the rat population was now relatively small, the French ended their control program.[87] By the beginning of the war, the rat population had recovered, but labor and materials were not available to carry out the same control program. During the 1944 outbreak, some 10,500 rats were caught, of which 3,501 were examined at the PID, where 65 were found to be infected with plague.[88]

As with vaccines, the Americans took a different approach to vector control from the French. The U.S. surgeon general sent in a rodent control officer, Captain Milton Buehler, to address the rodent problem in and around the American installations and to assist local authorities. Buehler's investigations showed that practically none of the buildings in Dakar were rat proof, and that there was an abundance of food for rodents to consume. Many warehouses contained foodstuffs; garbage was routinely thrown into the streets, and residents stored food at home in gourds, open cans, and boxes. Furthermore, a great many rats were found in traditional homes. On the other hand, very few rats were found within U.S. installations, and these had usually migrated from adjacent French or Senegalese property. Each U.S. organization had a sanitary technician who regularly trapped or poisoned with barium carbonate all rats within the area.

The Americans requested permission from their French hosts to conduct a general rat control campaign in Dakar. The French objected on the valid ground that killing rats in plague season might drive fleas to humans and increase plague incidence. When the Americans persisted in their request, the French agreed only for those areas where no plague cases had occurred and no infected rats had been found. The Americans employed Antu, a new rodenticide imported from the U.S.A., but the results proved disappointing. Although the pesticide was not toxic to all species of rats, it was lethal to dogs, cats, and possibly small children, and for these reasons, the program was stopped.

The truly revolutionary control measure of 1944 was the application of DDT, a new insecticide, against fleas. As with rat control, the French initially brushed aside the Americans' offer to assist in flea control. But after several demonstrations in June that DDT dust could be a significant instrument in the reduction of the flea population, Dr. Cheneveau, chief of the Dakar Health Service, gave his approval. He singled out the work of an American entomologist, Captain Dunn, who applied DDT against malaria-bearing mosquitoes, and of Lieutenant. T. Roy Young of the U.S. Navy, "with whom we enjoy both technical and friendly relations," who supervised the spraying of plague-bearing fleas in the Médina. Cheneveau added that the Médina's inhabitants were not initially cooperative, but quickly changed their minds after they had observed the immediate impact of DDT on insects.[89]

If the French medical officials were supportive of American offers of assistance, the Free French colonial administrators and the private sector were not. Early in January 1944, entomologists who were members of the large American medical contingent had conducted a malarial survey of the Yoff area, where their new airport was to be built.[90] The French protested that the American survey was "unauthorized." When it turned out that a French medical official in the Health Service had granted

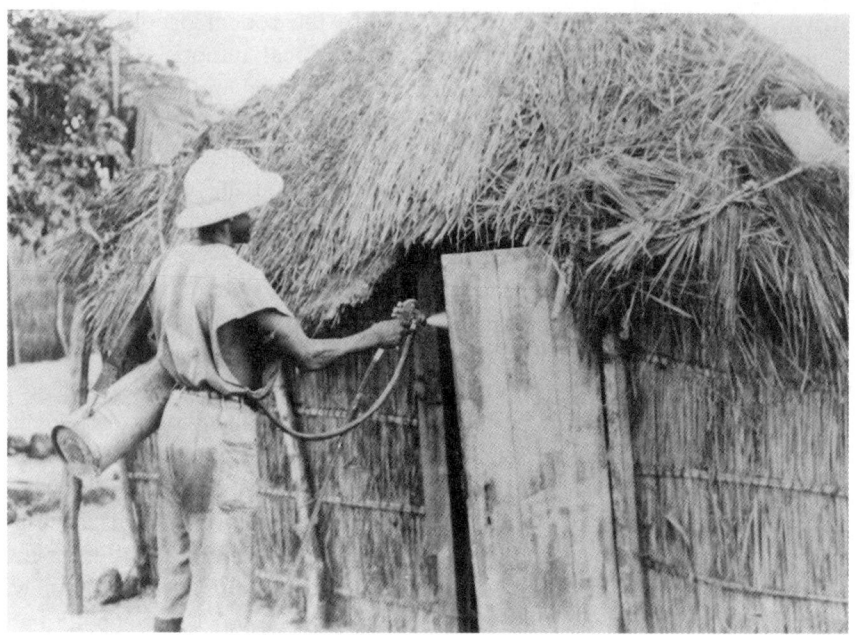

Photo 10.1 Crew Member Dusting a Médina Dwelling with DDT Powder, 1944. Courtesy of the family of the late Milton H. Buehler. All rights reserved.

approval, the French civilian government protested formally to the head of the American Mission that the medical official had no right to do so.[91] Subsequent offers by the Americans to help with the malaria survey were refused, and Young concluded that "malaria was not important to them" despite the American survey showing that of 1,000 schoolchildren in the Médina, 850 were infected with malaria. The indifference revealed by higher civilian officials, in contrast to the attitude of members of the Health Service who were "actively responsible for public health measures," was inexcusable, in Young's view.[92] Young and his fellow health officers persisted, and finally persuaded French officials that they were sincerely "trying to help rather than trying to take over [the French] colony." In June, the Americans proposed a cooperative program to treat plague areas with the new insecticide, DDT. French citizens wrote to their Health Service protesting against American dusting of their homes in infected areas. An article appeared in the local newspaper ridiculing the American efforts. Although the French medical personnel argued that the opposition came only from "cranks," in June

The Dakar Plague Epidemic of 1944

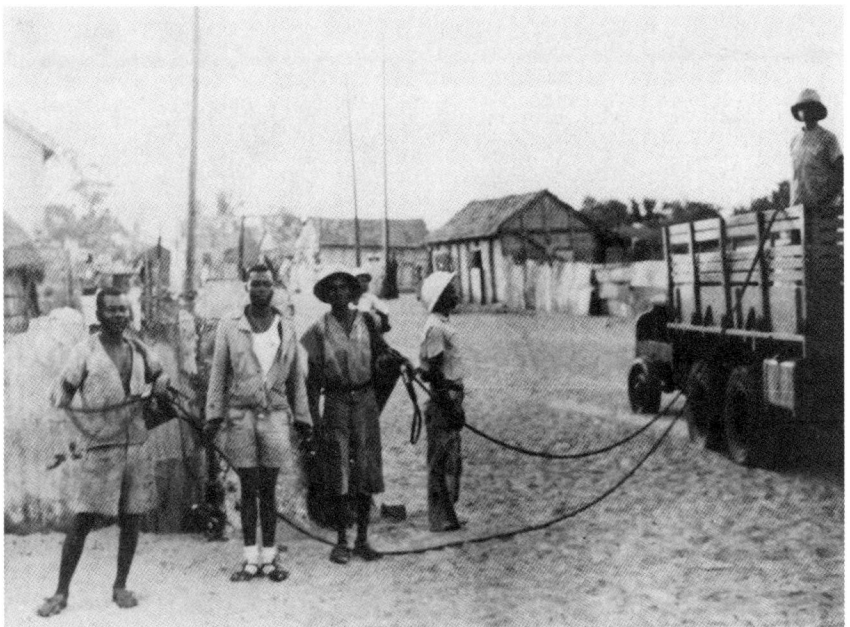

Photo 10.2 African Crew Members Preparing for DDT Dusting, Dakar Médina, 1944. Courtesy of the family of the late Milton H. Buehler. All rights reserved.

the Americans halted their DDT dusting program and declared that they would only resume it if French civil authorities made an official request. On 11 July, Young reported, the governor-general of French West Africa complied.[93]

DDT had been introduced to West Africa by the medical branch of the U.S. armed forces in the spring of 1944 as a means of controlling malaria, not bubonic plague. Malaria was recognized as far and away the greatest cause of lost man hours, and the U.S. Army had established military hospitals at Dakar, Accra (Ghana), and Robertsfield (Liberia), largely to treat malaria victims. The impact of DDT on *Anopheles gambiae*, the mosquito vector for falciparum malaria, was dramatic. By the close of 1944, malaria rates for army personnel at Dakar and Accra had been reduced to the lowest level ever known at these stations.[94] While the DDT program was extended in Dakar to include the plague emergency, it continued in 1945 against malaria, as well as against other insect borne diseases such as sleeping sickness, yellow fever, and filariasis.[95]

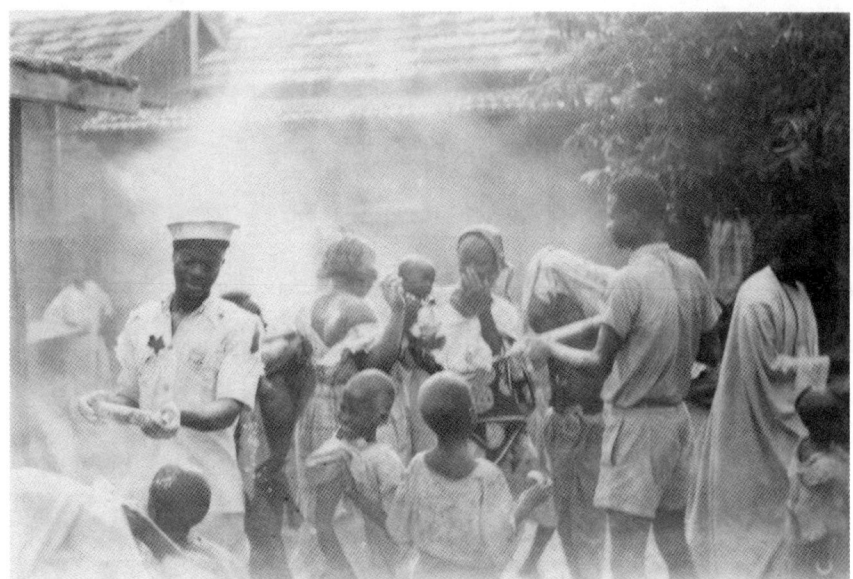

Photo 10.3 African Crew Members Dusting Women and Children, Dakar Médina, 1944. The DDT powder can be observed as a white cloud in the background. Courtesy of the family of the late Milton H. Buehler. All rights reserved.

The dusting of Dakar with DDT did not proceed without a political struggle. The Americans insisted on the need for a compulsory and complete dusting program. Beginning in June, they repeatedly requested, and were as often refused, permission to dust the mainly European residential areas of the Plateau. Finally, on 8 September, the Americans withdrew their dusting crews entirely, arguing that DDT use on a restricted scale was ineffective unless "a comprehensive [and] complete dusting program was approved."[96] For almost two months a stalemate persisted, partly because the French wanted to combine dusting with a mass inoculation project, to be delayed until December–January so that anti-plague protection would extend to the next year's plague season. After a further delay, the French finally agreed to proceed with the original plan and to let inoculation wait. The American compulsory dusting program for the Médina began on 24 October and ended on 10 November; the week after that, areas outside the Médina were included, so that the only area not dusted was the exclusively European district 7, south the of Avenue de la République. While dusting was made compulsory in

The Dakar Plague Epidemic of 1944 231

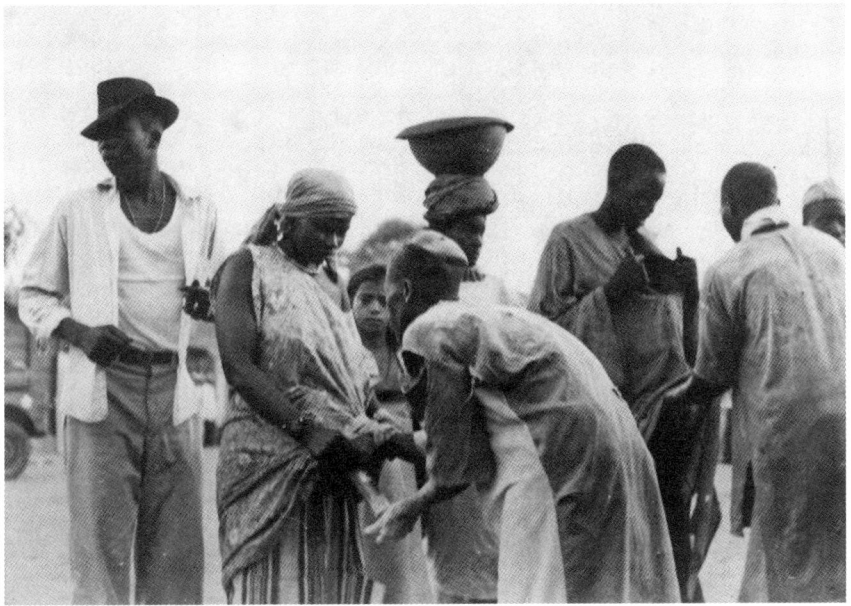

Photo 10.4 Women and Men Being Dusted with DDT, Dakar Médina, 1944. Courtesy of the family of the late Milton H. Buehler. All rights reserved.

all of the African sectors of Dakar, elsewhere it was only permitted on a voluntary basis.

The homes of Africans proved to be heavily flea-infested. Tests showed that DDT eliminated all fleas present and established a lethal barrier for varying periods ranging from one week to several weeks. The variables included the dosage and the amount of traffic in and out of the sand-floored houses. Although French authorities were delighted with the results, the Americans, in the absence of any scientific evidence of the effects of dusting, remained puzzled as to why some people died of plague in houses which had been dusted and sprayed on three occasions, and in which the flea population had been entirely destroyed. They concluded that human contacts had already been established in untreated areas, that some people were already incubating the disease, and that in fact the dusting team lagged behind the plague frontier by several days.

Just like earlier control efforts, the American DDT campaign of 1944 was coercive. Not only was it compulsory for Africans, although voluntary for Europeans, but some 200 to 300 gendarmes supplied by the

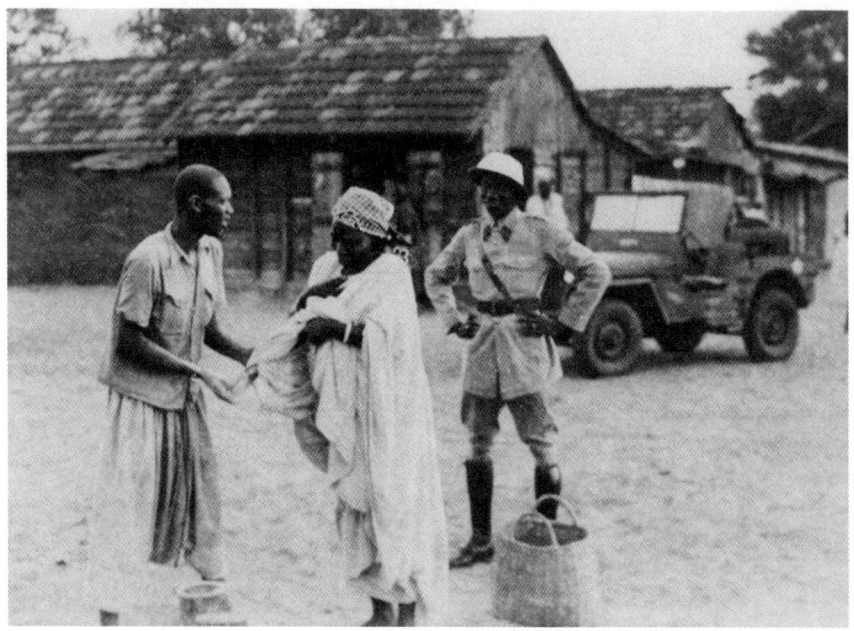

Photo 10.5 Woman Being Dusted with DDT Powder under the Watchful Eye of a Policeman, Dakar Médina, 1944. Courtesy of the family of the late Milton H. Buehler. All rights reserved.

French roped off each district to be treated. The district was selected the night before operations were to begin, in order to prevent any information being leaked to those wishing to avoid the dusting. The military *cordon* was put into place at 05:00 hours, and four or five outlet stations were established to release those Africans required to work outside the zone. Three or four African workers carried out the dusting using a small Hudson Plunger-type duster. The gendarmes lined up the subjects to be dusted; dusting began at the ankles, under varying layers of clothing, then continued to the waist, front and rear, then to the sleeves and neck, and finally to the hair. Roughly 9 grams of 10 percent DDT powder were used per person. Within the zone, an inner *cordon* isolated individual blocks, where house-by-house crews dusted floors, lower walls, and beds for fleas. The Americans estimated that as few as 5 percent of the African population of Dakar avoided these rigorous procedures, when "occasional misunderstanding by the gendarmes" allowed some to escape.[97] In all, an estimated 125,000 people were dusted. As a further safeguard for U.S. personnel, all public places likely to be frequented by Americans—cafés, restaurants, bars, brothels, and cinemas—were sprayed with a 5 percent DDT solution.

The Americans were pleased with the test results and the cooperation they received from Dakar residents. They observed that people "welcomed the treatment as a major contribution to their comfort and have usually called attention to any house that the dusting crews overlooked." Of 1,643 houses examined, only 33 or 2 percent had live fleas seven to eight weeks after the spraying. Of course, by then the flea season (and the plague season) was over and the Americans could not state whether DDT dusting had halted the plague or whether seasonal die-out had been involved.[98] Later research convinced them that DDT's effectiveness was virtually 100 percent against rat fleas, of both the *Synosternus pallidus* and *Xenopsylla cheopis* varieties.[99]

THE AMERICAN MEDICAL PRESENCE IN DAKAR

The American medical presence in Dakar represented the single most important new variable in public health since the medical reforms of the early 1920s. American medical preoccupations in West Africa were focused, with good reason, on malaria. That is not to say that bubonic plague was taken lightly. The Americans were well aware of the reputation of Dakar and its hinterland as a locus of endemic plague. During the 1943 epidemic in Senegal, for example, American consular reports monitored plague events closely.[100] Consul Barnes reported on the initial 1943 outbreak in the Tivaouane area, noting that while the plague never spread east of the rail line or north of Louga, it did advance toward the capital, penetrating the French *cordon sanitaire* and crossing into the Dakar region where a total of thirty-five cases and at least seventeen deaths occurred during the months of June and July. In replies by telegram from the State Department, the consulate was ordered to keep Washington "fully informed."[101] In January 1944, the new consul, John Goodyear, felt able to report that the 1943 plague epidemic had "definitely subsided" by December, leaving the clear implication that another season would see a recurrence of this scourge.[102]

The American attitude in 1944 turned rather quickly to concern, although in May, Barnes could telegraph the State Department that there had been six plague cases in April, but none since the first of May, so the French Health Service was relaxing its plague emergency measures. Barnes, like the French, while promising to continue to inform the State Department of developments, remained confident that "American Army and Navy physicians at this station have kept in touch with French medical authorities and are favorably impressed with the measures adopted."[103]

Beneath the surface of the polite dispatches, much more was going on between the French and the Americans than Washington was being told at the time. What makes this clear is an undated handwritten letter, probably composed in strict confidence around December 1944, by Lieutenant Roy Young, to provide background to the long report that he, Buehler, and Lewis had submitted.[104] Young made it clear at the outset that tensions were running high. "When I arrived in March of 1944 and contacted the French Health Authorities I found a definitely strained atmosphere between the French and the Americans. Many of the French officials were openly antagonistic and suspicious of our motives and aims in French West Africa."[105]

French resentment included not only the alleged "colonial" aims of the U.S.A., but also the abundance of their supplies and equipment, and the lack of finesse in their general behavior. When the American health specialists made their first offer to aid in malaria control, the variety of responses ranged from "mild lack of interest to intense antagonism." But Young did conclude on a less pessimistic note. As a result of the Americans' tactful behavior, this anti-American feeling had been "dissipated"; Young could now report in December 1944 that they were on "very friendly grounds" with the French medical people, and that "the civil authorities have written [sic] their appreciation of our work." Since the French were now grateful for all the U.S. aid and supplies they could receive, he asked that his remarks be kept confidential, and said that as the official report indicated, all was well that ended well.[106]

If Lieutenant Young had been disappointed by the reluctance of the French to accept American offers to help control malaria, his frustration only grew when the French adopted the same posture concerning bubonic plague:

> All our offers were summarily brushed aside, with the remark that the French were capable of handling their own problems and anyway, that plague was of no real concern, being merely a disease of natives. Pressure and ridicule were brought to bear on the American Consul General by the ranking French officials for us to stop meddling in their affairs, and as a result the American Consul General forbid [sic] us to enter into a control program.[107]

Meanwhile, within their own military installations, the Americans had no need to request French permission to introduce control measures. Indeed, they began anti-plague measures well before the official medical emergency was declared on 4 June.[108] On 6 May, they declared the entire waterfront "out of bounds" to American military and naval personnel with the exception only of those on indispensable business. All shore leave was canceled. Personnel entering the water front area were required to wear "protective clothing" consisting of leggings or mosquito boots, long trousers, and long-sleeved shirts, and to dust their clothing with an insect repellent, a powder with the brand name of Rotenone.

After 4 June, American medical officers extended their self-imposed *cordon* when they declared the entire city of Dakar off-limits not only to the U.S. Army and the merchant marine, but also to those they referred to as "contract-carrier people," that is, employees of American firms such as Socony-Vacuum Oil Company, Pan American Airlines, and American Export. On 7 June, Consul Barnes warned a company executive by telegram that civilians should think twice about sending their dependents to Dakar.[109] All Africans employed by Americans were either laid off or given plague vaccinations and obliged to dust their clothes and homes with 10 percent DDT powder. At the air base, for example, all Senegalese employees were laid off, and all work such as cooking, laundry, and guard duty was performed by soldiers, sailors, and airmen themselves.[110] Later, a camp was set up for those Senegalese willing to work at the American bases. They were confined to the bases, and all sanitation was strictly enforced by the army. Africans working at the U.S. Army station hospital were required to bathe and change clothes before work; in August, as the epidemic crested, Senegalese employees were quartered in and restricted to tents on the hospital compound. The homes and offices of all American personnel, including those leased to the State Department and the various contract companies, were treated with DDT. On 7 June, the U.S. naval air facility abandoned its quarters in Dakar and moved to the new army air base at the airstrip at Yoff, some 10 kilometers from the city.[111] When a case of plague developed ten days later next to the U.S. naval air facility at Bel-Air, the Americans closed this particular base and suspended the movement of U.S. naval aircraft through Dakar until 12 July, by which time it was felt that Bel-Air was again safe.[112] All other American emergency measures remained in effect until 4 December 1944.

French and American officials saw the Dakar plague epidemic of 1944 through their own particular lenses. Free French officials, if not the French medical community, were much more concerned about saving face than tackling what they had come to see as "merely a disease of natives." Obstructing the Americans at every turn, the Free French had become inured to the presence of plague in their colonies, did not regard it as a serious threat, and saw the American concern as alarmist in the extreme.

One particular incident in 1944 perhaps helps explain French frustration, and to a degree justifies their sensitivity, over their own dependent position. In June, the Navy Bureau of Medicine and Surgery in Washington requested permission from the governor-general of FWA to shoot an instructional film on plague control in Dakar. At a time when they were short of everything from uniforms to basic foodstuffs, the Free French must have viewed the request as the worst sort of conspicuous extravagance. Also contributing to the French attitude was the sense of embarrassment and indignity the French felt over their shoddy equipment and the shabbiness of large parts of their overcrowded African imperial capital. According to Young, initially, the chief of the French Health Service gave his enthusiastic support to the film project. But when the film crew arrived on 24 July, the general attitude had changed, and it seemed very questionable whether Americans should be allowed to photograph sanitary conditions in Dakar. As a compromise, it was agreed that the filming would proceed, but only under the direct supervision of a French colonel who had to be present at all times. He in turn told the Americans he could only spare thirty minutes a day for this activity. But the Americans persisted and "won him over."[113] The filming was completed with dispatch, but with no scenes allowed "which might reflect upon the colonial government." For example, filming the French improvisation of using garden sprinkling cans to spray disinfecting solution was not permitted.[114]

It can also be argued that, although they were more solicitous of Africans' health and their sufferings from plague, the Americans were also stern paternalists. They coerced their African employees to do their medical bidding on pain of dismissal, and they ruthlessly punished petty transgressions and crimes.

On balance, however, Free French *amour propre* failed to take into consideration the larger context in which the Americans were operating in 1944. American medical concerns about malaria and bubonic plague were linked to strategic issues. West Africa was an important link in the chain of air and sea traffic between North America and the Mediterranean theater of operations. Indeed, a few cases of plague did break out in Naples soon after the Dakar epidemic began; whether there was a connection cannot be determined but local opinion certainly believed there was. It was said that the American Medical Services, which had followed the plague very closely, succeeded in limiting the damage caused by plague in the Italian port.[115] But the occurrence of plague in Naples helps explain the very real concerns of the day. Once again a conjunction of war and plague can be seen to have been operating in the history of public health in Senegal.

RESPONSES TO THE 1944 EPIDEMIC

Resistance to plague control measures in 1944 was a pale imitation of the angry protest which had occurred some thirty years before. While some evidence of the public's continuing reluctance to cooperate with health officials does filter through the otherwise uninformative medical reports, no street demonstrations occurred, and, more notably, no confrontations with police or the military. While it is usually unwise to speculate on why historical events did not occur, two arguments can be advanced. First, the political context of the 1944 epidemic was vastly different from that of 1914. Second, after living through three decades of persistent intrusion by health officials, the population of Dakar and the plague zone in Senegal had come to accept plague control measures, like death and taxes, as an enduring feature of their lives.

In 1944, Senegalese political issues no longer centered on whether residents of the four communes were citizens, whether an African like Blaise Diagne could be elected deputy, or whether the Lebu had title to Dakar real estate. Instead, wartime politics turned on the restoration of African electoral rights which had been suspended by Vichy and on an nonarticulated desire for reform leading to equality with France once the war was ended. Although there were a variety of opinions, ranging from the conservative Islamic modernism of Abdel-Kader Diagne and his reformist group, "Fraternité Musulmane," to the radical claims for autonomy if not full independence advocated by Pierre Diagne or Amadou Ba, the two most important groupings were the Socialists under Lamine Guèye and a group of young Lebu militants centered around Thierno Amat Mbengue.[116]

Mbengue was the only Senegalese activist to make plague control measures a political issue. Calling his organization the "Young Lebu," Mbengue and his associates bombarded the Free French Administration with letters and complaints, with copies sent to the Allied missions in Dakar.[117] In addition to blaming the French administration for the shortages, inflation, and general immiseration brought on by the war, they also, in a manner eerily similar to 1914, held the municipality of Dakar responsible for a series of unpopular plague control measures: the forced removal of families from the center of town; the burning of goods and property; and the disrespect for Muslim burial practices. Some of the more militant Lebu, invoking the Atlantic Charter, went so far as to prepare a constitution for the "République du Cap-Vert," but autonomy or independence were never articulated as goals by Mbengue and his movement.[118]

A far more serious threat to the political *status quo* under the Free French came from Lamine Guèye and the Socialists.[119] Still on excellent terms with his French colleagues, Guèye, in October 1944, was preparing to run for mayor against Alfred Goux, a long-time Dakar businessman and amateur ethnologist.[120] French colonial reports of the day made it clear that they saw Guèye as the emerging successor to Blaise Diagne and Galandou Diouf as Senegal's political boss.[121] Elections were called for December 1944, but the tragedy of Thiaroye on 1 December, when French armed forces opened fire on a large contingent of demobilized veterans, intervened, and all elections were postponed until after the war's end.[122]

Deeply assimilationist, Lamine Guèye was even less likely than Blaise Diagne or Galandou Diouf before him to challenge the principles of Western biomedicine during a plague emergency. A doctor of law, a one-time circuit judge in the French Antilles, and political director since the mid 1930s of the Senegalese section of the French Socialist Party, the SFIO (Section Française de l'Internationale Ouvrière), Guèye strove for the full equality of the Senegalese before French Law. He would have been prepared to defend the rights of plague victims of the Dakar slums in court, but never on the streets.[123] He had defended the railroad strikers of 1938 in court, and did the same for the soldiers accused of mutiny in the Thiaroye affair, but he left it to his lieutenant, Léopold Sédar Senghor, to rub shoulders with the masses in the Médina of Dakar and in the countryside during the 1945 elections.[124] In short, while his socialist principles certainly called for a more humane colonialism leading to full integration within a larger French community, Guèye's commitment to Western and, specifically, to French culture was too strong for him ever to contemplate rejecting Western biomedicine and its methods, however imperfect, let alone leading resistance to plague control measures.

Of course, there were grievances against intrusive measures. Two of those which surfaced represented both continuity and change in the ongoing battle with bubonic plague, and help to illustrate how plague measures, and efforts to thwart them, had become a regular feature of Senegalese life. First, health officials continued to interfere with customary funeral and burial practices. Second, war shortages provided officials with the opportunity to link the distribution of ration books with proof from vaccination cards that individuals had received anti-plague injections. With regard to burial practices, the French health authorities did make a few concessions to African sensibilities. To avert clandestine burials, they permitted a few members of the bereaved family to accompany the truck taking the deceased to the cemetery.[125] Such small but symbolic gestures may explain the willingness of many to accept plague control measures as an ongoing aspect of their lives.

The ration book issue was another matter. In order to obtain compliance, the French linked vaccination to ration privileges. Old ration books were canceled in mid summer 1944 and new ones were issued only to those who could produce a certificate showing they had been vaccinated against plague. Of course, this did not prevent fraud, as some unscrupulous patrons sent their clients to several centers under assumed names to receive multiple vaccinations and as a result, multiple ration books. The ultimate result was more valuable products to sell on the black market.[126] Rumor had it that the *taalibé* of an unscrupulous *marabout* died of plague from these overdoses, as a result of which the *marabout* was imprisoned.[127]

The Levantine community protested against discriminatory control measures. One Syrian merchant wrote to complain that colonial officials unfairly required all "natives, Moroccans, Portuguese métis or Libano-Syrians," but not their French business competitors, to have an anti-plague vaccination card in order to obtain a new ration book or to travel from Dakar to the interior.[128] In a letter to the governor-general, the administrator of Dakar admitted that while no legislation linked the vaccination card to ration book distribution, he recommended that the practice be continued on the ground that it was leading to more people being immunized than would otherwise be the case.[129]

Another way of measuring response to the 1944 plague is to examine the role played by two of the medical researchers active at the time, the American medical officer Milton H. Buehler,[130] and the French microbiologist Georges Girard.

Buehler's role in the Dakar plague epidemic illustrates how rapidly and successfully the American military could bring its expertise to bear on the thorny public health problem of plague control. Before the war, Buehler had been an agent of the U.S. Fish and Wildlife Service, supervising some thirty men engaged in predatory animal and rodent control in Arizona. After graduating with a Bachelor of Science degree from the University of Arizona in 1941, Buehler became a commissioned officer in the U.S. Army, specializing in rodent control, early in 1942. He spent the next thirty-three months at military camps in California as sanitary control officer in charge of water purification, sewage disposal, mess sanitation, and insect and rodent control. In late August 1944, he received orders to report to Dakar, for temporary duty as an insect and rodent control specialist. From September to late December, Buehler was in Dakar supervising a crew of forty men assigned to dust people and houses with DDT. It was the first time bubonic plague had been controlled in this manner. Buehler also conducted field tests on the use of the rodenticide Antu. Buehler ended the war on six months' special assignment in Manila, where he supervised rodent control activities in the harbor area, and where he commanded the 211th Malaria Survey Detachment. Upon his discharge, Buehler was able to build a successful civilian career based upon his wartime assignments.[131]

Georges Girard had been director of plague research at the Pasteur Institute in Madagascar for over a decade. Together with Robic, he had developed the institute's live anti-plague E.V. vaccine, a much improved version of earlier preparations.[132] Based in Paris in 1944, Girard was ordered urgently to proceed to Dakar on 9 December 1994, to study the way in which the 1944 plague control campaign had been organized, and to make recommendations for future campaigns.[133] The historical record of the 1944 plague epidemic is greatly enhanced by his candid and detailed twenty-one-page assessment.[134] Arriving by plane in Dakar on 13 December, Girard spent six weeks in Senegal, mostly in Dakar, but also, in January 1945, paying a visit to the Mboro area where a few cases of plague flared up after the official emergency was over. He departed for Paris on 22 January 1945.[135]

An eminent specialist with no ties to the Dakar research community, Georges Girard was sometimes devastating in his criticisms. He left little doubt that he considered not only the Colonial Health Service but also the Dakar branch of the Pasteur Institute sorely wanting. He wrote:

> In examining the literature regarding plague in Dakar and in Senegal, the impression was given that the research followed no overall plan and was conducted by authors following their own personal tendencies. Superficial observations led to premature conclusions and original hypotheses were never confirmed. The rat was incriminated as the principal source of the infection, then it was man who was so labeled; the notion of healthy carriers was even accepted without discussion and cited in modern works as a classic given, even while these carriers were never found in any country, let alone Senegal. On the subject of fleas, researchers entirely ignored where the domain of *Synosternus pallidus* began and ended.[136]

Girard also noted that major research questions were rarely raised, and promising leads were not followed up. Why was it that plague followed the railway north but rarely east and never south? Why did plague never reach other colonies linked to Senegal by the railway? Could it be linked to the species of fleas found elsewhere? Only by understanding the flea population in a region would researchers begin to solve these problems.[137] With his fresh perspective, Girard argued that the sand and dirt found in the African dwellings of the Senegal coast, Dakar included, provided an excellent environment for fleas. Likewise, the numerous grain and peanut silos were excellent breeding grounds for fleas.

Yet another problem centered on the relationship that should have existed, but did not, between the Pasteur Institute and the Colonial Health Service. The colonial archives and records Girard examined suggested that the two units worked completely independently of each other. The Health Service generally waited far too long to call in the PID for assistance in plague diagnosis. Under the circumstances, and considering the fact that plague had been absent from Dakar for seven years, Girard excused the PID and its director, M. Durieux, for having become concerned with more immediate problems.[138]

Not everything was hopeless, of course. Girard did concede that significant practical improvements in sanitation in Dakar had occurred since the early days. Citing the "magisterial" Heckenroth report as something that health workers should always keep before them, Girard noted how far Dakar had come. The greatest improvements were in the port area, where the "mountains" of peanuts standing on the quay which he had observed during his brief passage through Dakar in 1935 had disappeared. Instead, peanuts were now stored in large cement silos of "rat proof" construction in the North Zone of the port. Unfortunately, the Médina still remained a "collection of hovels," even more dangerous in 1944 because its population had quintupled in fifteen years.

While not free of bias against Africans, Girard blamed the health authorities rather than the victims. He understood correctly that rat extermination was impossible, and that the Médina would not quickly become sanitized. He argued that while his vaccine, along with DDT, offered new hope of breaking the chain of transmission of plague, these new products were not enough. Only a change of political will by the French government leading to new investment in modern housing would eradicate the scourge of bubonic plague.[139]

Girard's linkage of structural change to public health was new to Senegal in 1944. More typical of an older approach was the report on the 1944 epidemic by Dr. Charles Robin, a military physician who practiced at the Hôpital Indigène and also served as medical inspector of schools.[140] Believing that coercion in the cause of medical science was always justified, Robin also argued that while a few *évolués* might accept modern hygiene, the African masses "will always be loyal to their ancestral customs and their anti-hygienic practices." Therefore, only severe public health measures in the spirit of urbanist policy would work. Robin called for the expulsion of the entire "floating population" and the creation of a special police force whose duties would be to watch over the movements of population and to irradicate vagabondage. To assure a supply of cooks, servants, and laborers, "workers' camps" should be built, and closely supervised by health officials. While supporting the new vaccination and sulfa drug therapies, Robin was completely out of touch with the changing political climate of Senegal. He was, in fact, advocating a form of severe urban residential segregation that only the Union of South Africa applied on the African continent, for a country where the assimilationist African political elite bristled at the mere hint of formal racial discrimination.[141]

CONCLUSION

Much that happened in the 1944 plague epidemic evoked sharp memories of 1914. As Eric Silla found with regard to French medical approaches to leprosy in Mali, French medical policy toward bubonic plague in Senegal continued to be authoritarian, parsimonious, and insensitive to African health perspectives and needs.[142] Quarantine, *cordons*, lazarettos, compulsory vaccination and restriction on travel, undignified burial, even a resettlement scheme for the homeless—all these had become familiar hardships to be endured. Some elements, however, were new in 1944. The linkage of vaccination cards to ration books bespoke wartime scarcity and a rather devious route to securing compliance with the immunization program. Second, and more importantly, the American military and medical presence helped assure the application of a dramatic, and demonstrably effective, new insecticide, DDT. Neither the Africans who saw its immediate results on their flea-ridden dwellings nor the French and American medical officials realized it then, but DDT, by breaking the chain of transmission of bubonic plague, probably was responsible for its disappearance from Senegal after 1945.

What was also different about 1944 was the relatively mild and muted resistance to anti-plague control measures. True, Thierno Amat Mbengue and his radical "Young Lebu" followers did decry the intrusive and culturally disrespectful aspects of anti-plague control, and they added these grievances to more fundamental ones about wartime suffering and misrule. But while in 1914, the Lebu took to the streets with knives and sticks to defend their homes, thirty years later Mbengue and his small band confined their protests to a letter-writing campaign. The emerging African power broker, moreover, was not the fiery Mbengue but the strongly assimilationist Lamine

Guèye, a man committed by temperament and training to Western legal and medical ideology.

Important though these differences were, a better explanation for the resigned nature of the Dakarois response to plague control in 1944 can be suggested. It is that bubonic plague, and the largely futile French control measures that accompanied it, had become a painful fact of life, to be endured in the same manner as drought, malaria, rule by foreigners, and wartime hardships. One French administrator put it well when he observed near the end of the war that "what preoccupied the [African] masses are the material difficulties of existence inherent in the colonial situation."[143]

NOTES

1. The best account of the Vichy interlude is James L. Giblin, "The Vichy Years in French Africa: A Period of African Resistance to Capitalism" (master's dissertation, McGill University, Montreal, 1978); see also Catherine Akpo-Vaché, *L'AOF et la Seconde Guerre mondiale (septembre 1939–octobre 1945)* (Paris: Karthala, 1996). Gaullists and their opponents, whether they viewed Boisson as a traitor or as a French patriot trying to preserve the empire from both the Germans and the British, agree that Boisson kept a tight hold on FWA during his term of office. See *Réveil* (Dakar), 3 November 1944, in "L'héritage Boisson"; Maurice Martin du Gard, *La carte impériale: Histoire de la France Outre-Mer, 1940–45* (Paris: A. Bonne, 1949), 138; Jean Suret-Canale, *French Colonialism in Tropical Africa, 1900–1945*, translated by Till Gottheiner (London: C. Hurst and Co., 1971); and William Cohen, *Rulers of Empire: The French Colonial Service in Africa* (Stanford, Calif.: Hoover Institution, 1971), 159.

2. The threat that Dakar might become a submarine and air base for the Germans had prompted Churchill to agree, with Free French and Polish troops aboard British ships, to attempt to seize the port. Plans went as far back as July 1940. In August the British cabinet approved the mission, and the expedition arrived off Dakar on 23 September. But the resistance was firm, the mission was impossible, and the force was recalled after two days. Winston S. Churchill, *Their Finest Hour*, vol. 2 (Boston: Houghton Mifflin, 1949), chapter 9; Giblin, "Vichy Years," 36–37.

3. Giblin, "Vichy Years," 236.

4. Giblin, "Vichy Years," 237, quoting from U.S. Department of State, Serial File 85lt. 01/70.

5. Roosevelt had long believed that Dakar was of strategic concern to the United States. In a radio address on 27 May 1941, before the Americans entered the war, he had pointed out that Dakar was only 1,700 miles from the bulge of Brazil, and "less than [the distance] from Washington to Denver—five hours for the latest type of bomber." Dakar in hostile hands would bring the war "very close to home." Cited in Milton Viorst, *Hostile Allies: FDR and Charles de Gaulle* (New York: Macmillan, 1965), 62.

6. Herbert Feis, *Churchill, Roosevelt, Stalin* (Princeton, N.J.: Princeton University Press, 1957), 121.

7. Giblin, "Vichy Years," 238, quoting from U.S. Department of State, Record Group 218, no. 334, Joint Chiefs of Staff Meeting, 15 November 1943, held to plan the Teheran Conference, 123–38. Later, in conversation with Stalin at Teheran, Roosevelt stated that the Soviet leader had agreed that "the French must pay for their criminal collaboration with Germany" by losing their colonies. Not wanting to establish a precedent for the reapportioning of colonial possessions, Eden expressed the more nuanced British view that French bases might stay under U.N. control, but some form of French sovereignty would continue. Giblin, "Vichy Years," 240, citing "Memorandum of Conversation, Evening, November 28, 1943," and "Memorandum of Marshall Stalin's Views, as Expressed during the Evening of November 28, 1943," in U.S. Department of State, Records of Harley A. Notter, 1939–1945, "Minutes of Meetings of President Roosevelt, Marshall Stalin and Prime Minister Churchill (November 28–December 1, 1943)."

8. Giblin, "Vichy Years," 240, referring to U.S. Department of State, Serial File 8515.00/108.

9. It is important to note that in 1944, as the Axis powers were thrown on the defensive, American interest in FWA waned, as its strategic importance diminished. The U.S.A. no longer saw FWA as an issue for which it was worth alienating the French and the British. Gaddis Smith, *American Diplomacy during the Second World War, 1941–1945* (New York: Wiley, 1965), 94. It was also the case that Roosevelt was not unequivocally liberationist. He observed paternalistically that "for a time at least there are many minor children among the peoples of the world who need trustees." Smith, *American Diplomacy*, 83.

10. Charles M. Wiltse, *United States Army in World War II. The Technical Services. The Medical Department: Medical Service in the Mediterranean and Minor Theaters* (Washington, D.C.: Office of the Chief of Medical History, Department of the Army, 1945), 66, 76–78. For the U.S./French protocol allowing the Americans to build the new airport at Yoff, see Archives of the United States Department of State, Washington, D.C. RG84, Foreign Service Posts of the Department of State, 1936–54. Senegal: Dakar Consulate General. Security-Segregated General Records, 1940–44. 1944, Box 2 (hereafter cited as RG84, Foreign Service Posts), Consul Maynard B. Barnes to Admiral William Glassford, Dakar to Washington, 26 May 1944. Barnes was evasive about the real reasons for abandoning Bargny, and would only remark that the old site was "no longer adequate."

The Yoff airfield was built by Pan American Airways, under U.S. government contract, with runways suitable for heavy bombers. An American geographer, Derwent Whittlesey, observed that the airfields displaced most of the fields of millet and vegetables that had supplied the local fishing communities and provided some surplus for Dakar. This led to a need for more imports at a time when the European population of Dakar had increased by 50 percent and the total population by nearly that much. Derwent Whittlesey, "Dakar Revisited," *Geographical Review* 38 (1948): 626.

11. ANS\2G43\15, Dakar, Annual Report on Health for 1943, no author or date listed.

12. The two French medical sources for the plague of 1944 were ANS\2G44\11, Dakar, Annual Report on Health for 1944, Dr. Jardon, 3 vols., 16 August 1945

(hereafter, Jardon Report for 1944); and ANS\1H79\163. Mission Report by Dr. Girard, Head of the Plague Service of the Pasteur Institute, Paris, "Peste à Dakar en 1944," 21 pp. + 3 attached, Paris, 6 March 1945 (hereafter, Girard Report). We also have a lengthy private report filed by U.S. Army physicians Major Paul M. Lewis, A.U.S., Captain Milton H. Buehler, Jr., A.U.S., and Lieutenant T. Roy Young, U.S.N.R., "A Report on Plague in Dakar, Senegal, F.W.A., 1944." 43 pp., graphs, 2 large maps and photographs, in U.S. Army Military History Institute, Carlisle, Pa., filed as Professional Papers, Box no. 68 (hereafter cited as Lewis, Buehler, and Young ms.).

13. An examination of the sailors' barracks revealed the presence of an abundance of rats. Girard Report. For speculation on the origins of the 1944 Dakar outbreak, see also Denise Bouche, "Dakar pendant la Seconde Guerre mondiale. Problèmes de surpeuplement," in *Le sol, la parole et l'écrit: Mélanges en hommage à Raymond Mauny*, vol. 2 (Paris: SFHOM et L'Harmattan, 1981), 971; and Adrien Ndiouga Benga, "L'évolution politique de la ville de Dakar de 1924 à 1960" (mémoire de maitrîse, Université Cheikh Anta Diop, Dakar, 1989), 109.

14. Jardon Report for 1944.

15. Lewis, Buehler, and Young ms.; Maurice Maillat, "Dakar sous la flamme de guerre" (ANS, unpublished memoirs of a former employee of the Chemin de Fer, no date, probably post 1968, 16 pages); hereafter cited as as Maillat, "La flamme."

16. Lewis, Buehler, and Young ms.

17. Jardon Report for 1944, but also Girard Report for number of cases at the station.

18. Lewis, Buehler, and Young ms.

19. RG84, Foreign Service Posts, Barnes to State Department, 19 June 1944.

20. Bouche, "Dakar," 971.

21. Lewis, Buehler, and Young ms.

22. ANS\1H1\1, Medical Inspector-General Ricou, General Director of Public Health for FWA, "Actualités épidémiologiques en Afrique occidentale française," for the Comité d'Hygiène et d'Épidémiologie de l'Empire, Session d'Octobre, 1944, Algiers (hereafter cited as Ricou Report).

23. Bouche, "Dakar," 971. Assane Seck, *Dakar, métropole ouest-africaine* (Dakar: IFAN, 1970), 115.

24. Ricou Report.

25. ANS\2G44\11, Senegal, Annual Report on Health for 1944, Dr. Tisseuil, Saint-Louis, 15 March 1945 (hereafter cited as Tisseuil Report for 1944).

26. Tisseuil Report for 1944.

27. Tisseuil Report for 1944. Unfortunately, none of the victims was ever identified by name in this report.

28. Of the 127, 91, or 72 percent were males. Lewis, Buehler, and Young ms. So little statistical information is supplied by the French that we need the American report to supplement findings regarding patients at the two hospitals. The gendered rate of hospitalization which favored males was probably significant.

A second question is the segregation by citizenship associated with hospital treatment. Of the seventeen treated in the French hospital, no less than sixteen were males in their thirties, fifteen were Africans, one a European, and one a Syrian. All these were males in their twenties; the lone woman was in her fifties. Ten bubonic cases were treated and all but one lived. Seven deaths resulted from the seven septicemic cases, so called. Some data of a statistical nature are also to be found in the Ricou Report.

29. Girard Report. Girard noted that for those patients admitted to the Dakar hospitals, the death rate was 63 percent.

30. It should be recognized that population figures during the war are estimates only, as no census was taken. I agree with Frederick Cooper that the figures (in Tables 10.2 and 10.3) have to be used very cautiously. See Frederick Cooper, *Decolonization and African Society: The Labor Question in French and British Africa* (Cambridge: Cambridge University Press, 1996), 164.

31. Spurred on by rapid postwar economic development, Dakar's population has continued to grow exponentially. The 1991 estimate of just under 2 million is ten times the size of the population of 1951. Seck, *Dakar*, 210–12; Charles Becker and Mohamed Mbodj, "Dynamiques régionales au XXè siècle," in *La population du Sénégal*, edited by Yves Charbit and Salif Ndiaye (Dakar-Paris: DPS-CERPAA, 1994), 467–486.

32. Tisseuil Report for 1944.

33. Whittlesey, "Dakar Revisited," 632.

34. The best source is Seck's magisterial study. He notes that in 1937, the Popular Front sponsored a preliminary study by the architect-urbanist Lopez on how to reorganize Dakar and the Cape Verde peninsula. The next year, the governor-general of FWA created an urbanism commission headed by Hoyez, an architect who in April 1940 produced a general report on a project to "reorganize and beautify Dakar." Immediately after the war, it was this plan that the government began to implement. Seck, *Dakar*, 140–41, and 144–90 generally.

35. From the mid 1920s onward, all French West African subjects over fifteen years of age needed an identity card issued by the central commissariat of Dakar in order to be legally employed within the Dakar urban area. Those found in the city without proof of residency could be arrested as "vagabonds" and jailed or deported to their rural residences. In practice, however, such regulations were easily circumvented. For one thing, casual employees, defined as those hired as day laborers, were exempted. For another, the penalties were both mild and rarely enforced. Bouche, "Dakar," 968. In 1943 and 1944, the numbers officially declared as vagabonds were 557 and 853 respectively. ANS\2G44\11, Circonscription of Dakar, General Report for 1944 M. Alessandri, n.d. Hereafter cited as Alessandri Report for 1944.

36. Located near the canal boundary of the Médina, the houses in this new quarter were surrounded by a small courtyard and contained three or four rooms, a kitchen, shower, and water closet. Although they were relatively inexpensive, only the rising middle-class sector of Senegalese society could afford such accommodation, the only new housing available until after the Second World War. Seck, *Dakar*, 115; Jean Dresch "Villes d'Afrique occidentale," *Cahiers d'Outre-Mer* (1950): 222.

37. Whittlesey, "Dakar Revisited," 631. A geography professor from Harvard who had traveled extensively in West Africa, Whittlesey first visited Dakar in 1936. For his account of this visit, see Derwent Whittlesey, "Dakar and the Other Cape Verde Settlements," *Geographical Review* 31 (1941): 609–38.

38. Whittlesey, "Dakar Revisited," 631.

39. ANS\1H15\1, report entitled "Assainissement de la ville de Dakar," 1924.

40. ANS\2G45\4, Dakar, Annual Report on Health for 1945, Dr. Cheveneau, 16 July 1946. See also Bouche, "Dakar," 968.

41. Bouche, "Dakar," 968.

42. ANS\2G45\4, Dakar, Annual Report on Health for 1945, Dr. Cheveneau, 16 July 1946.

43. ANS\2G44, Dakar, Annual Report on Health for 1944, no author listed, 16 August 1945.

44. Lewis, Buehler, and Young ms.

45. ANS\2G43\6, Dakar, Annual Report on Health for 1942, Dr. Jardon, Dakar, 25 August 1943. Hereafter as Jardon report for 1942. The second portion workers at Yoff numbered around 900. They were young males from colonies in the interior of FWA who had been conscripted to serve as a military reserve. In the 1930s and during the Second World War, some men of this reserve were drafted into military labor brigades to work on projects deemed to be in the public interest. Africans viewed this service, with considerable justification, as a disguised form of forced labor. See Myron Echenberg and Jean Filipovich, "African Military Labour and the Building of the *Office du Niger* Installations, 1925–1950," *Journal of African History* 27 (1986): 533–51; and Bouche, "Dakar," 971–72.

46. ANS\2G41, Dakar, Annual Report on Health for 1941, no author listed. Tuberculosis deaths increased from 121 in 1936 to 163 in 1941, malaria deaths from 55 to 64, and total recorded deaths from 1,459 to 1,923. The Health Service's figures for the total African population of Dakar were 86,126 and 92,803.

47. ANS\2G41, Dakar, Annual Report on Health for 1941, no author or date listed.

48. As an example, see ANS\2G41\15, Senegal, Annual Report on Health for 1941, Dr. Vogel, 21 March 1942 (hereafter cited as Vogel Report for 1941). Also see Jardon Report for 1942.

49. Jardon Report for 1942. For a review of colonial health policy toward sexually transmitted diseases in Senegal, see Charles Becker and René Collignon, "A History of Sexually Transmitted Diseases and AIDS in Senegal: Difficulties in Accounting for Social Logics in Health Policy," in *Histories of Sexually Transmitted Diseases and HIV/AIDS in Sub-Saharan Africa*, edited by Philip W. Setel, Milton Lewis, and Maryinez Lyons (Westport, Conn.: Greenwood Press, 1999), 65–77.

50. Jardon Report for 1942. The numbers would appear to be fanciful, even given the presence of French, American, and African troops in the city. Five brothels, each with thirty prostitutes turning fifty tricks a day, would make for over 50,000 sexual encounters in a week in a city where the combined military presence did not exceed 15,000 troops.

51. ANS\2G41, Dakar, Annual Report on Health for 1941, no author or date listed.

52. For a thorough discussion of the history of Dakar's potable water problems, see Whittlesey, "Dakar Revisited," 630, and Seck, *Dakar*, 216–17. Seck noted that over fifty years, Dakar's water consumption had doubled every decade, a rise which corresponded roughly to the population increase. To meet its needs by 1970, the city drew on a new source as far away as Pout.

53. ANS\2G44, Dakar, Annual Report on Health for 1944, no author listed, 16 August 1945.

54. ANS\2G43 and 2G44, Dakar, Annual Reports on Health for 1943 and 1944, no author listed.

55. Bouche, "Dakar," 965.

56. Seck, *Dakar*, 217; Dresch, "Villes," 221.

57. The Second World War initiated what Austen calls "accelerated neo-mercantilism," brought on by the sharp increase in world demand for African primary products. Immediately after the war, there was a huge increase in African demand for labor, services, and supplies, and large development investment increases from the metropoles. Ralph Austen, *African Economic History: Internal Development and External Dependency* (Portsmouth, N.H.: Heinemann, 1987), 200–204.

58. Cooper, *Decolonization*, 156.

59. A. G. Hopkins, *An Economic History of West Africa* (London: Longmans, 1973), graph on 175, and 267.

60. Alessandri Report for 1944.

61. Alessandri Report for 1944. Note that the ration cards required an African to present an identity card issued in his home *cercle* together with a certificate from a local employer proving he held a regular job. This drove the unemployed and casually employed into the black market.

62. Cooper, *Decolonization*, 156–57.

63. For example, in March 1944 Governor-General Cournarie was obliged to ask the Americans to increase their rice imports from 48,000 to 75,000 tons. RG84, Cournarie to Consul Barnes, 27 March 1944; and Consul Barnes to GG Cournarie, 15 April 1944. American corn also became available after 1942, as did a smaller quantity of such American processed foods as powdered eggs and condensed milk. Maillat, "La flamme," marveled at the abundance and ingenuity of American products, and at the versatility of the Senegalese peanut. The shells provided fuel, the kernels food, and the refined oil was used in diesel motors, factories, submarines, trains and buses, and electricity generators. In emulsions it was used as a grease, and its stalks were used for animal fodder.

64. Jardon Report for 1944.

65. As an temporary measure in June, contacts were dispatched to the lazaretto in Rufisque, some 40 kilometers away. Jardon report for 1944.

66. Lewis, Buehler, and Young ms.

67. Ricou Report.

68. ANS\1H1, Digo, Chef de Cabinet of Governor-General of FWA to Marcadier, 29 June 1944.

69. Jardon Report for 1944.

70. ANS\2G45, Dakar, Annual Report on Health for 1945, no author or date listed.

71. Jardon Report for 1944.

72. Maillat, "La flamme."

73. Archives of the Pasteur Institute, Dakar, Box 9, "Correspondance sur les vaccinations, 1944–45" (hereafter cited as P.I. Correspondence).

74. Maillat, "La flamme."

75. Jardon Report.

76. R. N. Hunter, "Plague in Kenya," *Kenya Medical Journal* 2 (1925–26): 83.

77. Lewis, Buehler, and Young ms.

78. The American formulation consisted of a suspension of 2,000 million killed plague bacilli per cc., whereas the French preparation was a virulent living vaccine with 1 billion bacilli per cc. After the Dakar plague outbreak began in April–May, the Americans ordered their personnel revaccinated with the same dosage of 0.5 cc. By mid June, the Americans added, on a voluntary basis, a 1 cc. dose of the Girard-Robic vaccine. Lewis, Buehler, and Young ms.

79. Lewis, Buehler, and Young ms.

80. Ricou Report. Sulfadiazine was very familiar to American forces. In tablet form it was part of every soldier's first aid kit, to be swallowed after being wounded. After May 1945, its use was terminated except under the supervision of Medical Department officers because it was ineffective in major bleeding wounds. See James F. Baxter, III, *Scientists against Time* (Boston: Little Brown, 1947), 338–340.

81. Ricou Report; Jardon Report for 1944.

82. Ricou Report.

83. The only American reference I have found came not from any of the medical officers but from Consul Barnes, who mentioned in late August that an air shipment of penicillin had been ordered from the U.S.A., to be tried on plague cases. He added that the physicians held out little hope for the usefulness of the new drug since it had been tried without success on plague cases in Cairo by U.S. Army medical officers there. RG84, Foreign Service Posts, Barnes to Secretary of State, 30 August 1944.

Barnes and his medical consultants were ignorant of the situation unfolding in the Mediterranean theater, where penicillin was being used with great success from 1943 onward by British and American medical officers to treat a variety of infections ranging from battlefield wounds to gonorrhea. See Peter Neushul, "Fighting Research: Army Participation in the Clinical Testing and Mass Production of Penicillin during the Second World War," in *War, Medicine and Modernity*, edited by Roger Cooter, Mark Harrison, and Steve Sturdy (England: Sutton Publishing, 1998), 216–18.

84. A more cynical assumption might be that penicillin's limited supply precluded its use in a remote setting to treat African colonial subjects. It is, however, worth noting that, although the new wonder drugs became available by 1950, Western biomedicine did not immediately discern their utility against plague. In a 1947 article on prevention and treatment, Ruegsegger and Gilchrist still maintained that streptomycin was "experimental" and hoped that sulfadiazine would become the drug of choice for plague. James M. Ruegsegger and Huntington Gilchrist, "Plague: A Study of Recent Developments in the Prevention and Treatment of the Disease," *American Journal of Tropical Medicine* 27 (1947): 683–89.

85. Lewis, Buehler, and Young ms. The debate over sulfa was moot, because the immediate future would witness the emergence of an entirely new generation of antibiotics, beginning with penicillin, all of which proved remarkably effective against *Yersinia pestis*.

86. Lewis, Buehler, and Young ms. The authors note with some embarrassment that "even on American merchant ships," rat shields were unavailable and that ships leaving the port of Dakar during the entire outbreak were "NOT fumigated" (their emphasis).

87. Girard Report.

88. Lewis, Buehler and Young ms. While the three major species of rats (Norwegian, Alexandrian, and Common) were found, there was also a much less common local large rodent, the Camtchouli rat, (*Crycetomys gambianus*). Only the Norwegian and Alexandrian rats were among those infected. Finally, two dead cats were examined and found to be infected with plague.

89. ANS\Senegal H79, Dr. Cheneveau, Colonel, Troupes Coloniales, and Head of the Health Service for Senegal, "Compte rendu sommaire sur l'expérimentation de la D.D.T. à Médina, les 11 et 12 juin 1944," 14 June 1944.

90. Malaria control was begun by Captain Dunn, and, from March onward, continued by Lieutenant Thomas Roy Young, the malaria control officer attached to the Naval Air Transport Facility. RG84, Foreign Service Posts, Barnes to State Department, 19 June 1944.

91. RG84, Foreign Service Posts, Young to Wilkinson, undated, but from context, December 1944 (hereafter cited as Young's letter). Running to ten handwritten pages, Young's letter constituted a personal history of his involvement in the Dakar anti-plague campaign from March to December 1944.

92. Young's letter.

93. Young's letter. His sequence and dating are not clear, because he states that although the Americans protested that "spot" dusting was not working, the French refused the repeated requests for compulsory dusting of at least the native area "on the grounds that a precarious political situation would not permit such action." Young states that the Americans halted their spraying on 8 September, and told the French they would only resume if the restrictions were lifted. The French finally gave the Americans permission to proceed in early October.

94. It seems that there were only two deaths of American service men in Dakar from malaria. When the remains of sixty-one U.S. servicemen were exhumed from the military cemetery in Dakar for reburial, only two were recorded as having died from malaria. Most had been killed in airplane crashes. RG84, Foreign Service Posts, Colonel Whitfield W. Watson to Hasell H. Dick, American Consul General, Dakar, 19 September 1947.

95. Wiltse, *United States Army*, 76–78, 91.

96. Lewis, Buehler, and Young ms.

97. Lewis, Buehler, and Young ms. Though the language is cautious, bribes and other considerations may have been included under "misunderstandings."

98. Lewis, Buehler, and Young ms.

99. E. D. Davis, "The Control of Rat fleas (*Xenopsylla Cheopis*) by DDT," *Public Health Reports* 60 (1945): 485–89; Leo Kartman, "On DDT Control of *Synosternus pallidus* Taschenberg (Siphonaptera, Pulicidae) in Dakar, Senegal, French West Africa," *American Journal of Tropical Medicine* 26 (1946): 841–48; and Leo Kartman, "Plague in Dakar," 30–35.

100. RG84, Foreign Service Posts, Consul Barnes to Secretary of State, letters of 27 May, 20 June, and 29 October 1943.

101. RG84, Foreign Service Posts, Barnes to Secretary of State, 27 May 1943.

102. RG84, Foreign Service Posts, Goodyear to Secretary of State, 13 January 1944.

103. RG84, Foreign Service Posts, Barnes to Secretary of State, 12 May 1944.

104. Young's letter.

105. Young's letter.

106. Young's letter.

107. Young's letter.

108. Lewis, Buehler, and Young ms. All medical references to Americans are from this one outstanding source. It should be noted that a precis of the longer unpublished report by the same authors was published as "Plague in Dakar," in the *Bulletin of the U.S. Army Medical Department,* 87 (1945): 13–16.

109. His telegram read, in part, that "American Medical opinion here now considers advent wives and children matter of grave responsibility and suggests medical advice should be sought prior embarkation." RG84, Foreign Service Posts, Barnes to State Department, 7 June 1994, for transmission to Herbert E. Rea, Socony-Vacuum Oil Company.

110. RG84, Foreign Service Posts, Barnes to State Department, 19 June 1944.

111. RG84, Foreign Service Posts, Barnes to State Department, 19 June 1944. The irony that this was the same Yoff which had been a plague hecatomb in 1914 was lost on most.

112. Lewis, Buehler, and Young ms.

113. Young's letter. This letter leaves open to speculation what sorts of special considerations may have been offered.

114. While the original film has, unfortunately, not been located, a similar instructional film entitled "Sandfly Control" demonstrated the procedures used in Sicily, where sandfly fever hit the Allied troops hard. The film heralded DDT, delivered in barrels, as the first weapon ever developed which effectively controlled the tiny sandflies. The crystals of DDT stayed on sprayed surfaces for weeks or even months. The sandflies absorbed DDT on their feet where it acted as a nerve poison; fifteen to thirty minutes of contact was deemed sufficient to deliver a lethal dose. The film depicted a soldier, without a mask, spraying walls and carrying a large cylinder on his back. See "Sandfly Control," produced by the U.S. War Department, for the U.S. Army Training and Doctrine Command, Training Material Support Division, Washington, D.C., 1946, 33 minutes, color, 16 mm.; consulted at the National Institute of Health (NIH), Bethesda, Md. See also "Prevention of the Introduction of Diseases from Abroad," produced by the Film Unit, Bureau of Medicine and Surgery, United States Public Health Service, Washington, D.C., 1946, 10 minutes, 16 mm., black and white; consulted at the NIH in Bethesda. This film depicts a U.S public health officer, wearing no mask, spraying DDT on people exposed to typhus, to kill lice. Hair, body, and clothing are declared to be "disinfested" in this manner. The recipients are naked; one closes his eyes to avoid the DDT powder.

115. Maillat, "La flamme."

116. Abdel-Kader Diagne had been an active opponent of Vichy, and had been arrested and sentenced to two years in prison at Clermont-Ferrand for having engaged in espionage with Allied forces based in the Gambia. Because Vichy had passed legislation curbing Qur'anic school freedoms, conservative Muslims and modernists like Diagne were united in their opposition to Vichy. But when these restrictions were lifted by the Free French, Diagne became isolated politically since the overwhelming majority of Senegalese Muslims were not prepared to abandon

their *shaykhs*. See Lucy C. Behrman, *Muslim Brotherhoods and Politics in Senegal* (Cambridge: Harvard University Press, 1970), 160–61.

Pierre Diagne led the small Mouvement Nationaliste Africain while Amadou Ba headed the still smaller Mouvement Autonomiste Africain. Ruth Schachter Morgenthau, *Political Parties in French-Speaking West Africa* (Oxford: Clarendon Press, 1964), 136.

117. Benga, "Ville de Dakar," 120, citing ANS\2G44\139, Circonscription de Dakar et Dépendances, Monthly Political Affairs, 1944.

118. 2G44\139, Circonscription de Dakar et Dépendances, Monthly Political Affairs, 1944.

119. It should also be noted that opposition to the colonial *status quo*, but opposition that Guèye and the Socialists would defeat, came from the "Groupe d'Études Communistes" or GEC, in Senegal. Communist efforts in French Africa, whether in Algeria or Senegal, were hampered by the French Communist Party, which viewed independence as premature and autonomy as a "nationalist deviation." Morgenthau, *Political Parties*, 23, 136.

A much weaker element in Senegal was composed of those nationalists who were prepared to seek autonomy if not full independence. This small minority had two advocates: Pierre Diagne, leader of the Mouvement Nationaliste Africain and publisher of a newspaper called *Communauté*; and Amadou Ba, leader of the still smaller Mouvement Autonomiste Africaine, who published a newspaper entitled *Le Sénégal*. Morgenthau, *Political Parties*, 136.

120. Goux was chief adviser to Galandou Diouf, dispenser of patronage to the Diouf party, and anathema to the younger elite. G. Wesley Johnson, "The Senegalese Urban Elite, 1900–1945," in *Africa and the West*, edited by Philip D. Curtin (Madison: University of Wisconsin Press, 1972), 182.

121. One report stated that Guèye and the Socialists were virtually "unchallenged in native circles." Alessandri Report.

122. For Thiaroye, see Myron Echenberg, *Colonial Conscripts: The Tirailleurs Sénégalais in French West Africa, 1857–1960* (Portsmouth, N.H.: Heinemann, 1991), 100–104; for the postponed elections, see Benga, "Ville de Dakar," 120. When the municipal elections were finally held on 1 July, 1945, Guèye and his "Bloc Africain" won a complete victory. Benga, "Ville de Dakar," 121.

123. For details of his early career, see G. Wesley Johnson, "The Impact of the Senegalese Elite upon the French, 1900–1940," in *Double Impact: France and Africa in the Age of Imperialism*, edited by G. Wesley Johnson. (Westport, Conn.: Greenwood Press, 1985), 173–74.

124. Edward Mortimer, *France and the Africans, 1944–1960: A Political History* (London: Faber and Faber, 1969), 45; Echenberg, *Colonial Conscripts*, 149.

125. Jardon Report for 1944.

126. Benga, "Ville de Dakar," 104.

127. Story cited in Maillat, "La flamme."

128. Excerpts from the merchant's letter were found in ANS\1H1\1, Digo Chef de Cabinet of Governor-General of FWA to Marcadier, Administer of Circonscription of Dakar, 29 June 1944.

129. ANS\1H1\1, Administrator of Circonscription of Dakar, Mercadier, to Governor-General of FWA, 29 June 1944.

130. Milton Henry Buehler, Jr., was born on 13 November 1914, and died on 26 March 1983. I am most grateful to his widow, Mrs. Coral Beth Buehler, since deceased, who very kindly gave me access to her private collection of documents and photographs dealing with Milton Buehler's career, and who granted me a personal interview at her home in McMinnville, Oregon, on 20 April 1998.

131. Upon his discharge, Buehler for a time was an instructor in biology at Gonzaga University in Spokane, where he worked as the business manager of a sanitorium. In August 1949 he joined the U.S. Public Health Service as a commissioned officer, on loan to the Oregon State Board of Health as an insect and rodent control consultant. An experienced specialist in both insect and rodent control, Buehler gained national recognition when he successfully eliminated all rats from the small town of Halsey, Oregon, by means of a new rodenticide, Warfarin. His success led the state to adopt a statewide rat control program. The *Wall Street Journal* of 28 January 1952 included the following headline: "Modern Pied Piper of Hamelin Forsakes Flute for Warfarin. Armed with Drug, Federal Health Man Rids Oregon Town of Rodents." *Newsweek*, 24 December 1951, gave less flamboyant coverage to the same story.

132. For a laudatory view of Girard and the vaccine, see Dr. Robert Pirot, "Cinquante années d'endémies tropicales," *Compte-Rendus Mensuels des Séances de l'Académie des Sciences d'Outre-Mer*, 30 (1970): 98–105. For a balanced view, see Fabian L. Hirst, *The Conquest of Plague: A Study of the Evolution of Epidemiology* (Oxford: Clarendon Press, 1953), 441–45; and James R. Busvine, *Disease Transmission by Insects: Its Discovery and 90 Years of Effort to Prevent It* (Berlin: Springer-Verlag, 1993), 198–99.

133. Paris wanted Dakar's agreement that the FWA would pay for the Girard mission out of the FWA budget. P.I. Correspondence, Telegram of 17 October 1944 from Minister of Colonies to Governor-General of FWA.

134. Girard Report.

135. Girard Report. He is silent on why he had not been sent out earlier, although Paris was not liberated until August. Plague in Dakar may not have had as high a priority as other pressing matters related to the war.

136. Girard Report.

137. It seemed to Girard as if researchers in Senegal never drew comparisons with any other part of the globe. Their reports were written as if they were the first people ever to be visited by plague. Girard did admit that some of the research had value, such as the work of Casanove and Advier, who identified the presence of "free-standing" *Xenopsylla cheopis* fleas in cereal dust. Together, their findings corroborated those in India of Hirst, King, and Pandit, who, by first discovering "free-standing" *X. cheopis* fleas, opened a new chapter in plague epidemiology. Girard's research team in Madagascar had benefited from this.

138. Girard Report.

139. Girard put it this way: "The day when cement has replaced sand everywhere, in the streets as well as in houses, and when light is able to penetrate inside homes, the flea, whether of rats or of humans, will not be able to develop. The rat will not have disappeared, that's true, but its reproduction rate will have dropped below a critical level, and the complex plague pathogen will have become disassociated from its hosts." Girard Report.

140. ANS\2G45\6, Report on Medical Inspection of Schools for the school year 1944–45, by Dr. Charles Robin, Lieutenant-Colonel des Troupes Coloniales, "Considérations épidémiologiques et prophylactiques sur la peste à Dakar," 16 pages, Dakar, 26 October 1944 (hereafter cited as Robin Report).

141. Robin Report.

142. Eric Silla, *"People Are Not the Same": Leprosy and Identity in Twentieth Century Mali* (Portsmouth, N.H.: Heinemann, 1998), 115.

143. Alessandri Report.

11

THE PLAGUE'S RETREAT AFTER 1945

SMALLPOX AND BUBONIC PLAGUE IN 1945

Neither the French nor the Americans had any way of knowing that the 1944 outbreak would be Dakar's last experience with bubonic plague.[1] Although 1945 saw four confirmed deaths from plague in Dakar, these were regarded as the final convulsions of 1944. The cases were separated by several weeks. On 10 January 1945, a boy of ten, Débe Dieng, died in the Gouye-Salam quarter of the Médina. On 21 February, after fourteen days of illness, a forty-three-year-old male, Saer Lo, of 12, rue Calmette in the Plateau, succumbed. Four days later, a sixty-year-old woman from Gouye-Salam, Coumba Sarr, passed away. The last confirmed death from bubonic plague in Dakar was that of another Médina resident, Mohamed Saloum Fall, forty-four years old, who expired on 18 March.[2]

Plague also made a curtain call in rural Senegal early in 1945. Georges Girard witnessed a small rural epidemic in January 1945, in the village of Ngappo in Diourbel cercle. He was able to observe at first hand the futility of engrained French plague control practices. After an inquiry determined that three deaths had occurred before the Health Service's arrival, the village was burned and the people relocated. Girard noted, however, that the relatives and friends who had visited the sick patients had some time earlier returned to other villages, where they might easily have created new foci of infection. Ten such cases had indeed sprung up. Even though it was the dry season, the French team found enough fleas in Ngappo to allow for plague transmission. Rats were of course plentiful in the village, where the silos were bursting with millet. Enough fleas remained active that the microclimate effect could persist even in the dry season.[3]

Even if plague seemed to be temporarily in hiding in 1945, it cannot be said that health authorities had cause for celebration. For the first time in years, a serious smallpox epidemic struck Dakar, with 46 fatalities among its 386 cases. An unrecorded number of deaths also occurred among 97 cases of diphtheria that same year. Civil authorities blamed these outbreaks on immigration, but it was a breakdown in immunization programs because of the war that was clearly responsible. While smallpox had a long-standing presence in Africa, the 1945 diphtheria outbreak was attributed by health officials to European children coming to join their fathers and attending school without medical certificates.[4]

The general health and well-being of a society cannot be assessed from the perspective of one infectious disease but has to be seen in a larger context. To take one example, in 1944, the subdivision of Tivaouane in Senegal, which had been haunted by recurring plague epidemics, had no single case of bubonic plague for the first time in thirty years; nor from that time forward did epidemic plague ever recur there. Yet people in the region had little reason to celebrate the condition of their public health. Some 169 cases of smallpox were reported that year for the first time in a decade. Wartime shortages and financial constraints meant that both medication and medical workers were in short supply at the various colonial clinics scattered throughout the region. Very few women, moreover, received immediate pre- or postnatal maternity care. In short, although plague was absent, the road to better public health in Tivaouane and in Senegal remained long and treacherous.[5]

BRAZZAVILLE

The Brazzaville Conference of January–February 1944 has become, through hindsight, regarded as a watershed in the history of French Colonialism in Africa. Convened by General de Gaulle, who opened proceedings on 30 January, and hosted by Governor-General Félix Éboué of French Equatorial Africa, the gathering's original purpose was for French colonial officials to assess the modest, internal reforms in Africa required to maintain colonial peace. In the changing international arena in 1945–46, however, when France now confronted unrest and rebellion in Algeria and Indochina, Brazzaville became the symbol of a new French colonialism which could only survive if it moved away from its highly authoritarian past. The conference thus became the beginning of the process in which forced labor and polygyny would be abolished, trade union rights extended, and a new African development plan launched.[6]

In reality, Brazzaville in 1944 gathered together forty-four conservative-minded colonial officials, Gaullist politicians, a few French trade unionists, and even a Roman Catholic bishop, most of whom were not yet committed to significant change. There were only two nonwhite delegates, one of whom was Éboué himself, at the conference, although a few African *évolués* attended as observers.[7] Most of the delegates still believed it desirable that Africans remain as rural peasants, but they now acknowledged the existence of permanent city dwellers, and were prepared to expand the political participation of African elites. When the political reforms ushering in the new French Union were announced in 1946, they were modest, and disappointing to the African elite, who, as Cooper puts it, proved surprisingly willing "to settle for so little."[8]

If political and labor issues were predominant, education and health were also on the agenda at Brazzaville. The seven-man subcommittee on health was chaired by Dr. Vaucel, chief physician in the Colonial Health Service, and included a second colonial physician and five civilian governors.[9] Not surprisingly, given the conference locale, the health panel was deeply concerned with the "dominant diseases in the African pathology," which had plagued French Equatorial Africa, and aimed at health reforms that would assure the "repopulation of Africa."[10] To combat such "social diseases" as syphilis, which Vaucel complained had been neglected in favor of the more publicized sleeping sickness, medical officials would be required to place greater emphasis on epidemiology and demography through vaccination campaigns, surveillance of hygiene in villages, and increased inspection of schools. In fact, the health panel recommended few novel reforms, and instead urged a major increase in health budgets in order to meet the health goals originally outlined in the 1920s by Sarraut and Carde: the expansion of the AMI network through the recruitment of additional personnel, the building of more installations, including a pharmacy and a psychiatric center at Thiès, and a better administrative framework to be supplied by a new director of Public Health for FWA, who would be equipped with a new research institute for social hygiene and preventive medicine.[11]

One measure of the lack of innovation at Brazzaville was the failure to provide for structural change. Apart from the rhetorical statement by the health panel that a modification in living conditions was also required to reverse Africa's demographic stagnation, colonial officials did not yet recognize the fact that the African elite was no more prepared to accept inferior status in the health sector than it was in politics or the civil service. Thus the Brazzaville Conference in plenary session approved the creation of a federal medical school which would eventually create 2,000 African doctors each year, with a training and status inferior to European physicians. There would also be more local recruitment and training of nurses, and an increase in the number of African midwives. It would take almost a decade before the Faculty of Medicine in Dakar opened its doors. By the 1950s, however, African elites were no longer prepared to accept what they perceived as a subordinate and inferior form of training and insisted on an educational curriculum that matched those of the medical schools in the metropole.[12]

Despite these shortcomings, the symbolism of Brazzaville as a new dawn prevailed in the health sector as it did in other realms of life in the French African colonies. In his major report on the Dakar plague epidemic of 1944, Georges Girard took up the theme of what he called the "spirit of Brazzaville." If the Brazzaville Conference had accepted the point that a permanent urban African labor force was no longer something to be avoided, the living conditions and health needs of the urban workers needed to be addressed more directly than before. When the new transfusion of health funding arrived, Girard urged that "Dakar should become the first African city to benefit from this new resolution."[13]

THE LEGACY OF BUBONIC PLAGUE AFTER 1945

In many respects, Girard's expectations were fulfilled. Postwar colonial budgets were dramatically bolstered by the Fonds pour l'Investissement et le Développement Économique et Social (FIDES), a large transfusion of metropolitan funds for colonial development approved by the French National Assembly in 1946.[14] FIDES sought to provide large capital spending to improve colonial infrastructure, and Dakar and Senegal both benefited. A 1946 urban plan for Dakar used 10.2 billion francs from FIDES to transform the city into a military stronghold, to extend the port facilities, and to begin to turn the federal capital into a model multiracial city.[15] From 1946 through 1950, Senegal's general budget rose from 584 million to 3.16 billion francs, and the health budget from 70 to 407 million francs; throughout this period health expenditures represented from 8 to 13 percent of the total budget.[16] There was also an effort to keep salaries for personnel from eating up the totality of the increases. In 1947, the health budget for Senegal was able to limit salaries to 60 percent of total expenditure.[17]

Not only was there more money to spend, but the ending of plague endemicity made more funds available to address other much-needed and neglected items. One measure of this shift can be observed in the declining number of anti-plague vaccinations performed, which dwindled to 563 in 1947, 199 in 1948, and 48 in 1949.[18] Plague, in any event, had ceased to be a life-threatening disease with the advent of antibiotics. By 1950 French therapy had shifted dramatically to the use of sulfa drugs for those in contact with pulmonary plague patients, and to the administration of streptomycin with 100 percent cure rates for those infected.[19] Similarly, the use of DDT as a pesticide expanded dramatically from the experimental days of 1944.[20] In Dakar, the PID director, Durieux, stated as early as 1947 that his institute had ended all plague research in Senegal and was monitoring plague only in Mauritania.[21] Mauritania's last cases of plague were noted in 1953 in the remote oasis of Azib-Aftassa, east of Fort-Gouraud and some 100 kilometers from the border separating Mauritania from Rio de Oro.[22]

It cannot be said that all were sanguine about plague's disappearance, or about the general health of the population. In an official publication in 1949, Dr. M. Peltier, director of public health in FWA, continued to sound the alarm in language reminiscent of the days of Marcel Léger.[23] Beginning with Léger's dubious proposition that Senegalese plague epidemics did not begin with epizootics as was the norm internationally, Peltier stressed the need for vigilance, and for continuing urban improvements such as paving all the streets in the Médina and further extending the sewer system. If plague were temporarily in retreat, it could reappear without warning. In addition, tuberculosis now threatened to become widespread among the overcrowded population. Despite the efforts of the commission of urban architects and planners, Dakar remained a disease-ridden city "unworthy of the French Community."[24]

Almost a decade later, in 1957, Dr. Kovacs, chief medical officer for Dakar, saw no reason to rejoice over public health conditions in the city. He complained bitterly over the decision to close the lazaretto on the Front de Terre road, which left the city without any means to isolate suspects in the event of another epidemic. In 1957, the number of typhoid cases had risen from 36 to 121, and over the same period smallpox cases had jumped from 6 to 196. Only 81 percent of a total population estimated at 230,579 in 1957 had their residences sprayed against insects. In a voice that echoed those of his predecessors, Dr. Kovacs noted that while 2,167 summonses for health infractions were issued in 1957, morale was low among health inspectors because no more than 1 percent of the fines were in fact ever paid.[25]

In the postwar era, Dakar continued to be a city where income and not race dictated residential patterns. For French expatriates, and for the growing African middle class, urban improvements made the city one of the most pleasant on the West African coast. One historian, Denise Bouche, has argued in fact that 1945 marked the end of Dakar as a small colonial city and the true beginning of its vocation as an imperial capital.[26] To house the growing number of Africans gaining middle-rank positions in the civil service and in the private sector, French urban planners, beginning in 1952 developed a new suburb, known by the acronym SICAP, for Société Immobilière du Cap-Vert. Modeled after the suburbs of Scandinavia, SICAP illustrated the continuing tendency to import Western architecture and urban planning principles into a colonial setting.[27]

If the middle class was expanding, so too was the work force, fueled as in the past by a large number of new immigrants to the city. Dakar's population grew exponentially after 1945, doubling every ten years or less.[28] Major changes in organized labor had occurred quickly after the war. By 1948, 40 percent of workers in Dakar belonged to trade unions, mainly to the radical Confédération Générale du Travail (CGT), and their new militancy manifested itself in strike action, especially the major railroad strike of 1947–48.[29] Meanwhile, an important shift took place in colonial labor ideology. Adopting a policy they called "stabilization," the French no longer opposed the migration of women to join their husbands as permanent residents of the colonial city.[30]

For the majority of Dakarois, finding affordable and decent accommodation was a continuing struggle, just as it had been before and during the war. To cope with the rapidly expanding population of greater Dakar, two new neighborhoods, Grand Dakar and Pikine, sprang up some 15 kilometers from the city center and well beyond the overcrowded Médina. Their initial inhabitants were new arrivals from the countryside in search of a better life than they could expect in rural Senegal, as well as persons displaced by the latest efforts at urban renewal within the city core.[31] Beginning with a handful of residents in 1952, Pikine by 1960 accommodated 30,000 inhabitants; by the mid 1970s, its population had swollen to over 200,000, one-quarter of the entire population of the Cape Verde peninsula. The sociologist Fatou Sow, who conducted extensive interviews in Pikine, found that 60 percent of her informants were wage earners.[32] Less than a decade later, Pikine housed 30 percent of the 1 million people living in the peninsula.[33]

Health infrastructure investments in Dakar were badly skewed in favor of the wealthier residents. Pikine in the early 1980s may have had 30 percent of the population but it counted only three major health facilities compared to over 200 in Dakar. Similar disparities prevailed in educational facilities, water supply, and waste management.[34] Nor did the situation improve after the coming of independence in 1960. The government of Léopold Sédar Senghor continued the late colonial urban policy of beautifying the core area of Dakar, even at the expense of the underprivileged. Arguing that itinerant peddlers and beggars in the core of the city were "eyesores" who had a deleterious effect on tourism, public order, and safety, Senghor's government in the 1970s fined, removed, and jailed street vendors, and even people with physical disabilities, as vagrants.[35]

CONCLUSION

Unfortunately, in its attitude toward the poor, and toward public health in general, the modern postcolonial state in Senegal harkens back to colonial times rather than to a new and better future. Blaming victims, imposing health measures from above, and denigrating local therapies reveal only a few of the lessons that have not been learned. More fundamentally, the political will to address the structural issues that lie behind epidemic disease is still lacking. People in Senegal thus remain at risk, not only from such recent scourges as HIV/AIDS, but from malaria, which has been present for millennia, or from yellow fever, which has been around for centuries but can be controlled by vaccination so long as regular inoculation programs for infants are sustained.

The postcolonial state's inclination to blame victims has an unfortunate ring of familiarity. As the colonial state went about its construction of epidemic plague, it preferred to substitute scapegoating for structural change. When they sought out scientific explanations, health officials too often sought simple ones based on the presumed inadequacies of the African population, rather than the more difficult multifactor explanations which better accounted for the complexity of a zoonosis like bubonic plague.

Nor was scapegoating limited to one side of the colonial equation. Some Africans also exhibited uncharitable behavior brought on by the stress of medical crises. During the course of urban epidemics in Dakar, migrant workers were often treated badly. Lacking relatives to take responsibility for nursing them, or burying them according to accepted custom, such "strangers" were overrepresented among the corpses ignominiously abandoned in the streets of the city.[36] In rural Senegal, plague lazarettos served to identify but also to stigmatize both the afflicted and their kin. The oral testimony of Thérèse Tisa Mbengue stressed the shabby treatment she received at the hands of her fellow villagers for years afterward.[37]

Too often, French colonial health officials combined the political paternalism of ruler over subject with the medical paternalism of doctor over patient. They imposed plague control measures in an authoritarian manner, with no appreciation for local environmental or empirical knowledge. Instead of seeking local cooperation in their elaborate campaigns against plague, they chose coercion and constraint. As school principal Abdoulaye Yaré Fall wryly observed, when French authorities did seek local input during the rat catching campaigns, they were attracted by labor at low cost even as they risked the health of schoolchildren.

One way of evaluating the contrasting French and Senegalese responses to bubonic plague is to borrow Gramsci's notion of hegemony, his term for the way in which the bourgeoisie achieved predominance through the consent of other classes or groups. In their introduction to a series of essays which explore the utility of "colonial hegemony," Dagmar Engels and Shula Marks draw on the contributions of David Arnold and Megan Vaughan to show that, whereas in India, the public health measures of the Raj had hegemonic intent and potential and were successful, in Nyasaland, on the other hand, British health policy was coercive, meager, and not directed toward manufacturing consent.[38] French public health measures directed toward bubonic plague fall between these two poles. Health measures in Senegal certainly included a large degree of coercion, and generated tenacious resistance, but colonial officials gradually sought the consent of a westernized minority of privileged African elites, who came to embrace Western biomedicine as a symbol of modernity.

The urge to segregate residential neighborhoods in the towns of Senegal resonated throughout the thirty years of endo-epidemic plague. What made Dakar and the other communes of Senegal different from virtually every other urban setting in Africa, however, was the ability of African citizens to use the law and, if necessary, the streets, to resist forced relocation. Their success was a remarkable achievement, and can best be understood within the context of epidemic plague.

The changing disease ecology in Senegal remains an intriguing variable in the reconstruction of the past and in prognoses about the future. Whether bubonic plague is still a threat remains more than a hypothetical question. Although antibiotics provide sound therapy, when widespread ecological disruption is accompanied by political breakdown, such as in wartorn Southeast Asia in the 1970s, human epidemics of bubonic plague can materialize.[39] In the former plague zone of Senegal, the same microclimatic conditions which produced thirty years of endo-epidemic plague still prevail, with the critical exception of the presence of *Yersinia pestis*. In fact, modern agro-engineering efforts to create an oasis at Richard-Toll, at the mouth of the Senegal River above Saint-Louis, have actually created conditions conducive to a new plague zone in Senegal. The reintroduction of the plague bacillus, or the emergence, for example, of a less complicated vector than the rat-flea combination, would be sufficient to launch a new epidemic.[40]

Given the worldwide existence today of extensive reservoirs of enzootic plague, and the possibility that a wild rodent reservoir of plague might still exist in Senegal, celebration of plague's disappearance would be premature.[41]

NOTES

1. For example, Georges Girard, while hopeful about his vaccine and about DDT, felt that the "overpopulation of Dakar, with its 150,000 inhabitants, cannot help but cause deep disquiet." ANS\1H79\163, Mission Report by Dr. Girard, Head of the Plague Service of the Pasteur Institute, Paris, "Peste à Dakar en 1944," 21 pp. + 3 attached, signed Paris, 6 March 1945 (hereafter cited as Girard Report).
2. ANS 2G45\4, Dr. Cheneveau, Annual Health Report for 1945, Dakar, 16 July 1946 (hereafter cited as Cheneveau Report for 1945).
3. Girard Report.
4. Cheneveau Report for 1945.
5. ANS 2G44\124 and 2G45\101: Annual Reports for Tivaouane Cercle for 1944 and 1945. As Randall Packard has shown for South Africa, no dramatic breakthroughs in public health could really be expected without structural changes in society. Randall Packard, *White Plague, Black Labor: Tuberculosis and the Political Economy of Health and Disease in South Africa* (Berkeley: University of California Press, 1989). More than simply the ending of colonialism was required for this condition to be realized.
6. There is an extensive bibliography. A generally positive view of Brazzaville can be found in a collection of articles by leading French historians, Institut Charles-de-Gaulle, eds. *Brazzaville, janvier–février 1944: Aux sources de la décolonisation* (Paris: Plon, 1988). This collection includes a chapter on health issues by Danielle Domergue-Cloarec, "Les problèmes de santé à la conférence de Brazzaville," 157–69. For a negative view of the Brazzaville reforms, see Jean Suret-Canale, *French Colonialism in Tropical Africa, 1900–1945*, translated by Till Gottheiner (London: C. Hurst and Co., 1971), 484–88. See also Catherine Akpo-Vaché, *L'AOF et la Seconde Guerre mondiale (septembre 1939–octobre 1945)* (Paris: Karthala, 1996), 207–26; Edward Mortimer, *France and the Africans, 1944–1960: A Political History* (London: Faber and Faber, 1969), 48–52; and Frederick Cooper, *Decolonization and African Society: The Labor Question in French and British Africa* (Cambridge: Cambridge University Press, 1996), 178–82.
7. Cooper, *Decolonization*, 178.
8. Cooper, *Decolonization*, 182.
9. Dr. David, a medical lieutenant-colonel, was head of the Health Service in Cameroun. Domergue-Cloarec, "Les problèmes de santé," 167.
10. Domergue-Cloarec, "Les problèmes de santé," 159. For the demographic crisis in French Equatorial Africa, see Dennis D. Cordell, "Extracting People from Precapitalist Production: French Equatorial Africa from the 1890s to 1930s," in *African Population and Capitalism: Historical Perspectives*, edited by Dennis D. Cordell and Joel W. Gregory (Boulder, Colo.: Westview Press, 1987), 137–52.
11. For more on psychiatry in Senegal and in FWA in general, see two articles by René Collignon, "Quelques propositions pour une histoire de la psychiatrie au Sénégal,"

Psychopathologie africaine 12 (1976): 245–73, and "Folie et ordre colonial. Les difficultés de mise en place d'une assistance psychiatrique au Sénégal et en Afrique Occidentale," in *AOF: Réalités et héritages. Sociétés ouest africaines et ordre coloniale, 1895–1960*, vol. 2, edited by Charles Becker, Saliou Mbaye, and Ibrahima Thioub (Dakar: Direction des Archives du Sénégal, 1997), 1151–63.

12. Domergue-Cloarec, "Les problémes de santé," 168–69.

13. Girard Report.

14. Cooper, *Decolonization*, 176, 194–95.

15. For urban planning that transformed Dakar between 1946 and 1961, see Assane Seck, *Dakar, métropole ouest-africaine* (Dakar: IFAN, 1970), 115–20, and 140–48. The postcolonial government of Senegal also saw urbanization as an aspect of social and economic progress. Seck argues that a genuine effort was made to provide decent accommodation for new arrivals. Seck, *Dakar*, 147.

16. ANS\2G50\15, Senegal, Annual Report on Health for 1950, Dr. Mondain, 15 October 1951 (hereafter cited as Mondain Report for 1950).

17. ANS\2G47\13, Senegal, Annual Report on Health for 1947, Dr. Guillaume, 2 June 1948.

18. Mondain Report for 1950. In 1950, the number of anti-plague vaccinations rose to 212 to protect health workers destined for Mauritania, where a small plague epidemic broke out that year.

19. ANS\1H79\163, Dr. Mercier, Report on Tananarive Plague Therapy, no date. One French observer, well aware of the important changes in international health measures against plague, triumphally gave credit to a long line of French researchers from Yersin and Simond to Georges Girard, including Marcel Baltazard and his "Iranian school," but studiously avoiding any mention of non-French researchers, let alone the role played by the U.S. Army in Dakar in 1944. See Dr. Robert Pirot, "Cinquante années," 92.

20. In 1957, for example, over 7,000 kilograms of DDT were applied to over 38,000 buildings in Dakar and its suburbs. ANS\2G57\33, Dakar, Annual Report on Health for 1957, Dr. Kovacs, no date (hereafter cited as Kovacs Report for 1957).

21. Archives of the Pasteur Institute, Dakar, Box 9, "Correspondence sur les vaccinations, 1944–45" (hereafter cited as P. I. Correspondence).

22. P. I. Correspondence, Report by Dr. Carrière, Head of Public Health for Senegal and Mauritania, to Head of Public Health in Dakar, entitled "Épidémie de peste à Mauritanie," 23 March 1953.

23. M. Peltier, "La pathologie de la presqu'île du Cap-Vert," *Études Sénégalaises* 1 (1949): 209–38.

24. Peltier, "La Pathologie," 238.

25. Kovacs Report for 1957.

26. Denise Bouche, "Dakar pendant la Seconde Guerre mondiale. Problèmes de surpeuplement," in *Le sol, la parole et l'écrit: Mélanges en hommage à Raymond Mauny*, vol. 2 (Paris: SFHOM et L'Harmattan, 1981), 975.

27. A. A. Ousmane Wane, "La croissance urbaine au Sénégal: Urbanisation et extension de Dakar," in *Mondes en Développement* 13 (1985): 560–61; Jacques Bugnicourt, "Dakar without Bounds," in Aga Khan Foundation, ed., *Reading the Contemporary African City* (Singapore: Concept Media, 1982), 32–33.

28. Seck, *Dakar*, 211–13. See also S. L. Diop, "La situation démographique et son évolution," *Dakar en devenir*, edited by M. Sankalé, L. V. Thomas, and P. Fougeyrollas (Paris: Présence Africaine, 1968), 78–94.

29. Frederick Cooper, "'Our Strike': Equality, Anticolonial Politics and the 1947–48 Railway Strike in French West Africa," *Journal of African History* 37 (1996): 88.

30. The British adopted a similar policy. Cooper, *Decolonization*, 2.

31. Seck, *Dakar*, 131; Fatima Sow, "Pikine, Senegal: A Reading of a Contemporary African City," in Aga Khan Foundation, ed., *Reading the Contemporary African City* (Singapore: Concept Media, 1982), 47.

32. Sow, "Pikine, Senegal," 50–51, 54.

33. Thiècouta Ngom, "Appropriate Standards for Infrastructure in Dakar," *African Cities in Crisis*, edited by Richard E. Stren and Rodney R. White (Boulder, Colo.: Westview Press, 1989), 189.

34. Ngom, "Appropriate Standards," 189–94. For a thorough recent study, see Gérard Salem, *La santé dans la ville: Géographie d'une petit espace dense: Pikine (Sénégal)* (Paris: Karthala, 1998).

35. René Collignon, "La lutte des pouvoirs publics contre les 'encombrements humains' à Dakar," *Revue Canadienne des Etudes Africaines* 18 (1984): 574–78. For more on the efforts of people to cope with poor living conditions in contemporary Dakar, see Harold Lubell and Charbe Zarour, "Resilience amidst Crisis: The Informal Sector of Dakar," *International Labour Review* 129 (1990): 387–96.

36. Elikia Mbokolo, "Peste et société urbaine à Dakar: L'épidèmie de 1914," *Cahiers d'Études Africaines* 22 (1982): 31.

37. Interview with Thérèse Tisa Mbengue.

38. See Dagmar Engels and Shula Marks, eds., *Contesting Colonial Hegemony: State and Society in Africa and India* (London: British Academic Press, 1994), 12–13. In the same collection, see David Arnold "Public Health and Public Power: Medicine and Hegemony in Colonial India," 131–51; and Megan Vaughan, "Health and Hegemony: Representation of Disease and the Creation of the Colonial Subject in Nyasaland," 173–201.

39. Andrew Learmonth, *Disease Ecology: An Introduction* (Oxford: Basil Blackwell, 1988), 141–42; and Peter Curzon and Kevin McCracken, *Plague in Sydney: Anatomy of an Epidemic* (Kensington, N.S.W.: New South Wales University Press, 1989), 4, listing 16,500 cases in southeast Asia in the 1970s with a case fatality rate of almost 4 percent as antibiotics were often not immediately available.

40. Personal communication from Mme. Mariama Sène, research biologist at ORSTOM, Dakar, Senegal, 19 February 1994.

41. Interview with Mariama Sène, who stated that no investigation of the presence of *Yersinia pestis* in wild rodents has taken place in Senegal since the early 1950s.

APPENDIX:
THE STATISTICAL PICTURE

A number of caveats need to be mentioned regarding statistical portraits of endo-epidemic plague death in Senegal from 1914 to 1945. First, plague deaths were seriously underreported for reasons that have been elaborated upon elsewhere in the text. The hiding of corpses and their secret burial was universal, as Africans tried desperately to avoid intrusive health inspectors, fines, destruction of property, and most importantly, cultural invasion of their private burial rites. Because the rural areas were only lightly policed by the colonial authorities, it might be assumed that plague death in rural Senegal was more seriously underestimated than in urban areas. On the other hand, plague epidemics took heavier tolls when populations were crowded into substandard urban housing. Particularly in the opening weeks of an epidemic, as was the case in 1914, unreported urban deaths may have been significant. There is no way of knowing the actual count. Nevertheless, official statistics may have an internal consistency of error, and they do permit general magnitudes to be grasped.

A second problem arises for the war years from 1915 to 1917. The official medical story is that plague did not appear anywhere in Senegal until a small outbreak occurred in the *cercles* of Tivaouane and Diourbel late in 1917. Yet, because France was at war and personnel were being recalled everywhere to participate in the war effort, few physicians remained in the countryside to take cognizance of any unusual medical developments. As long as the urban centers and smaller towns remained untouched, it is entirely possible that hundreds if not thousands of plague cases went unrecorded during the war. This seems all the more probable when it is recognized (Table A.1) that the first decade of plague in Senegal, and especially the years from 1918 to 1921, saw the largest numbers of deaths registered.

Table A.1 Urban and Rural Plague Deaths, 1914–45

Year	Dakar	Rufisque	Saint-Louis	Urban	Rural	Total
1914	1,480	144	0	1,624	3,742	5,366
1915	4	0	0	0	133	137
1916	0	0	0	0	0	0
1917	0	0	58	58	872	930
1918	0	36	1,097	1,133	1,700	2,833
1919	712	437	257	1,406	2,964	4,370
1920	122	99	197	418	5,462	5,880
1921	899	12	0	901	1,285	2,186
1922	30	0	0	30	508	538
1923	7	245	0	252	801	1,053
1924	0	0	0	0	1,503	1,503
1925	0	0	0	0	229	229
1926	0	3	0	3	481	484
1927	184	133	0	317	1,585	1,902
1928	0	57	0	57	1,121	1,178
1929	244	4	314	562	1,159	1,721
1930	333	0	0	333	1,030	1,363
1931	361	42	0	403	212	615
1932	75	68	0	143	61	204
1933	91	0	0	91	10	101
1934	508	76	0	584	220	804
1935	59	27	0	86	121	207
1936	9	0	0	9	15	24
1937	0	0	0	0	8	8
1938	0	0	0	0	2	2
1939	0	0	0	0	0	0
1940	1	0	0	1	6	7
1941	0	0	0	0	0	0
1942	0	0	0	0	6	6
1943	26	0	0	26	226	252
1944	512	0	0	512	60	572
1945	4	0	0	4	42	46
	5,651	1,383	1,923	8,953	25,568	34,521

Sources: Annual Reports of the Dakar and Senegal Health Services, 1914-45, Archives Nationales du Sénégal.

In those four short years, over 15,000 deaths were counted, roughly 44 percent of the losses for the entire thirty-year period.

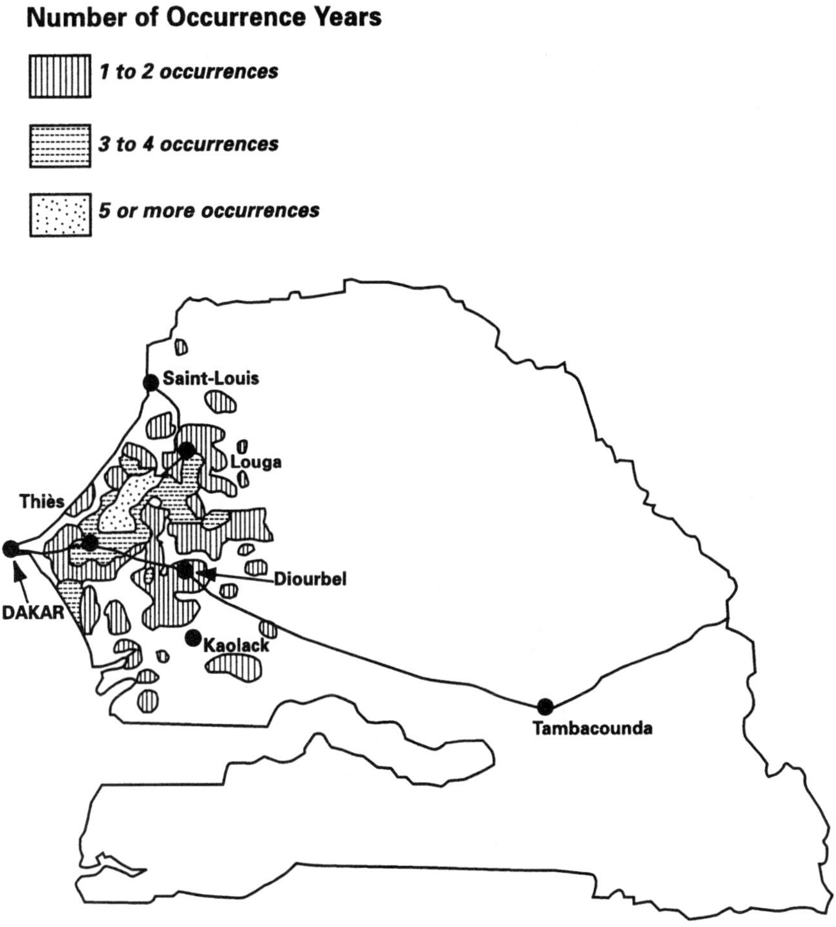

The Statistical Picture 269

Number of Occurrence Years

- 1 to 2 occurrences
- 3 to 4 occurrences
- 5 or more occurrences

Map A.1 Plague in Senegal, Overview, 1922–37. Taken from Annual Reports on Health in Archives Nationales du Sénégal, 1922–37.

A third difficulty is that urban, peri-urban and rural jurisdictions shifted during this lengthy period. Redefinitions of the *cercles* of Thiès and Tivaouane, right in the heart of the plague zone, occurred several times. Furthermore, calling plague death outside the three centers of Dakar, Saint-Louis, and Rufisque "rural" overlooks the existence of significant plague death in such important provincial towns as Tivaouane, Thiès, or, for example, the subdivision of Bargny. Bargny was part of the *cercle* of Thiès until 1927, when it was attached to the commune of Rufisque. The area of

Rufisque itself was attached to greater Dakar in 1937. Finally, in 1928, the *cercle* of Tivaouane was disbanded and its territory made a subdivision of the *cercle* of Thiès.[1] Since most of the plague deaths occurred before the major redistributions, there is some value in the categories I have used, but they cannot be taken as definitive. Perhaps the breakdown of plague in the distribution map (Map A.1), which deals with villages and subdivisions, solves this problem best.

Bearing in mind their limitations, the statistical data suggest the following conclusions:

1. In the thirty-year period of endo-epidemic plague, the second and third decades of the century were the worst. Death rates in the four years from 1918 to 1921 accounted for 44 percent of the grand total of recorded deaths.
2. The years 1920 and 1914 recorded the highest yearly totals, but 1919 was close behind. In terms of distribution of deaths, 1919 brought significant losses to each of the three communes and to rural Senegal as well.
3. For Dakar, the worst years were 1914, 1921, 1934, and 1944, with intervals therefore of seven years, thirteen years, and ten years, respectively. The plagues of 1919 and 1929 lingered for three years while the others died out more rapidly. There was no correlation with rural plague. Sometimes, as in 1914, the plague originated in Dakar and spread to the rural areas. In 1943, the countryside was hit, and then contaminated Dakar the following year.
4. In Saint-Louis, plague was a less frequent visitor. Indeed, apart from significant losses beginning in 1917 and continuing to 1920, 1929 was the only other year in which plague occurred. Clearly, Saint-Louis, lying to the north of the plague zone, was sufficiently removed from the microclimate most favorable to plague to have been spared its heaviest impact.
5. Everywhere, plague death fell off dramatically in the 1930s and 1940s. The years 1943 and 1944 were almost a decade removed from previous epidemics.
6. Expressed in percentages, Dakar absorbed 16 percent of Senegal's total deaths, and Saint-Louis and Rufisque a combined 10 percent, with rural plague accounting for just under 75 percent of all deaths. The great majority of all rural deaths occurred within the boundaries of the plague zone, that is, within the *cercles* of Tivaouane and Thiès.

NOTE

1. For a guide to the many shifts in regional boundaries, see the excellent article by Charles Becker and Victor Martin, "Les divisions administratives coloniales," in *L'atlas national du Sénégal*, edited by Régine Nguyen Van Chi (Paris: Institut Géographique National, 1977), 62–63.

SOURCES

INTERVIEWS CONDUCTED IN SENEGAL BY THE AUTHOR

Ciss, Adama and Mor Daga, 11 November 1990. Translated by Thomas Gana Diouf. Adama and Mor are brothers. Adama, the older, was born in 1904 at Loukhousse, in the compound of Gan Seck. Mor was born in the same village in 1917, and performed his military service as a Tirailleur Sénégalais in 1937.

Dieng, Cheikh, with Ibrahima Dieng, his younger brother, and Mandione Dieng, his wife. Toukar, 4 October 1990. Translated by Aissatou Pouye. Cheikh Dieng was *diaraf* or chief of Toukar at the time of the interview.

Diop, Ngor Laba (called "Goudi"). Ndiambour, 14 October 1990. Translated by Guedj Faye. The informant was a *saltigi* or healer.

Diouf, Coumba Ndoffène. Ngayokhème, 14 October 1990. Grandson of the *buur siin*, ruler of Sereer, of the same name.

Diouf, Ko. Toukar, 4 October 1990. Translated by Aissatou Pouye. Over 80 years old when interviewed, this informant was an adolescent at the time of the First World War. He was renowned throughout Siin as a powerful healer.

Diouf, Marie-Anne Yaayo, Tiwigne Diassa, first interview, 28 October 1990; second interview, 11 November 1990. Translated by Thomas Gana Diouf, her son. This informant was a mourner and composer of Sereer funeral dirges.

Diouf, Sitor, with his son Amad Diouf. Ngonin, 14 October 1990. Translated by Guedj Faye. Village chief of Ngonin when interviewed, Sitor Diouf lived at Toukar during the plague years and remembered how plague infected the region.

Diouf, Tekheye. Niakhar, 4 October 1990. Medical assistant, head of Sereer therapeutic center for the mentally ill.

Faye, Étienne, with Dièn Dione. Ngayokhème, 4 October 1990. Translated by Guedj Faye. Aged 70, the informant never personally saw plague cases but remembered the crisis.

Faye, Gaye. Daga, 11 November 1990. Translated by Thomas Gana Diouf. Informant claimed to be 103 years old.

Faye, Guedj. Ngayokhème, 3 October 1990. The informant was an interpreter and assistant during various medical projects among the Sereer of Siin.

Faye, Wali. Ngayokhème, 4 October 1990. Translated by Aissatou Pouye.

Gaye, Aissatou. Darou Alfa, 28 October 1990. Translated by Thomas Gana Diouf. Over 80 years of age when interviewed, she was afflicted by plague as a child. Among the first inhabitants of Darou Alfa, formerly called Danigal, she first contracted plague at Tiwigne Tangor.

Gaye, Coumba. Darou Alfa, 28 October 1990. Translated by Thomas Gana Diouf. A woman afflicted by plague as a child, the informant carried a scar on the inside of her left leg. She was a mourner and composer of Sereer funeral dirges.

Mbengue, Dauda. Darou Alfa, 28 October 1990. Translated by Thomas Gana Diouf. Born in 1926, the informant was afflicted by plague as a child of three or four.

Mbengue, Pierre Bangoné. Tiwigne Tangor, 28 October 1990. Translated by Thomas Gana Diouf.

Mbengue, Thérèse Tisa. Tiwigne Tangor, 28 October 1990. Translated by Thomas Gana Diouf. A woman of over 70 years of age, she remembered plague outbreaks.

Sine, Diatta. Ngayokhème, 4 October 1990. Translated by Guedj Faye.

Thiombane, Al Hajj Serigne Malik. Darou Alfa, 28 October 1990. Translated by Thomas Gana Diouf. Spiritual leader of the community and son of the village's founder, Malik was born in 1927. While he never personally witnessed plague, he remembers his parents discussing it frequently. He also recalls that the first wife of his father died of plague.

Yat, Dié. Toukar, 14 October 1990. Translated by Guedj Faye. The informant was a woman of around 60 years of age who had been afflicted by the plague.

ARCHIVES AND FILMS

Archives of the Congrégation du Saint-Esprit, Chevilly-Larue, France. "Dossier 262A, Correspondance Sénégambie."

Archives of the Government of French West Africa, housed in the Archives Nationales du Sénégal (ANS), Dakar, Senegal.

Archives of the Pasteur Institute, Dakar, Senegal.

Archives of the United States Department of State, Washington, D.C. RG84, Foreign Service Posts of the Department of State, 1936–54. Senegal: Dakar Consulate General. Security-Segregated General Records, 1940–44. 1944. Box 2.

Film Collection, National Institute of Health, Bethesda, Md. 1. "Prevention of the Introduction of Diseases from Abroad." Documentary produced by the Film Unit, Bureau of Medicine and Surgery, United States Public Health Service, Washington, D.C., 1946. 10 minutes, 16 mm., black and white. 2. "Sandfly Control." Documentary produced by the United States War Department for the U.S. Army Training and Doctrine Command, Training Material Support Division, Washington, D.C. 1946. 33 minutes, color, 16 mm.

NEWSPAPERS AND GOVERNMENT PUBLICATIONS

AOF, L'. Dakar: 1914.
Bulletin du Comité de l'Afrique française. Paris: 1914–1939.
Conseil Général, procès-verbal des délibérations: sessions of October 1914, October 1915 December 1918, December 1920 and June 1929, Published in Paris and Saint-Louis: Imprimerie du Gouvernement, 1915, 1919, 1921, 1930.
Démocratie, La. Dakar: 1914.
Journal Officiel du Sénégal. Saint-Louis: Imprimerie du Gouvernement, 1893, 1904, 1909, 1912.
Petit Sénégalais, Le. Dakar: 1916.

BOOKS AND ARTICLES

Abdalla, Ismail H. "Diffusion of Islamic Medicine into Hausaland." In *The Social Basis of Health and Healing in Africa*. Edited by Steven Feierman and John M. Janzen. Berkeley: University of California Press, 1992, 177–94.
———. *Islam, Medicine and Practitioners in Northern Nigeria*, Lewiston, N.Y.: Edwin Mellen Press, 1997.
Abun-Nasr, Jamil M. *The Tijaniyya: A Sufi Order in the Modern World*. London: Oxford University Press, 1965.
Advier, Marcel. "Sur l'épidémie de la peste au Sénégal." *Bulletin de la Société de Pathologie Exotique* 26 (1933): 465–74.
———. "Étude expérimentale du rôle du *Synosternus pallidus* dans la transmission de la peste," *Bulletin de la Société de Pathologie Exotique* 30 (1937): 643–46.
Advier, Marcel, and A. Diagne. "Observations épidémiologiques sur la peste à Dakar (décembre 1932)." *Bulletin de la Société de Pathologie Exotique* 26 (1933): 388–89.
Akpo-Vaché, Catherine. *L'AOF et la Seconde Guerre mondiale (septembre 1939–octobre 1945)*. Paris: Karthala, 1996.
Alexiou, Margaret. *The Ritual Lament in Greek Tradition*. Cambridge: Cambridge University Press, 1974.
Allen, Pauline. "The 'Justinianic' Plague." *Byzantion* 49 (1979): 5–20.
Anderson, D. M. and D. H. Johnson, eds. *Revealing Prophets: Prophecy in Eastern African History*. London: James Currey, 1995.
Angrand, Armand-Pierre. *Les Lébous de la presqu'île du Cap-Vert, Essai sur leur histoire et leurs coutumes*. Dakar: La Maison du livre, 1946.
Arnold, David. *Colonizing the Body: State Medicine and Epidemic Disease in Nineteenth Century India*. Berkeley: University of California Press, 1993.
———. "Public Health and Public Power: Medicine and Hegemony in Colonial India." In *Contesting Colonial Hegemony: State and Society in Africa and India*. Edited by Dagmar Engels and Shula Marks. London: British Academic Press, 1994, 131–51.
Austen, Ralph. *African Economic History: Internal Development and External Dependency*. Portsmouth, N.H.: Heinemann, 1987.

Bado, Jean-Paul. *Médecine coloniale et grandes endémies en Afrique, 1900–1960: Lèpre, trypanosomiase humaine et onchocercose.* Paris: Karthala, 1996.
Bahmanyar, M., and D. C. Cavanaugh. *Plague Manual.* Geneva: World Health Organization, 1976.
Balandier, Georges. *Afrique ambigüe.* Paris: Plon, 1957.
Ballard, Charles. "Drought and Economic Distress: South Africa in the 1800s." *Journal of Interdisciplinary History* 17 (1986): 359–78.
Bantam Medical Dictionary. Revised Edition. New York: Bantam Books, 1990.
Baxter, James F., III. *Scientists against Time.* Boston: Little Brown, 1947.
Bean, J. "Plague, Population and Economic Decline in England in the Later Middle Ages." *Economic History Review*, 2nd series, 15 (1962–63): 423–37.
Becker, Charles. "La Sénégambie à l'époque de la traite des esclaves." *Revue Française d'Histoire d'Outre-Mer* vol. 46 (1977): 203–24.
———. "Notes sur les conditions écologiques en Sénégambie aux 17e et 18e siècles." *African Economic History* 14 (1985): 167–216.
———. "La représentation des Sereer du Nord-Ouest dans les sources européennes (XVe–XIXe siècle)." In *Worso, mélanges offerts à Marguerite Dupire, Journal des Africanistes* 55 (1985): 165–85.
———. "Conditions écologiques, crises de subsistance et histoire de la population à l'époque de la traite des esclaves en Sénégambie (17e–18e siècle)." *Revue Canadienne des Études Africaines*, 20 (1986): 357–76.
———. "L'apparition du SIDA et la gestion des épidémies du passé au Sénégal." In *Les sciences sociales face au Sida en Afrique. Cas africains autour de l'exemple ivoirien.* Edited by Jean-Pierre Dozon and Laurent Vidal. Abidjan: GIDIS-CI-ORSTOM, 1993, 71–98.
———. *Vestiges historiques, témoins matériels du passé dans les pays sereer.* Dakar: ORSTOM, 1993.
Becker, Charles, and René Collignon. "A History of Sexually Transmitted Diseases and AIDS in Senegal: Difficulties in Accounting for Social Logics in Health Policy." In *Histories of Sexually Transmitted Diseases and HIV/AIDS in Sub-Saharan Africa.* Edited by Philip W. Setel, Milton Lewis, and Maryinez Lyons. Westport, Conn.: Greenwood Press, 1999, 65–96.
Becker, Charles, and Victor Martin. "Les divisions administratives coloniales." In *L'atlas national du Sénégal.* Edited by Régine Nguyen Van Chi. Paris: Institut Géographique National, 1977, 62–63.
———. "Kayor and Baol: Senegalese Kingdoms and the Slave Trade in the Eighteenth Century." In *Forced Migration: The Impact of the Export Slave Trade on African Societies.* Edited by J. E. Inikori. London: Hutchinson, 1982, 100–125.
———. "Rites de sépulture préislamiques au Sénégal et vestiges protohistoriques." *Archives Suisses d'Anthropologie Générale*, Génève, 46 (1982): 261–93.
Becker, Charles, Victor Martin, Jean Schmitz, and Monique Chastanet (with the collaboration of Jean François Maurel and Saliou Mbaye). *Les premiers recensements au Sénégal et l'évolution démographique. Partie I, Présentation des documents.* Dakar: ORSTOM, 1983.
Becker, Charles, and Mohamed Mbodj. "Dynamiques régionales au XXè siècle." In *La population du Sénégal.* Edited by Yves Charbit and Salif Ndiaye. Dakar-Paris: DPS-CERPAA, 1994, 467–86.

Behrman, Lucy C. *Muslim Brotherhoods and Politics in Senegal.* Cambridge: Harvard University Press, 1970.
Bell, Heather. *Frontiers of Medicine in the Anglo-Egyptian Sudan, 1899–1940.* Oxford: Clarendon Press, 1999.
Benedict, Carol. *Bubonic Plague in Nineteenth-Century China.* Stanford, Calif.: Stanford University Press, 1996.
Benga, Ndiouga Adrien. "Du modèle dégradé au contre-modéle, la question municipale: Rufisque (Sénégal, 1926–1960)." In *La ville européenne outre-mer: Un modèle conquérant? (XVè-XXè siècles).* Edited by Catherine Coquery-Vidrovitch and Odile Goerg. Paris: L'Harmattan, 1996, 261–79.
Bentley, Jerry H. "Hemispheric Integration, 500–1500 C.E." *Journal of World History* 9 (1998): 237–54.
Bernard, Noël. *Yersin: Pionnier-savant-explorateur (1863–1943).* Paris: Albin Michel, 1961.
Betts, Raymond F. *Assimilation and Association in French Colonial Theory, 1890–1914.* New York: Columbia University Press, 1961.
———. "The Problem of the Medina in the Urban Planning of Dakar, Senegal." *Urban African Notes* 4 (1969): 5–15.
———. "The Establishment of the Medina in Dakar, Senegal, 1914." *Africa* 41 (1971): 143–52.
———. "Dakar, ville impériale." In *Colonial Cities: Essays on Urbanism in a Colonial Context.* Edited by Robert Ross and Gerard J. Telkamp. Dordrecht, Holland: Martinus Nijhoff Publishers, 1985, 193–206.
Bibel, David J., and T. H. Chen. "Diagnosis of Plague: An Analysis of the Yersin-Kitasato Controversy." *Bacteriological Review* 40 (1976): 633–51.
Biraben, Jean-Noël. *Les hommes et la peste en France et dans les pays européens et méditerranéens.* Vol. 1. *La peste dans l'histoire.* Paris: Mouton, 1975; Vol. 2. *Les hommes face à la peste.* Paris: Mouton, 1976.
Bloch, Maurice. *Placing the Dead: Tombs, Ancestral Villages, and Kinship Organization in Madagascar.* London: Seminar Press, 1971.
Boccaccio, Giovanni. *The Decameron.* Translated by G. H. McWilliam, 1972. Harmondsworth, England: Penguin, 1972.
Boilat, L'Abbé. *Esquisses sénégalaises.* Paris: P. Bertrand, 1853; reprinted, Paris: Karthala, 1984.
Bouche, Denise. "Le retour de l'Afrique dans la lutte contre l'ennemi aux côtés des alliés." *Revue d'Histoire de la Deuxième Guerre Mondiale,* no. 114 (1979): 41–68.
———. "Dakar pendant la Seconde Guerre mondiale. Problèmes de surpeuplement." In *Le sol, la parole et l'écrit: Mélanges en hommage à Raymond Mauny.* Vol. 2. Paris: SFHOM et L'Harmattan, 1981, 961–76.
Brink, André. *The Wall of the Plague.* London: Fontana, 1985.
Brooks, George. "The Signares of Saint-Louis and Gorée: Women Entrepreneurs in Eighteenth Century Senegal." In *Women in Africa.* Edited by Edna Bay and Nancy Hafkin. Stanford, Calif.: Stanford University Press, 1976, 19–44.
Bugnicourt, Jacques. "Dakar without Bounds." In *Reading the Contemporary African City.* Edited by the Aga Khan Foundation. Singapore: Concept Media, 1982, 27–42.

Busvine, James R. *Disease Transmission by Insects: Its Discovery and 90 Years of Effort to Prevent It.* Berlin: Springer-Verlag, 1993.
Butler, Thomas C. *Plague and Other Yersinia Infections.* New York: Plenum Medical Book Co., 1983.
Calhoun, J. B. *The Ecology and Sociology of the Norway Rat.* Baltimore: U.S. Public Health Service, 1963.
Campbell, A. M. *The Black Death and Men of Learning.* New York: AMS Press, 1931.
Camus, Albert. *The Plague.* Translated by Hamish Hamilton. Harmondsworth, England: Penguin, 1960.
Carmichael, Ann G. *Plague and the Poor in Renaissance Florence.* New York: Cambridge University Press, 1986.
———. "Bubonic Plague." In *The Cambridge World History of Human Disease.* Edited by Kenneth Kiple. New York: Cambridge University Press, 1992, 628–31.
Carrière, Charles, M. Courdurié, and F. Rebuffat. *Marseille, ville morte: La peste de 1720.* Marseille: Éditions Jean-Michel Garçon, 1988.
Carson, Rachel. *Silent Spring.* Boston: Houghton Mifflin, 1962.
Cazanove, Franck. "Recherches sur les causes de la persistance de la peste au Sénégal." *Bulletin de l'OIHP* 22 (1930): 2103–7.
———. "Le problème du rat dans le territoire de Dakar et dépendances." Extraits du Rapport à la 2e conférence internationale du rat et de la peste, Paris, 7–12 octobre 1931. *Annales de Médecine et de Pharmacie Coloniales* 30 (1932): 108–144.
———. "Le rat de ville et le rat de champs à Dakar." *Outre-Mer* 5 (1933): 64–76.
Churchill, Winston S. *Their Finest Hour.* Vol. 2. Boston: Houghton Mifflin, 1949.
Cipolla, Carlo. *Cristofaro and the Plague: A Study in the History of Public Health in the Age of Galileo.* Berkeley: University of California Press, 1973.
———. *Public Health and the Medical Profession in the Renaissance.* Cambridge: Cambridge University Press, 1976.
———. *Fighting the Plague in Seventeenth-Century Italy.* Madison: University of Wisconsin Press, 1981.
Cissoko, Sékéné-Mody. "Famines et épidémies à Tombouctou et dans la boucle du Niger du XVè au XVIIIè siècle." *Bulletin de l'I.F.A.N.* 30B (1968): 806–21.
Clark, Andrew. "Environmental Decline and Ecological Response in the Upper Senegal Valley, West Africa, from the Late Nineteenth Century to World War I." *Journal of African History* 36 (1995): 197–218.
Cohen, William. *Rulers of Empire: The French Colonial Service in Africa.* Stanford, Calif.: Hoover Institution, 1971.
———. "Health and Colonialism in French Africa." In *Études africaines offertes à Henri Brunschwig.* Edited by Jan Vansina et al. Paris: Éditions de l'École des Hautes Études en Sciences Sociales, 1982.
———. "Malaria and French Imperialism." *Journal of African History* 24 (1983): 23–36.
Collignon, René. "Quelques propositions pour une histoire de la psychiatrie au Sénégal." *Psychopathologie Africaine* 12 (1976): 245–73.

———. "La lutte des pouvoirs publics contre les 'encombrements humains' à Dakar." *Revue Canadienne des Études Africaines*, 18 (1984): 573–82.

———. "Folie et ordre colonial. Les difficultés de mise en place d'une assistance psychiatrique au Sénégal et en Afrique Occidentale." In *AOF: Réalités et héritages. Sociétés ouest africaines et ordre coloniale, 1895–1960*. Vol. 2. Edited by Charles Becker, Saliou Mbaye, and Ibrahima Thioub. Dakar: Direction des Archives du Sénégal, 1997, 1151–63.

Collignon, René, and Charles Becker (with the collaboration of Ellen Brickwedde, Didier Fassin, and Christine Henry). *Santé et population en Sénégambie des origines à 1960: Bibliographie annotée*. Paris: Institut National d'Études Démographiques, 1989.

Collomb, Huot, and Lecomte. "Note sur l'épidémie de peste au Sénégal en 1914." *Annales de Hygiène et de Médecine Coloniales* 19 (1921): 38–72.

Comaroff, Jean. "The Diseased Heart of Africa: Medicine, Colonialism, and the Black Body." In *Knowledge, Power, and Practice: The Anthropology of Medicine and Everyday Life*. Edited by Shirley Lindenbaum and Margaret Lock. Berkeley: University of California Press, 1993, 305–29.

Commoner, Barry. *Making Peace with the Planet*. New York: Pantheon, 1990.

Conklin, Alice L. *A Mission to Civilize: The Republican Idea of Empire in France and West Africa, 1895–1930*. Stanford, Calif.: Stanford University Press, 1997.

Conrad, Lawrence I. "The Arab-Islamic medical tradition." In *The Western Medical Tradition, 800 B.C. to A.D. 1800*. Edited by Lawrence I. Conrad et al. Cambridge: Cambridge University Press, 1995, 93–138.

Cooper, Frederick. *Decolonization and African Society: The Labor Question in French and British Africa*. Cambridge: Cambridge University Press, 1996.

———. "'Our Strike': Equality, Anticolonial Politics and the 1947–48 Railway Strike in French West Africa." *Journal of African History* 37 (1996): 81–118.

Cooper, Frederick, and Ann Stoler, eds. *Tensions of Empire: Colonial Cultures in a Bourgeois World*. Berkeley: University of California Press, 1997.

Copans, Jean. *Les marabouts de l'arachide*. Paris: Le Sycomore, 1980.

Cordell, Dennis D. "Extracting People from Precapitalist Production: French Equatorial Africa from the 1890s to 1930s." In *African Population and Capitalism: Historical Perspectives*. Edited by Dennis D. Cordell and Joel W. Gregory. Boulder, Colo.: Westview Press, 1987, 137–52.

Cordell, Dennis D., Joel W. Gregory, and Victor Piché. "The Demographic Reproduction of Health and Disease: Colonial Central African Republic and Contemporary Burkina Faso." In *The Social Basis of Health and Healing in Africa*. Edited by Steven Feierman and John M. Janzen. Berkeley: University of California Press, 1992, 39–70.

Courtet, M. *Étude sur le Sénégal*. Paris: Challamel, 1903.

Couvy, L. "La tuberculose à Dakar." *Bulletin de la Société de Pathologie Exotique* 20 (1927): 228–32.

Crawfurd, Raymond. *Plague and Pestilence in Literature and Art*. London: Oxford University Press, 1914.

Crosby, Alfred W. *The Columbian Exchange: Biological and Cultural Consequences of 1492*. Westport, Conn.: Greenwood Press, 1972.

———. *Ecological Imperialism: The Biological Expansion of Europe, 900–1900*. Cambridge: Cambridge University Press, 1986.
———. *America's Forgotten Pandemic: The Influenza of 1918*. New Edition. New York: Cambridge University Press, 1989.
Cruise O'Brien, Donal. *The Mourides of Senegal: The Political and Economic Organization of an Islamic Brotherhood*. Oxford: Clarendon Press, 1971.
Cruise O'Brien, Rita. *White Society in Black Africa: The French of Senegal*. London: Faber and Faber, 1972.
Cunningham, Andrew. "Transforming Plague: The Laboratory and the Identity of Infectious Disease." In *The Laboratory Revolution in Medicine*. Edited by Andrew Cunningham and Perry Williams. Cambridge: Cambridge University Press, 1992, 209–244.
Curtin, Philip D. *Economic Change in Pre-colonial Africa: Senegambia in the Era of the Slave Trade*. Madison: University of Wisconsin Press, 1975.
———. "Medical Knowledge and Urban Planning in Tropical Africa." *American Historical Review* 90 (1985): 594–613.
———. *Disease and Empire: The Health of European Troops in the Conquest of Africa*. Cambridge: Cambridge University Press, 1998.
Curzon, Peter, and Kevin McCracken. *Plague in Sydney: Anatomy of an Epidemic*. Kensington, N.S.W.: New South Wales University Press, 1989.
Danforth, Loring. *The Death Rituals of Greece*. Princeton, N.J.: Princeton University Press, 1982.
Davis, E. D. "The Control of Rat Fleas (*Xenopsylla cheopis*) by DDT." *Public Health Reports* 60 (1945): 485–89.
Dawson, Marc H. "Disease and Social Change: Smallpox in Kenya, 1880–1920." *Social Science and Medicine* 13B (1979): 245–51.
———. "Disease and Population Decline of the Kikuyu of Kenya, 1890–1925." In *African Historical Demography*. Vol.2. Edited by Christopher Fyfe and David McMaster. Edinburgh: Centre for African Studies, University of Edinburgh, 1981, 121–38.
———. "Health, Nutrition, and Population in Central Kenya, 1890–1945." In *African Population and Capitalism*. Edited by Dennis D. Cordell and Joel W. Gregory. Boulder, Colo.: Westview Press, 1987, 201–17.
Defoe, Daniel. *A Journal of the Plague Year*. Harmondsworth, England: Penguin, 1966. Original edition, 1722.
Diagne, A., L. Michel, P. Koite, and D. Veyret. "Note préliminaire sur l'emploi du dicoumarol comme raticide en A.O.F." *Bulletin Médical de l'AOF* 9 (1952): 185–87.
———. "Sur l'emploi des dérivés de la coumarine comme raticide à Dakar." *Bulletin Médical de l'AOF*, 9 (1952): 273–300.
Diagne, Pathé. "Les royaumes sérères: Les institutions traditionnelles du Sine-Saloum." *Présence Africaine* 54 (1965): 142–72.
Dieng, Amady Aly. *Blaise Diagne, premier député africain*. Paris: Éditions Chaka, 1990.
Diop, S. L. "La situation démographique et son évolution." In *Dakar en devenir*. Edited by M. Sankalé, L. V. Thomas, and P. Fougeyrollas. Paris: Présence Africaine, 1968, 78–94.

Domergue-Cloarec, Danielle. *La santé en Côte d'Ivoire, 1905–1958*. Toulouse-Le Mirail: Association des Publications Universitaires, 1986.

———. "Les problémes de santé à la conférence de Brazzaville." In *Brazzaville, janvier–février 1944: Aux sources de la décolonisation*, edited by Institut Charles-de-Gaulle. Paris: Plon, 1988, 157–69.

Dozon, Jean-Pierre. "Quand les Pastoriens traquaient la maladie du sommeil." *Sciences Sociales et Santé* 3 (1985): 27–56.

———. "À propos de l'ouvrage de Danielle Domergue-Cloarec: La santé en Côte d'Ivoire 1905–1958." *Psychopathologie Africaine* 31 (1986–87): 211–17.

———. "D'un tombeau à l'autre." *Cahiers d'Études Africaines* vol. 121–22, 31 (1991): 135–57.

Dresch, Jean. "Villes d'Afrique occidentale." *Cahiers d'Outre-Mer* (1950): 200–30.

Dubois, Jean-Paul. "Les Serer et la question des terres neuves au Sénégal." *Cahiers de l'ORSTOM*, sér. Sciences Humaines, 12 (1975): 81–120.

Dupire, Marguerite. "Chasse rituelle, divination et reconduction de l'ordre socio-politique chez les Serer du Sine (Sénégal)." *L'Homme* 16 (1976): 5–32.

———. "Funérailles et relations entre lignages dans une société bilinéaire: Les Serer (Sénégal)." *Anthropos* 72 (1977): 376–400.

———. "La tabatière et les réseaux de l'amitié chez les Sereer: Extrait d'objets et mondes." *Revue du Musée de l'Homme* 23 (1983): 143–54.

——— "Les 'tombes de chiens': Mythologies de la mort en pays Serer (Sénégal)," *Journal of Religion in Africa* 15 (1985): 201–15.

———. " L'ambiguité structurale du fosterage dans une société matri-virilocale (Sereer Ndut, Sénégal)." *Anthropologie et Sociétés* 12 (1988): 7–24.

———. *Sagesse sereer: Essais sur la pensée sereer ndut*. Paris: Karthala, 1994.

Dupire, Marguerite, André Lericollais, Bernard Delpech, and Jean-Marc Gastellu. "Résidence, tenure foncière, alliance dans une société bilinéaire (Serer du Sine et du Baol, Sénégal)." *Cahiers d'Études Africaines* 55 (1974): 417–52.

Duplantier, Jean-Marc, and Laurent Granjon. *Les rongeurs du Sénégal*. Dakar: ORSTOM, 1993.

Echenberg, Myron. *Colonial Conscripts: The Tirailleurs Sénégalais in French West Africa, 1857–1960*. Portsmouth, N.H.: Heinemann, 1991.

———. " 'Scientific Gold': Robert Koch and Africa, 1883–1906." In *Agency and Action in Colonial Africa: Essays for John E. Flint*. Edited by Chris Youé and Tim Stapleton. London: Palgrave, 2001, 34–49.

Echenberg, Myron, and Jean Filipovich. "African Military Labour and the Building of the *Office du Niger* Installations, 1925–1950." *Journal of African History* 27 (1986): 533–51;

Eldredge, Elizabeth. "Famine and Disease in Nineteenth-Century Lesotho." *African Economic History* 16 (1987): 61–93;

Engels, Dagmar, and Shula Marks, eds. *Contesting Colonial Hegemony: State and Society in Africa and India*. London: British Academic Press, 1994.

"Enquête sur la peste en Afrique et sur le rôle des rongeurs sauvages et domestiques dans sa population." *Bulletin de l'OIHP* 26 (1934): 830–84.

Esoavelomandroso, Faranirina. "Maladie et politique en situation coloniale: La peste à Madagascar." *Annales ESC* 36 no. 2 (1981): 168–90.

Esquier, A. "La deuxième épidémie de peste à Dakar." *Archives de Médecine et de Pharmacie Navales*, 110 (1920): 187–213.
Fanon, Frantz. "Medicine and Colonialism." In *A Dying Colonialism*. New York: Grove Press, 1965, 121–45.
Feierman, Steven. "Struggles for Control: The Social Roots of Health and Healing in Modern Africa." *African Studies Review* 28 (1985): 73–147.
———. *Peasant Intellectuals: Anthropology and History in Tanzania*. Madison: University of Wisconsin Press, 1990.
Feierman, Steven and John M. Janzen, eds. *The Social Basis of Health and Healing in Africa*. Berkeley: University of California Press, 1992.
Feis, Herbert. *Churchill, Roosevelt, Stalin*. Princeton, N.J.: Princeton University Press, 1957.
Foucault, Michel. *Madness and Civilization: A History of Insanity in the Age of Reason*. Translated by Richard Howard. Toronto: New American Library of Canada, 1965. Original edition, Paris: Plon, 1961.
———. *The Birth of the Clinic: An Archaeology of Medical Perception*. Translated by A. M. Sheridan Smith. New York: Pantheon, 1973. Original edition, Paris: Presses Universitaires de France 1963.
———. *The History of Sexuality*. Vol. 1. *An Introduction*. Translated by Robert Hurley. New York: Pantheon, 1978. Original edition, Paris: Gallimard, 1976.
Gado, Boureima Alpha. *Une histoire des famines au Sahel*. Paris: L'Harmattan, 1993.
Gallagher, Nancy. *Medicine and Power in Tunisia, 1780–1900*. Cambridge: Cambridge University Press, 1983.
Giblin, James L. "Famine and Social Change during the Transition to Colonial Rule in Northeastern Tanzania, 1880–1896." *African Economic History* 15 (1986): 85–105.
———. "Trypanosomiasis Control in African History: An Evaded Issue?" *Journal of African History* 31 (1990): 59–80.
———. *The Politics of Environmental Control in Northeastern Tanzania, 1840–1940*. Philadelphia: University of Pennsylvania Press, 1992.
Gifford, Prosser, and Timothy Weiskel. "African Education in a Colonial Context: French and British Styles." In *France and Britain in Africa: Imperial Rivalry and Colonial Rule*. Edited by Prosser Gifford and William Roger Louis. New Haven, Conn.: Yale University Press, 1971, 663–711.
Goerg, Odile. "From Hill Station (Freetown) to Downtown Conakry (First Ward): Comparing French and British Approaches to Segregation in Colonial Cities at the Beginning of the Twentieth Century." *Canadian Journal of African Studies* 32 (1998): 1–31.
Gottfried, Robert S. *The Black Death: Natural and Human Disaster in Medieval Europe*. New York: The Free Press, 1983.
Guèye, Lamine. *Itinéraire africain*. Paris: Présence Africaine, 1966.
Guiart, Jules, Charles Garin, and Marcel Léger. *Précis de médecine coloniale. Maladies des pays chauds*. Paris: J. B. Baillère, 1929.
Harrison, Mark. *Public Health in British India: Anglo-Indian Preventive Medicine 1859–1914*. Cambridge: Cambridge University Press, 1994.

Hartwig, Gerald W., and K. David Patterson, eds. *Disease in African History: An Introductory Survey and Case Studies*. Durham, N.C.: Duke University Press, 1978.
Headrick, Daniel. *Tools of Empire: Technology and European Imperialism in the Nineteenth Century*. Oxford: Oxford University Press, 1981.
―――. *The Tentacles of Progress: Technology Transfer in the Age of Imperialism, 1850–1940*. New York: Oxford University Press, 1988.
Headrick, Rita. *Colonialism, Health and Illness in French Equatorial Africa, 1885–935*. Atlanta: African Studies Association Press, 1994.
Hirst, Fabian L. *The Conquest of Plague: A Study of the Evolution of Epidemiology*. Oxford: Clarendon Press, 1953.
Hochschild, Adam. *King Leopold's Ghost: A Story of Greed, Terror, and Heroism in Colonial Africa*. Boston: Houghton Mifflin, 1998.
Holst-Warhaft, Gail. *Dangerous Voices: Women's Laments and Greek Literature*. London: Routledge, 1992.
Hopkins, A. G. *An Economic History of West Africa*. London: Longmans, 1973.
Howard-Jones, Norman. "Kitasato, Yersin, and the Plague Bacillus." *Clio Medica* 10 (1975): 23–27.
―――. *The Scientific Background of the International Sanitary Conferences, 1851–1938*. Geneva: WHO, 1975.
Hunter, R. N. "Plague in Kenya." *Kenya Medical Journal* 2 (1925–26), 75–85.
Hunwick, John. *Literacy and Scholarship in Muslim West Africa in the Pre-colonial Period*. Lagos: University of Nigeria Press, 1974.
Idowu, E. B. *Olodumare: God in Yoruba Belief*. London: Longmans, 1962.
Iliffe, John. *The African Poor, a History*. Cambridge: Cambridge University Press, 1987.
―――. *Africans: The History of a Continent*. Cambridge: Cambridge University Press, 1995.
―――. *East African Doctors: A History of the Modern Profession*. Cambridge: Cambridge University Press, 1998.
Institut Charles-de-Gaulle, eds. *Brazzaville, janvier–février 1944: Aux sources de la décolonisation*. Paris: Plon, 1988.
Janzen, John. *The Quest for Therapy: Medical Pluralism in Lower Zaire*. Berkeley: University of California Press, 1978.
―――. *Ngoma: Discourse of Healing in Central and Southern Africa*. Berkeley: University of California Press, 1992.
Johnson, G. Wesley. *The Emergence of Black Politics in Senegal: The Struggle for Power in the Four Communes, 1900–1920*. Stanford, Calif.: Stanford University Press, 1971.
―――. "The Senegalese Urban Elite, 1900–1945." In *Africa and the West*. Edited by Philip D. Curtin. Madison: University of Wisconsin Press, 1972, 139–87.
―――. "William Ponty and Republican Paternalism in French West Africa, 1866–1915." In *African Proconsuls: European Governors in Africa*. Edited by L. H. Gann and P. Duignan. Stanford, Calif.: Hoover Institution, 1978, 127–56.
―――. "The Impact of the Senegalese Elite upon the French, 1900–1940". In *Double Impact: France and Africa in the Age of Imperialism*. Edited by G. Wesley Johnson. Westport, Conn.: Greenwood Press, 1985, 155–78.

Jojot, C. *Dakar. Essai de géographie médicale et d'ethnographie.* Montdidier, France: Grau-Radenez, 1907.

Jorge, Ricardo. *Les faunes régionales des rongeurs et des puces dans leurs rapports avec la peste. Résultats de l'enquête du comité permanent de l'Office International d'Hygiène Publique, 1924–27.* Paris: Masson, 1928, 53–54.

Kartman, Leo. "A Note on the Problem of Plague in Dakar, Sénégal, French West Africa." *Journal of Parasitology* 32 (1946): 30–35.

———. "On DDT Control of *Synosternus pallidus* Taschenberg (Siphonaptera, Pulicidae) in Dakar, Senegal, French West Africa." *American Journal of Tropical Medicine* 26 (1946): 841–48.

Kerharo, Joseph. *La pharmacopée sénégalaise traditionnelle. Plantes médicinales et toxiques.* Paris: Éditions Vigot frères, 1974.

Kermorgant, Alexandre. "Instructions adressées à nos colonies de la côte occidentale d'Afrique, au sujet des mesures à prendre en cas de peste." *Annales d'Hygiène et de Médecine Coloniales* 2 (1899): 497–509.

———. *Hygiène coloniale.* Paris: Masson, 1911.

———. "L'épidémie de peste qui a sévi à Dakar et au Sénégal d'avril 1914 à février 1915." *Bulletin de l'Academie de Médecine* 76 (1916): 126–33.

King, H., and C. Pandit. "Summary of Rat-Flea Survey of Madras Presidency." *Indian Journal of Medical Research* 19 (1931): 357–92.

Kirk, Joyce F. *Making a Voice: African Resistance to Segregation in South Africa.* Boulder, Colo.: Westview Press, 1998.

Klein, Ira. "Plague, Policy and Popular Unrest in British India." *Modern Asian Studies* 22 (1988): 755.

Klein, Martin A. *Islam and Imperialism: Sine Saloum 1847–1914.* Stanford, Calif.: Stanford University Press, 1968.

———. *Slavery and Colonial Rule in French West Africa.* Cambridge: Cambridge University Press, 1998.

Kuhnke, LaVerne. *Lives at Risk: Public Health in Nineteenth Century Egypt.* Berkeley: University of California Press, 1989.

Laberge, Marie-Paule. "Les Instituts Pasteur du Maghreb: Le recherche scientifique médicale dans le cadre de la politique coloniale." *Revue Française d'Histoire d'Outre-Mer* 74 (1987): 27–42.

Labouret, Henri. "Main d'oeuvre dans l'ouest africain." *L'Afrique Française* (1930): 240–50.

Lafont, André. "Une épidémie de peste humaine à Dakar (avril 1914–février 1915)." *Bulletin de la Société de Pathologie Exotique* 8 (1915): 660–80.

Learmonth, Andrew. *Disease Ecology: An Introduction.* Oxford: Basil Blackwell, 1988.

Le Borgne, Jean. *La pluviomètrie au Sénégal et en Gambie.* Dakar: ORSTOM, 1988.

Lefrou, Gustave. "L'épidémie de peste de 1929 à Saint-Louis du Sénégal." *Annales de Médecine et de Pharmacie Coloniales* 30 (1932): 599–602.

Léger, Marcel. "La tuberculose au Sénégal. Étude historique." *Bulletin du Comité d'Études Historiques et Scientifiques de l'AOF,* 5 (1922): 529–48.

———. "Considérations sur l'épidémiologie de la peste. L'homme peut, comme le rat, être réservoir de virus." *Revue de Médecine et d'Hygiène Tropicales* 15 (1923): 209–10.

———. "Souche pesteuse isolée des porteurs sains humains et sa virulence comparée." *Bulletin de la Société de Pathologie Exotique* 16 (1923): 54–57.

---. "La peste au Sénégal de 1914 à 1924." *Annales de Médecine et de Pharmacie Coloniales* 24 (1926): 289–318.

---. "Rôle non exclusif des rats réservoirs de la peste." *Bulletin de la Société de Pathologie Exotique* 23 (1930): 564–68.

---. "La peste à la conquête de l'Afrique." Communiqué présenté à l'Académie des Sciences Coloniales, séance du 3 janvier 1934. *Revue Coloniale de Médecine et de Chirurgie* (1934): 354–64.

Léger, Marcel, and A. Baury. "Porteurs sains de bacilles pesteux." *Compte-Rendu de l'Académie des Sciences* 175 (1922): 734–36.

Lewis, I. M. *Ecstatic Religion: An Anthropologic Study of Spirit Possession and Shamanism.* Harmondsworth, England: Penguin Books, 1971.

Lewis, Paul M., Milton H. Buehler, and T. Roy Young, Jr. "Plague in Dakar." *Bulletin of the U.S. Army Medical Department* 87 (1945): 13–16.

Low, Bruce. *Reports on Public Health and Medical Subjects, no. 3: The Progress and Diffusion of Plague, Cholera and Yellow Fever throughout the World, 1914–1917.* London: Ministry of Health, 1920.

Lubell, Harold, and Charbe Zarour. "Resilience amidst Crisis: The Informal Sector of Dakar." *International Labour Review* 129 (1990): 387–96.

Lunn, Joe. *Memoirs of the Maelstrom: A Senegalese Oral History of the First World War.* Portsmouth, N.H.: Heinemann, 1999.

Lyons, Maryinez. *The Colonial Disease: A Social History of Sleeping Sickness in Northern Zaire, 1900–1940.* Cambridge: Cambridge University Press, 1992.

---. "The Power to Heal: African Medical Auxiliaries in Colonial Belgian Congo and Uganda." In *Contesting Colonial Hegemony: State and Society in Africa and India.* Edited by Dagmar Engels and Shula Marks. London: British Academic Press, 1994, 202–23.

Manchuelle, François. *Willing Migrants: Soninke Labor Diasporas, 1848–1960.* Athens, Ohio: Ohio University Press, 1997.

Manning, Patrick. *Slavery, Colonialism and Economic Growth in Dahomey, 1640–1960.* Cambridge: Cambridge University Press, 1982.

Marcandier, André. "Note sur les vaccinations contre la peste faites pendant et après l'épidémie de Dakar (1914–1915–1916)." *Bulletin de la Société de Pathologie Exotique* 9 (1916): 592–600.

---. "La peste à Dakar (1914–15)." *Archives de Médecine Navale* 106 (1918): 125–45; 191–219.

Marchoux, E., A. Salimbeni, and P. L. Simond. "La fièvre jaune." *Annales de l'Institut Pasteur* 17 (1903): 665–731.

Marcovich, Anne. "French Colonial Medicine and Colonial Rule: Algeria and Indochina." In *Disease, Medicine and Empire: Perspectives on Western Medicine and the Experience of European Expansion.* Edited by Roy MacLeod and Milton Lewis. London: Routledge, 1988, 103–17.

Marone, Ibrahima. "Le Tidjanisme au Sénégal." *Bulletin de l'IFAN* 32, sér.B (1970): 136–215.

Martin, M. "Le médecin colonial." In *Histoire des médecins et pharmaciens de marine et des colonies.* Edited by Pierre Pluchon. Paris: Éditions Privat, 1985, 257–79.

Martin du Gard, Maurice. *La carte impériale: Histoire de la France Outre-Mer, 1940–45.* Paris: A. Bonne, 1949.

Marty, Paul. *Études sur l'Islam au Sénégal*. Vol.1. Paris: Ernest Leroux, 1917.
Mathis, Constant. *L'oeuvre des Pastoriens en Afrique noire, Afrique occidentale française*. Paris: Presses Universitaires de France, 1946.
Mathis, Constant, and Marcel Advier. "Considérations épidémiques sur la peste au Sénégal." *Bulletin de la Société de Pathologie Exotique* 25 (1932): 941–44.
Mbokolo, Elikia. "Peste et société urbaine à Dakar: L'épidémie de 1914." *Cahiers d'Études Africaines* 22 (1982): 13–46.
McClain, Charles J. *In Search of Equality: The Chinese Struggle against Discrimination in Nineteenth Century America*. Berkeley: University of California Press, 1994.
McNeill, William H. *Plagues and Peoples*. New York: Doubleday Anchor, 1976.
Meyer, K. F., D. Cavanaugh, O. Bartelloni, and J. Marshall. "Plague Immunization I. Past and Present Trends." *Journal of Infectious Diseases* 129 (Supplement) (1974): 513–18.
Michel, Marc. *L'appel à l'Afrique: Contributions et réaction à l'effort de guerre en AOF, 1914–1919*. Paris: Publications de la Sorbonne, 1982.
———. "Le corps de santé des troupes coloniales." In *Histoire des médecins et pharmaciens de marine et des colonies*. Edited by Pierre Pluchon. Paris: Editions Privat, 1985, 185–212.
Miller, Joseph. "Demographic History Revisited: Review Article," *Journal of African History* 25 (1984): 93–96.
Mollaret, Henri, and Jacqueline Brossolet. *Alexandre Yersin, le vainqueur de la peste*. Paris: Fayard, 1985.
Monnais-Rousselot, Laurence. *Médecine et colonisation: L'aventure indochinoise, 1860–1939*. Paris: Éditions CNRS, 1999.
Moore, Henrietta, and Megan Vaughan. *Cutting down Trees: Gender, Nutrition, and Agricultural Change in the Northern Province of Zambia, 1890–1990*. London: James Currey, 1994.
Moreau, N. "Note sur le service médical du lazaret de Saint-Louis (Sénégal) pendant l'épidémie de peste de 1929." *Annales de Médecine et de Pharmacie Coloniales* 28 (1930): 218–35.
Morgenthau, Ruth Schachter. *Political Parties in French-Speaking West Africa*. Oxford: Clarendon Press, 1964.
Mortimer, Edward. *France and the Africans, 1944–1960: A Political History*. London: Faber and Faber, 1969.
Moulin, Anne-Marie. "Patriarchal Science: The Network of the Overseas Pasteur Institutes." In *Science and Empires: Historical Studies about Scientific Development and European Expansion*. Edited by Patrick Petitjean, Catherine Jami, and Anne-Marie Moulin. Dordrecht, Holland: Kluwer, 1992, 307–21.
———. "Tropical without the Tropics: The Turning-Point of Pastorian Medicine in North Africa." In *Warm Climates and Western Medicine: The Emergence of Tropical Medicine, 1500–1900*. Edited by David Arnold. Atlanta: Rodopi B.V., 1996, 160–80.
Mudimbe, Valentin Y. *The Invention of Africa: Gnosis, Philosophy, and the Order of Knowledge*. Bloomington: Indiana University Press, 1988.
Nelkin, Dorothy, and Sander L. Gilman. "Placing Blame for Devastating Disease." *Social Research* 55 (1988): 361–78.

Neushul, Peter. "Fighting Research: Army Participation in the Clinical Testing and Mass Production of Penicillin during the Second World War." In *War, Medicine and Modernity*. Edited by Roger Cooter, Mark Harrison, and Steve Sturdy. England: Sutton Publishing, 1998, 203–24.

Ngom, Thiécouta. "Appropriate Standards for Infrastructure in Dakar." In *African Cities in Crisis*. Edited by Richard E. Stren and Rodney R. White. Boulder, Colo.: Westview Press, 1989, 177–202.

Nguyen Van Chi, Régine, ed. *L'atlas national du Sénégal*. Paris: Institut Géographique National, 1977.

Nikiforuk, Andrew. *The Fourth Horseman: A Short History of Epidemics, Plagues, Famine and Other Scourges*. Toronto: Viking Penguin, 1991.

1991 Red Book, The: Report of the Committee on Infectious Diseases. 22nd edition. Elk Grove, Ill.: American Academy of Pediatrics, 1991.

Nossal, G.V.J. *Antibodies and Immunities*. Second edition. New York: Basic Books, 1978.

Osborne, Michael A. "Resurrecting Hippocrates: Hygienic Sciences and the French Scientific Expeditions to Egypt, Morea and Algeria." In *Warm Climates and Western Medicine: The Emergence of Tropical Medicine, 1500–1900*. Edited by David Arnold. Atlanta: Rodopi B.V., 1996, 80–98.

Packard, Randall. "Maize, Cattle and Mosquitoes: The Political Economy of Malaria Epidemics in Colonial Swaziland." *Journal of African History* 25 (1984): 189–212.

———. *White Plague, Black Labor: Tuberculosis and the Political Economy of Health and Disease in South Africa*. Berkeley: University of California Press, 1989.

Park, Katharine. "Black Death." In *The Cambridge World History of Human Disease*. Edited by Kenneth Kiple. New York: Cambridge University Press, 1992, 612–16.

Pasquier, Roger. "Villes du Sénégal au XIXe siècle." *Revue Française d'Histoire d'Outre-Mer* 47, nos. 168/69 (1960): 387–426.

Patterson, K. David, "Bibliographic Essay." In *Disease in African History: An Introductory Survey and Case Studies*. Edited by Gerald W. Hartwig and K. David Patterson. Durham, N.C.: Duke University Press, 1978, 238–50.

Patton, Adell, Jr. *Physicians, Colonial Racism, and Diaspora in West Africa*. Gainsville: University Press of Florida, 1996.

Pélissier, Paul. *Les paysans du Sénégal*. Saint-Yrieix, France: Imprimerie Fabrègue, 1966.

Peltier, M. "La pathologie de la presqu'île du Cap-Vert." *Études Sénégalaises* 1 (1949): 209–38.

Phillips, Howard. *"Black October": The Impact of the Spanish Influenza Epidemic of 1918 on South Africa*. Pretoria: Government Printer, 1990.

Pirot, Dr. Robert. "Cinquante années d'endémies tropicales." *Compte-Rendus Mensuels des Séances de l'Académie des Sciences d'Outre-Mer* 30 (1970): 98–105.

Pluchon, Pierre, ed. *Histoire des médecins et pharmaciens de marine et des colonies*. Paris: Éditions Privat, 1985.

Pollitzer, R. *Plague*. Geneva: WHO, 1954.

Porter, Roy. *The Greatest Benefit to Mankind: A Medical History of Humanity from Antiquity to the Present.* London: Harper Collins, 1997.
Prins, Gwyn. "But What Was the Disease? The Present State of Health and Healing in African Studies." *Past and Present*, no. 124 (1989): 158–79.
Pyenson, Lewis. *Civilizing Mission: Exact Science and French Overseas Expansion, 1830–1940.* Baltimore: Johns Hopkins Press, 1993.
Ramsey, George H. "Yellow Fever in Senegal, with Special Reference to 1926 and 1927 Epidemics." *American Journal of Hygiene* 13, no. 1 (1931): 129–63.
Ranger, Terence O. "Godly Medicine: The Ambiguities of Medical Mission in Southeastern Tanzania, 1900–1945." In *The Social Basis of Health and Healing in Africa.* Edited by Steven Feierman and John M. Janzen. Berkeley: University of California Press, 1992, 256–82.
Remlinger, P. "La peste au Maroc." *Revue d'Hygiène et de Police Sanitaire* 35 (1913): 11–24.
Ribot, Georges and Robert Lafon. *Dakar. Ses origines, son avenir.* Bordeaux: G. Delmas, 1908.
Risse, Guenter B. "History of Western Medicine from Hippocrates to Germ Theory." In *The Cambridge World History of Human Disease.* Edited by Kenneth Kiple. Cambridge: Cambridge University Press, 1993, 11–19.
Roberts, Richard. "Text and Testimony in the *Tribunal de Première Instance*, Dakar, during the Early Twentieth Century." *Journal of African History* 31 (1990): 447–63.
Robinson, David. *The Holy War of Umar Tal: The Western Sudan in the Mid-Nineteenth Century.* Oxford: Clarendon Press, 1985.
Rodenwaldt, Ernst and Helmut J. Jusatz, eds. *Welt-Seuchen Atlas (World Atlas of Epidemic Disease).* Hamburg: Falk-Verlag, 1961, Vol. 2, 47–48; and Vol. 3, 86–87.
Rosenberg, Charles E. "What Is an Epidemic? AIDS in Historical Perspective." *Daedalus* 118 (1989): 1–17.
Rosenblatt, P. C., R. Walsh, and A. Jackson. *Grief and Mourning in Cross-Cultural Perspective.* New Haven, Conn: Human Relations Area File Press, 1974.
Rouamba, Étienne-Goama. "La vie d'un infirmier du services des grandes endémies." In *La Haute-Volta coloniale: Témoignages, recherches, regards.* Edited by Gabriel Massa and Y. Georges Madiéga. Paris: Karthala, 1995, 385–93.
Rousseau, Paul. "Au sujet de la peste du Sénégal." *Journal des Praticiens* 31 (1917): 738–44.
Ruegsegger, James M., and Huntington Gilchrist. "Plague: A study of Recent Developments in the Prevention and Treatment of the Disease." *American Journal of Tropical Medicine* 27 (1947): 683–89.
Sabatier, Peggy. "Did Africans Really Learn to be French? The Francophone Elite of the Ecole William Ponty." In *Double Impact: France and Africa in the Age of Imperialism.* Edited by G. Wesley Johnson. Westport, Conn.: Greenwood Press, 1985, 179–87.
Salem, Gérard. *La santé dans la ville: Géographie d'une petit espace dense: Pikine (Sénégal).* Paris: Karthala, 1998.
Sankalé, Marc. *Médecins et action sanitaire en Afrique noire.* Paris: Présence Africaine, 1969.
Sarraut, Albert. *La mise en valeur des colonies françaises.* Paris: Payot, 1923.

Savonnet, Georges. "Une ville neuve du Sénégal: Thiès." *Cahiers d'Outre-Mer* (1956): 70–93.
Schmidt, Elizabeth. *Peasants, Traders and Wives: Shona Women in the History of Zimbabwe, 1870–1939.* Portsmouth, N.H.: Heinemann, 1992.
Schneider, William. *Quality and Quantity: The Quest for Biological Regeneration in Twentieth-Century France.* Cambridge: Cambridge University Press, 1990.
Schwabe, Calvin W. *Veterinary Medicine and Human Health.* Third Edition. Baltimore: Williams and Wilkins, 1984.
Sebire, A. *Les plantes utiles du Sénégal.* Paris: Baillière, 1895.
Seck, Assane. *Dakar, métropole ouest-africaine.* Dakar: IFAN, 1970.
Seck, Papa Ibrahima. *La stratégie culturelle de la France en Afrique: L'enseignement colonial (1817–1960).* Paris: L'Harmattan, 1993.
Silla, Eric *"People Are Not the same": Leprosy and Identity in Twentieth Century Mali.* Portsmouth, N.H.: Heinemann, 1998.
Sinn, Elizabeth. *Power and Charity: The Early History of the Tung Wah Hospital.* Hong Kong: Oxford University Press, 1989.
Sinou, Alain. *Comptoirs et villes coloniales du Sénégal: Saint-Louis, Gorée, Dakar.* Paris: Karthala, 1993.
Slack, Paul. *The Impact of Plague in Tudor and Stuart England.* Oxford: Clarendon Press, 1985.
Smith, Gaddis. *American Diplomacy during the Second World War, 1941–1945.* New York: Wiley, 1965.
Snyder, Francis. "Health Policy and the Law in Senegal." *Social Science and Medicine* 8 (1979): 11–28.
Sorel, F.P.J. "La fièvre jaune chez les indigènes à Dakar en 1927." *Bulletin de la Société de Pathologie Exotique* 21 (1928): 509–11.
———. "L'épidémie de fièvre jaune à Dakar." *Compte-Rendu de l'Académie des Sciences* 12 (1932): 545–55.
Sorel, F.P.J., and M. Armstrong. "La lutte préventive contre la peste dans la circonscription de Dakar et dépendances durant l'année 1928." *Annales de Médecine et de Pharmacie Coloniales* 27 (1929): 64–72.
Sow, Fatima. "Pikine, Senegal: A Reading of a Contemporary African City." In *Reading the Contemporary African City.* Edited by the Aga Khan Foundation. Singapore: Concept Media, 1982, 45–60.
Suret-Canale, Jean, *French Colonialism in Tropical Africa, 1900–1945.* Translated by Till Gottheiner. London: C. Hurst and Co., 1971.
Sutphen, Mary. "Not What, but Where: Bubonic Plague and the Reception of Germ Theories in Hong Kong and Calcutta." *Journal of the History of Medicine and Allied Sciences* 52 (1997): 81–113.
———. "Rumoured Power: Hong Kong, 1894 and Cape Town, 1901." In *Western Medicine as Contested Knowledge.* Edited by Andrew Cunningham and Bridie Andrews. Manchester: Manchester University Press, 1997.
Swanson, Maynard. "The Sanitation Syndrome: Bubonic Plague and Urban Native Policy in the Cape Colony, 1900–1909." *Journal of African History* 18 (1977): 387–410.

Sylla, Assane. *Le peuple Lébou de la presqu''le du Cap-Vert*. Dakar: Les Nouvelles Éditions Africaines du Sénégal, 1992.
Tuchman, Barbara W. *The Guns of August*. New York: Dell, 1962.
Turshen, Meredeth. *The Political Ecology of Disease in Tanzania*. New Brunswick, N.J.: Rutgers University Press, 1984.
Vaillant, Janet G. *Black, French and African: A Life of Léopold Sédar* Senghor. Cambridge: Harvard University Press, 1990.
Van Heyningen, Elizabeth. "Cape Town and the Plague of 1901." In *Studies in the History of Cape Town*. Vol. 4. Edited by Christopher Saunders, Howard Phillips, and Elizabeth van Heyningen. Cape Town: University of Cape Town, 1981, 66–107.
Vaughan, Megan. *Curing their Ills: Colonial Power and African Illness*. Stanford, Calif.: Stanford University Press, 1991.
———. "Health and Hegemony: Representation of Disease and the Creation of the Colonial Subject in Nyasaland." In *Contesting Colonial Hegemony: State and Society in Africa and India*. Edited by Dagmar Engels and Shula Marks. London: British Academic Press, 1994, 173–201.
Villalon, Leonardo A. *Islamic Society and State Power in Senegal: Disciples and Citizens in Fatick*. Cambridge: Cambridge University Press, 1995.
Viorst, Milton. *Hostile Allies: FDR and Charles de Gaulle*. New York: Macmillan, 1965.
Waite, Gloria. "Public Health in Pre-colonial East-Central Africa." In *The Social Basis of Health and Healing in Africa*. Edited by Steven Feierman and John M. Janzen. Berkeley: University of California Press, 1992, 212–31.
Wakil, A. W. *The Third Pandemic of Plague in Egypt: Historical Statement and Epidemic Remarks on the First Thirty-Two Years of Its Prevalence*. Cairo: Egyptian University, 1932.
Wane, A. A. Ousmane. "La croissance urbaine au Sénégal: Urbanisation et extension de Dakar." *Mondes en Développement* 13 (1985): 553–580.
Wassilieff, Alexandre. "Observations sur les puces de la région de Cayor." *Bulletin de la Société de Pathologie Exotique* 23 (1930): 474–78.
———. "Recherches sur l'épidémiologie pesteuse au Sénégal en 1929. Les reservoirs du virus (suite)." *Bulletin de la Société de Pathologie Exotique* 23 (1930): 737–47.
Webb, James. *Desert Frontier: Ecological and Economic Change along the Western Sahel, 1600–1850*. Madison: University of Wisconsin Press, 1995.
White, Luise. "Vampire Priests of Central Africa: African Debates about Labor and Religion in Colonial Northern Zambia." *Comparative Studies in Society and History* 35 (1993): 746–72.
———. "Tsetse Visions: Narratives of Blood and Bugs in Colonial Northern Rhodesia." *Journal of African History* 36 (1995): 219–45.
Whittlesey, Derwent. "Dakar and the Other Cape Verde Settlements." *Geographical Review* 31 (1941): 609–38.
———. "Dakar Revisited." *Geographical Review* 38 (1948): 626–32.
Willis, Roy. "Magic and 'Medicine' in Ufipa." In *Culture and Curing: Anthropological Perspectives on Traditional Medical Beliefs and Practices*. Edited by Peter Morley and Roy Willis. London: Peter Owen, 1978, 139–51.

Wiltse, Charles M. *United States Army in World War II. The Technical Services. The Medical Department: Medical Service in the Mediterranean and Minor Theaters.* Washington, D.C.: Office of the Chief of Medical History, Department of the Army, 1945.

Wondji, Christophe. "La fièvre jaune à Grand-Bassam, 1899–1903." *Revue Française d'Histoire d'Outre-Mer* 59 (1972): 204–39.

Worboys, Michael. "The Emergence of Tropical Medicine: A Study in the Establishment of a Scientific Specialty." In *Perspectives on the Emergence of Scientific Disciplines.* Edited by Gérard Lemaine et al. The Hague: Mouton, 1976, 75–98.

Wylie, Diana. "The Changing Face of Hunger in Southern African History, 1880–1980." *Past and Present*, no. 122 (1989): 159–99.

———. *Starving on a Full Stomach: Hunger and the Triumph of Cultural Racism in Modern South Africa.* Charlottesville: University Press of Virginia, 2001.

Yersin, Alexandre. "La peste bubonique à Hong Kong." *Annales de l'Institut Pasteur* 8 (1894): 662–67.

Ziegler, Philip. *The Black Death.* Harmondsworth, England: Penguin, 1970.

UNPUBLISHED MATERIAL

Becker, Charles. "Les Serer Ndut: Études sur les mutations sociales et réligieuses." Mémoire de l'École Pratique des Hautes-Etudes, Paris, 1970.

Benga, Ndiouga Adrien. "L'évolution politique de la ville de Dakar de 1924 à 1960." Mémoire de maitrîse, Université Cheikh Anta Diop, Dakar, 1989.

Ciss, Ismaila. "Les Sereer du Nord-Ouest." Mémoire de maitrîse, Université de Dakar, Dakar, 1981–82.

Dawson, Marc Harry. "Socio-Economic and Epidemiological Change in Kenya, 1880–1925." Ph.D. dissertation, University of Wisconsin, Madison, 1983.

Dieng, Mamadou Moustapha. "Les épidémies au Sénégal au XIXe siècle: Méthodologies et perspectives de recherches." Rapport de D.E.A. en Histoire, Université de Dakar, October, 1984.

Diop, Angélique. "Santé et colonisation au Sénégal, 1895–1914." Thèse de troisième cycle, Université de Paris I, Paris, 1982.

Diouf, Tekheye. Six-page manuscript on traditional healing in Siin, Niakhar, 17 June 1989. Provided by Charles Becker.

———. "Traditions du Sine." Manuscript, unnumbered pages, with sixteen topics. Provided by Charles Becker.

Elshafei, Shereef. "Municipal Council in Turn of the Century Alexandria: The Politics of Urban Autonomy." Master's research paper, McGill University, Montreal, 1999.

Fall, Rokhaya. "Le Royaume du Bawol du XVIè au XIXè siècle: Pouvoir wolof et rapports avec les populations Séreer." Thèse de troisième cycle, Université de Paris I, Paris, 1983.

Gaye, Papa Amadou. "La diffusion institutionnelle du discours sur le microbe au Sénégal au cours de la Troisième République française (1870–1940)." Thése de doctorat, Université de Paris VII, Paris, 1997.

Giblin, James L. "The Vichy Years in French Africa: A Period of African Resistance to Capitalism." Master's dissertation, McGill University, Montreal, 1978.

Grimaud, Aimée (née Houémavo). "Les médecins africains en A.O.F.: Étude sociohistorique sur la formation d'une élite coloniale." Mémoire de maitrîse, Université de Dakar, Dakar, 1979.

Heckenroth, Ferdinand. "Le problème de la salubrité publique à Dakar." Dakar, Gouvernement-Général de l'AOF, 1921, 436 pp. duplicated report, located in ANS\H22, but with pages 123–269 missing.

Lewis, Major Paul M. Lewis, A.U.S., Captain Milton H. Buehler, Jr., A.U.S., and Lieutenant T. Roy Young, U.S.N.R. "A Report on Plague in Dakar, Senegal, F.W.A., 1944. 43 pp., graphs, two large maps, and photographs. Available at U.S. Army Military History Institute, Carlisle, Pa. Filed as Professional Papers, Box no. 68.

Maillat, Maurice. "Dakar sous la flamme de guerre." No date, probably post 1968. 16 pages. Unpublished memoirs of former employee of chemin de fer and sometime reservist in 6e RAC.

Malowany, Maureen. "Medical Pluralism: Disease, Health, and Healing on the Coast of Kenya, 1840–1940." Ph.D. dissertation, McGill University, Montreal, 1997.

Moitt, Bernard. "Peanut Production and Social Change in the Dakar Hinterland: Kajoor and Bawol, 1840–1940." Ph.D. dissertation, University of Toronto, 1985.

Musambachime, M. C. "The Bubonic Plague Epidemic in Karonga (Northern Malawi) and the North East Luangwa Valley (Eastern Zambia) between 1916 and 1920." Unpublished paper, Department of History, University of Namibia, 1999.

Ngalamulume, Kalala J. "City Growth, Health Problems, and Colonial Government Response: Saint-Louis (Senegal) from Mid-Nineteenth Century to the First World War." Ph.D. dissertation, Michigan State University, East Lansing, 1996.

Pheffer, Paul E. "Railroads and Aspects of Social Change in Senegal, 1878–1933." Ph.D. dissertation, University of Pennsylvania, Philadelphia, 1975.

Roberts, Jonathan. "The Black Death in the Gold Coast: African and British Responses to the Bubonic Plague Epidemic of 1908." Master's research paper, McGill University, Montreal, 1998.

Ross, Eric. "Cités sacrées du Sénégal: Essai de géographie spirituelle." Mémoire de maitrîse, Université de Québec à Montréal, Montreal, 1989.

Salleras, Bruno. "La politique sanitaire de la France à Dakar de 1900 à 1920." Mémoire de maitrîse, Paris X, Université de Nanterre, Paris, 1980.

———. "La peste à Dakar en 1914: Médina, ou les enjeux complexes d'une politique sanitaire." Thèse de troisième cycle, Université de Paris, École des Hautes Études en Sciences Sociales, Paris, 1984.

Sankalé, Marc. "La peste au Sénégal (1914–1938): Données épidémiologiques et cliniques." Thèse de Médecine, Université de Montpellier, Montpellier, 1944.

Searing, James F. "Accommodation and Resistance: Chiefs, Muslim Leaders, and Politicians in Colonial Senegal, 1890–1934." Ph.D. dissertation, Princeton University, Princeton, 1985.

Simond, Marc. "Le dépistage de l'infection pesteuse en pratique coloniale." Thèse de Médicine, Université de Montpellier, Montpellier, 1944.
Sinou, Alain. "Idéologies et pratiques de l'urbanisme dans le Sénégal colonial." Thèse de troisième cycle, Université de Paris, École des Hautes Études en Sciences Sociales, Paris, 1985.
Thiam, Iba Der. "L'évolution politique et syndicale du Sénégal colonial de 1840 à 1936." Nine volumes. Thèse d'état, Université de Paris I, Paris, 1982–83.

INDEX

Abdu, Muhammad, 151
ACSE (Archives of the Congrégation du Saint-Esprit), 8
ADs (African Auxiliary Doctors), 201–2
Advier, Marcel, 195
African medical assistants, 27
Aita, Demba, 61–62
Alexandria, Egypt, 117
Alexis, M., 188
Algeria, 7, 148, 203, 256
Allied Forces: in FWA, 213; in Normandy, 215; in North Africa, 213
AMI (Assistance Médicale Indigène), 27, 207 n.50, 257
Anglo-Egyptian Sudan, 4, 6
Aniodol (commercial antiseptic), 99, 105–6
ANS (Archives Nationales du Sénégal), 8
Antibiotics: as therapy for bubonic plague, 19, 21. *See also* Penicillin; Streptomycin; Sulfa drugs
Anti-plague vaccination, 21, 40 n.28, 66–67, 69, 78–79, 96–98, 103–5, 121, 126, 163, 169, 181 n.66, 185, 192, 224–25, 258–59. *See also* E.V. 76 (Madagascar) vaccine; Girard-Robic vaccine; Haffkine's vaccine

Antonetti, Raphaël, 64, 73, 78, 81–83, 85 n.27, 123, 125, 131
Antu (rodenticide), 227, 240
AOF, L' (newspaper), 35, 59–60, 66, 99, 131
Applied School of Medicine (L'École pratique de médecine), 201
Arnold, David, 262
Assimilation, as French colonial doctrine, 35, 198
Association, as French colonial doctrine, 198
Austen, Ralph, 248 n.57

Ba, Amadou, 237
Baba, Cheikh Sidia, 151
Bacteriophage, as therapy against bubonic plague, 226
Bado, Jean-Paul, 8
Bambara, 122
Bambey, town of, 217
Bargny (district of Rufisque), 188, 214, 269
Barnes, Maynard B., (American Consul in Dakar), 215–16, 233
Barros, Dr., 54, 109 n.6
Barthélémy, Georges, 199
Bawol, kingdom of, 121, 143
Becker, Charles, 8, 145

Bel-Air, 235; lazaretto in, 95, 123, 185–86, 191
Bell, Heather, 4, 6
Bello, Muhammad, 158 n.71
Beriberi, 98
Betts, Raymond, 73, 86 n.49
Bilharzia, 18
Black Death, 16, 19. See also Bubonic plague, second pandemic of
BLFWA (Bacteriological Laboratory of French West Africa), 31, 54, 91, 102, 106–7, 109, 124, 192–93. See also PID
Boilat, Abbé, 25
Boisson, Pierre, 213
Bordeaux trading houses, 34, 36, 37
Bouche, Denise, 259–60
Boutrais, Father J., 177; and bubonic plague in Mont-Roland, 145–47
Brazzaville Conference, and health reforms in French Africa, 256–58
Bubonic plague: and Africa, 16; and Cape Town, 7; and China, 16; control measures against, 223–33; disappearance and legacy of, 242, 258–61, 262–63; etiology of, 17–19, 139–42; and Europe, 16; financial costs of, 123–27; first pandemic of, 16; and Grand-Bassam, Ivory Coast, 24; and India, 16, 18, 21; and Indonesia, 16; and Madagascar, 7; and Manchuria, 11 n.8; and Mauritania, 259; and Naples, 236; second pandemic of, 16, 20; in Senegal, 20–21, 40 nn.25, 28, 117–20, 122–24, 137, 142; and South America, 16; third pandemic of, 16, 92; and Tunisia, 7. See also Black Death; Justinian's Plague; Statistics; *Yersinia pestis*
Buehler, Captain Milton H., Jr., 237; and vector control in Dakar, 1944, 239–40
Bulletin du comité de l'Afrique française, 68
Burial, and plague control, 101–2, 224–25

Burkina Faso, 8. See also Upper Volta

Caland, M., 63, 106, 109 n.6
Calmette, Albert, 110 n.7
Cambérène (district of Dakar), 92, 116, 118, 120
Cape Manuel (Dakar), lazaretto for Europeans and *originaires* at, 185, 224
Cape Town, 4, 117
Cape Verde Peninsula, 10, 92–93, 98, 116, 118, 121, 260; *cordons sanitaires* in, 93; and the plague zone, 141
Carde, Jules (Governor-General), 198, 201, 257
Carmichael, Ann, 16
Carpot, François, 35–37, 197
Ceddo, 143, 139
Central African Republic, 8
CGT (Confédération Générale du Travail), 260
Chambres (*kompe xoore*), 199
Cheneveau, Dr., 227
Children's diseases in Senegal, 221
Cholera, 5, 7, 11 n.7, 23–24, 41 n.31, 124, 169, 181 n.64
Chronic diseases in Senegal, 221
Churchill, Winston, 214, 243 n.2
Ciss, brothers Adama and Mar, 170–71, 173
Cohen, William, 7–8
Collignon, René, 8
Collomb, Dr., 188
Colonial Health Brigades, 108, 110 n.7, 169, 188, 191, 224
Comaroff, Jean, 6
Congrégation du Saint-Esprit (Pères Spiritains), 145–46
Congrégation du Saint-Joseph de Cluny (Sisters of), 24
Conklin, Alice, 27
Conspiracy theories and the Dakar plague of 1914, 65–68
Cooper, Frederick, 90, 246 n.30, 257
Coppet, J. M. de, (Governor-General), 150

Index

Cor, Henri, (Governor of Senegal), 35, 36, 60
Cordell, Dennis, 8
Cordon sanitaire, 59–60, 78, 92–94, 118–19, 121, 126, 224; harmful results of, 97–98; in the plague zone, 168; in Rufisque, 187
Creoles, 33, 34, 37, 46 n.120
Crespin, Georges, 35
Cricetomys gambiae (giant rat), 107. *See also* Rodents
Crocidura stampflii (African wild rodent), 113 n.77. *See also* Rodents
Crowd control, and bubonic plague, 224
Curtin, Philip, 6

Dagana, 24, 149
Dahomey, 201
Dakar, 4–5, 10–11, 24, 27–29, 31–32, 53–56, 70–71, 82, 92, 106, 108, 115–16, 142, 144, 149–51, 184–87, 190–91, 199, 222–24, 256, 258–60, 262; plague control measures, 223–33; and plague outbreak of 1914, 58–84; and plague outbreak of 1944, 211–18
Dakar Health Committee, 56, 58–59, 68–69, 80, 82, 92–93, 103, 185
Dakar Health Service, 53–54, 125, 199, 220, 221, 224, 227
Dakar Municipal Council, 60, 63, 100
Dakar-Niger railway station, 215
Dakar-Saint-Louis railway line, 141, 144; and bubonic plague, 192, 215–16
Darou Alfa, village of, 147, 174
DDT (Dichloro-diphenyl-trichlorothane), 11, 21–22, 41 n.38, 211, 259; in the Dakar plague outbreak of 1944, 227–33
De Gaulle, Charles, 213, 256
Démocratie, La (newspaper), 30, 34, 61, 65, 77, 197. *See also Ouest-Africain Français, L'*
Devès, François, 112 n.56, 123, 189
Devès, Justin, 35–36
Diagne, Abdel-Kader, 237

Diagne, Adolphe, 47 n.145, 194
Diagne, Blaise, 15, 30, 33–37, 51, 62, 65, 67, 75–77, 81, 98, 131–32, 138, 151, 187, 194, 197–98, 238
Diagne, Pierre, 237
Diagnism. *See* Diagne, Blaise
Dieng, Cheikh, 167
Diop, Ngo Laba, 163–64
Diop, Papa Mar, 34
Diop, Thiécouta, 34
Dior, Lat, 144
Diouf, Chief Coumba Ndoffène, 163, 167, 208 n.53
Diouf, Galandou, 34–35, 66, 76, 81–82, 188, 198, 238
Diouf, Ko, 164
Diouf, Marie-Anne Yaayo, 168, 170, 174–78, 181 n.66
Diouf, Tekheye, 171
Diourbel, 27, 101, 116, 119, 122, 142, 146, 164, 217, 255
Diphtheria, 256
Disease ecology, 5, 6, 262–63
Disinfection, and plague control, 95, 99, 100, 191–92, 224
Domergue-Cloarec, Danielle, 8
D'Oxoby, Daramy Jean, 34, 36, 63
Dozon, Jean-Pierre, 8
Drought, 218, 222
Duguay-Clédor, Amadou, 34, 62, 189
Dupire, Marguerite, 138 n.1, 160, 163, 173
Durieux, M., 241, 259
Dysentery, in Senegal, 17

Éboué, Félix, 256–57
École Faidherbe, 201
Economic impact of Second World War on Senegal, 223
Eden, Anthony, 214
Egypt, 151
Engels, Dagmar, 262
Esoavelomandroso, Faranirina, 7
Esquier, A., 185, 187
E.V. 76 (Madagascar) anti-plague vaccine, 21
Évolués, 257–60. *See also Originaires*

Eyam (Derbyshire, England), as a plague hecatomb, 97

Faculty of Medicine in Dakar, 258
Fall, Abdoulaye, Yaré, 197, 200–1, 262
Fanon, Frantz, 7, 130
Fatick, town of, 149
Faye, Guedj, 138 n.1
FEA (French Equatorial Africa), 8, 256–57
Feierman, Steven, 165
Fez (Morocco), 148–49
FIDES (Fonds pour l'Investissement et le Développement Économique et Social), 258
First World War, 69, 73–75, 109, 149
Fleas, 5, 17, 106–8, 192, 200, 228–33, 241. *See also Xenopsylla astia; Xenopsylla cheopis; Synosternus pallidus*
Foucault, Michel, 90, 196, 207 n.47
Fourmeaux, M., 63–64
France, bubonic plague cases in, 127, 134 n.43
Free French in Senegal, 213–14, 227, 234–36. *See also* Gaullists
French colonialism, 256–57; and indigenous healers, 150, 161; and public health in Senegal, 26–32, 108, 124, 257–58, 262
French expatriates in Senegal, 119, 228, 259
French Navy and bubonic plague in Senegal, 68, 95–97, 108, 120, 185, 215
French physicians in Senegal, 27, 90, 102, 110 n.7, 221
Front de Terre (district of Dakar), 244, 259
Funeral dirges, 174–79, 183 n.99
Fuulbe, 129–30, 141–42, 144, 158 n.71
FWA (French West Africa), 108–9, 141, 211, 213, 236

Gallagher, Nancy, 7, 11 n.2
Gaullists, 10, 211, 257
Gaye, Coumba, 174, 178–79, 182 n.66

Gaye, Papa Amadou, 151
General Council of Senegal, 73, 123, 188–90, 198
Gender. *See* women
Giblin, James, 6–7
Gilman, Sander L., 130
Girard, Georges, 196, 206 n.45, 218, 239–42, 255, 258, 263 n.1
Girard-Robic anti-plague vaccine, 225, 240
Glassford, Rear-Admiral William O., 213–14
Goerg, Odile, 6
Goodyear, John, U.S. Consul in Dakar, 233
Gorée, 24, 28, 201
Goux, Alfred, 238
Gramsci, Antonio, 262
Grand Dakar (district of Dakar), 262
Gregory, Joel, 8
Griot, 66, 174
Gris-gris (charms), 164
Guélor, village of, 116, 121–22
Guet Ndar (district of Saint-Louis), 189
Gueule Tapée (district of Dakar), 218
Guèye, Aly, 78–79
Guèye, Lamine, 34, 214, 237–38
Guèye, Samba, 78
Guèye, Shaykh Youssou Bamar, 35, 81

Haffkine, Waldemar, 20
Haffkine's anti-plague vaccine, 21, 41 n.35
Hann (district of Dakar), 92, 95, 121
Hann beach (Dakar), 214
Headrick, Rita, 8
Healers, 25, 26, 202; demonized by French health officials, 9, 26; in precolonial public health systems, 24, 43 n.58. *See also* Saltigi
Health budgets in Senegal, 123, 133 n.26, 258–59
Heckenroth, Dr. Ferdinand, 91, 185, 188, 190–93, 241
Heimburger, Henri, 35–37, 51
Henry, M., 186
HIV/AIDS, 261

Index

Hivernage, 119
Hock (district of Dakar), 70
Hong Kong, 16, 20, 117
Hospitals, 25, 52, 102, 115, 119, 185, 220, 241
Housing, 29–30, 218–20, 241
Hunter, Dr. R. N., 196, 225
Huot, Dr. L., 9, 56, 91, 98, 109 n.6, 118, 121

Incineration, and plague control, 99–100
India, 16, 18, 21, 262
Indochina, 256
Influenza, 6, 10
Insects, as disease vectors, 92. *See also* Fleas
ISC (International Sanitary Conferences), 20
Islam: and medicine in Senegal, 25, 151–52; and popular opposition to plague controls, 102–03
Ivory Coast, 8, 24, 108

Janzen, John, 24
Jojot, C., 29
Justinian's Plague, 16

Kajoor, kingdom of, 30, 36, 107, 142, 144, 148–49
Kane, Abdou Salam, 190
Kaolack, town of, 116, 122–23, 149, 152
Kébémer, 141, 217
Kenya, 196, 225
Kerharo, Joseph, 162
Kermorgant, Dr. Alexandre, 27, 91, 104–5, 118–19
Keur Daouda Ciss, village of, 147
Keur-Gallo-Isser, village of, 116, 118, 121
Khaldun, Ibn, 158 n.70
Khombole, town of, 121
Kirk, Joyce, 7
Kitasato, Shibasaburo, 20
Koch, Robert, 20, 41 n.30
Kooxa dooma ka (acute headaches), 9, 137, 138 n.1, 162

Kovacs, Dr., 259

Lafont, Dr. André, 54–55, 59, 91, 97, 101, 103, 118, 124–25
Laptot (African sailor), 96, 103, 107, 120, 215
Lazarettos, 20, 40 n.26, 121, 164, 166, 168, 181 n.60; in Dakar, 95, 125, 185, 191, 244, 259; in Rufisque, 188, 224, 248 n.65; in Saint-Louis, 189
Lebu, 28–29, 35, 74, 97, 119, 128–30, 141, 144, 162, 237; and land ownership in Dakar, 30, 36, 131; protest against plague controls, 60–62, 77–83, 185–86; relocation of, 70–72
Lefrou, Dr. G., 190
Léger, André, 109 n.5
Léger, Marcel, 109 n.5, 195–96, 259
Leopold II, King of Belgium, 27
Leprosy, in Mali, 8, 242
Lévecque, Governor Fernand, 186
Louga, town of, 28, 126, 141–42, 149, 233
Lyons, Maryinez, 6

Madagascar, 171, 182 n.91, 196, 225, 240
Maillat, Maurice, 225
Maison Peyrissac, 52, 61
Makka, Lake, 168, 181 n.60
Malaria, 8, 18, 40 n.23, 92, 221, 229; in Senegal, 17, 23, 124, 227–28, 250 n.94, 261
Malawi, 134 n.41, 262
Mali, 8, 242
Malika, village of, 215
Manchuelle, François, 197
Manchuria, 107
Manson, Patrick, 41 n.30
Marabouts, 9, 112 n.53, 149–50, 190, 239; as healers, 25, 152
Marcandier, Dr. André, 53, 82, 91–92, 96–97, 102–4, 108, 110 n.11, 115, 118–20, 127
Marcovitch, Anne, 8
Market boycott of 1914, 60–61

Marks, Shula, 262
Marsat, Fernand, 35, 47 n.132
Marseille, 97
Masson, Émile, 35, 37, 47 n.132, 52, 60–61, 63, 109 n.6
Matam, town of, 24
Mathis, Constant, 109 n.5, 195
Maurel, Dr., 24
Maurel et Prom, 47 n.132, 62–63, 216
Mauritania, 259
Mauritanians, 217
Mbacké, Ahmadu Bamba, 36, 128, 148, 150
Mbaye, Ndéné, 66
Mbaye, Serigne Sangoné, 148
Mbengue, Khayar, 190
Mbengue, Thérèse Tisa, 160, 181 n.53, 261
Mbengue, Thierno Amat, 237
Mbokolo, Elikia, 7–8, 125, 134 n.33, 135 n.51
McNeill, William H., 11 n.7
Mecca, 148
Meckhé, village of, 141
Medical crisis in Africa, 127
Medical pluralism in Senegal, 165
Medical researchers in Senegal, 91
Médina (district of Dakar), 71–73, 95, 123, 132, 185, 193, 197, 201, 215–16, 219, 224, 227–28, 230, 255, 260; unsanitary condition of, 126, 131, 222, 241, 259
Mérina, village of, 121, 182 n.91
Merlin, Governor-General Martial, 186–87, 198, 201
Michel, Marc, 74, 85 n.35, 110 n.7
Midwives, 25, 201
Migration, rural, 122; urban, 5, 22, 29, 119, 130, 155 n.23, 190, 199, 218, 261
Military labor brigades, 247 n.45
Monnais-Rousselot, Laurence, 8
Mont-Roland (villages of), 10, 141, 144–47, 154 n.15, 159, 168, 174. *See also* Tiwigne, village of; Tiwigne Diassa, village of; Tiwigne Tangor

Moroccans, in Senegal, 99, 101, 112 n.57, 130, 185, 239
Morocco, 108, 119, 213, 226
Moulin, Anne-Marie, 8
Mourid brotherhood, 36, 148–51
Mudimbe, Valentin, 90

Nayas, Al-Hajj Abdullah, 149
Ndiaganiao, village of, 116, 121–22
Ndiaye, Iba, 51–54, 61
Ndoye, Amadou Assane, 34–35
Nelkin, Dorothy, 130
Ngalamulume, Kalala J., 25, 157 n.63
Niakhar, village of, 154 n.22, 159, 181 n.64
Niayes (dunes), 141–44
Nicolle, Charles, 193, 206 n.39
Noc, Fernand, 109 n.5
Nurses, 202, 209 n.71
Nyasaland. *See* Malawi

Occupations, and susceptibility to bubonic plague, 190, 216, 218
Onchocerciasis, 8
Originaires, 33, 36, 51, 100, 131–32, 257–60. *See also* Évolués
Osborne, Michael, 8
Ouakam (district of Dakar), 78, 144, 214
Ouest-Africain Français, L' (newspaper), 197–98. *See also* Démocratie, La

Packard, Randall, 5, 263 n.5
Parc à Fourrages (district of Dakar), 80–82, 96, 103
Pasteur, Louis, 20, 102
Pasteur Institute. *See* PI
Pasteur Institute of Dakar. *See* PID
Patterson, David, 5
Pax Gallica, 5, 150
Peanuts, 144, 150, 241
Pellegrin, Louis, 35
Peltier, Dr. M., 259
Penicillin, 226, 249 n.83
Petit Sénégalais, Le (newspaper), 62
Pharmacists' assistants, 201
Phillips, Howard, 6

Index 301

Piché, Victor, 8
PI (Pasteur Institute), 8, 103, 105–6, 193, 196, 203, 226, 240
PID (Pasteur Institute of Dakar), 109 n.4, 193–97, 225–26, 240–42, 259. *See also* BLFWA
Pikine (district of Dakar), 260
Pinet-Laprade, Governor, 24
Pire, village of, 148–49
Plague zone, 10, 94, 140–42, 155 n.23, 269–70
Plateau (district of Dakar), 52, 184, 197, 214, 230, 255
Pneumonic plague. *See* Pulmonary plague
Podor, town of, 24
Ponty, Governor-General William, 28, 33, 35, 51, 53, 60–62, 64–65, 74–77, 79, 81, 83, 123, 130–31
Port Elizabeth (South Africa), 4
Pout, village of, 116, 118, 121, 144, 154 n.22
Prostitution, 221–22
Pulmonary plague, 19, 133 n.16

Qadiriyya brotherhood, 151, 156 n.51
Quarantine, and plague control, 92, 185, 191
Qur'an, 152

Randoulène (district of Thiès), 28
Ration books, and anti-plague vaccination, 239
Rats, 5, 18, 21, 106–8, 167, 226, 250 n.88. *See also* Rodents; *Rattus norvegicus*; *Rattus rattus*
Rattus norvegicus, 18
Rattus rattus, 18
Reform movements in Senegal, 237
Residential segregation: elsewhere in Africa, 6–7; in Dakar, 27–28, 69–73, 128, 187, 219, 241
Richard-Toll (Senegal Valley), 262
Robic, J., 196, 240
Robin, Dr. Charles, 241–42
Rodents, 17, 39 n.14, 107, 141, 192, 200–1, 216, 227. *See also*

Cricetomys gambiae; *Crocidura stampflii*; Rats; *Xerus erythropus*
Roman Catholics, 145–47, 149, 160
Roosevelt, Franklin D., 214
Rosenberg, Charles, 67
Roume, Governor-General Émile, 26–27, 33
Rousseau, Dr. Paul, 92, 101, 125–27
Roux, Émile, 41 n.30, 77
Rufisque, 24, 27, 28, 62, 66, 98–99, 116, 121, 125, 141, 144, 149– 50, 187–89, 224, 248 n.65
Rufisque Municipal Council, 188
Rural plague in Senegal, 120–23, 159– 83, 255–56, 269–70

Saint-Louis, 23–25, 27–28, 31, 34, 132, 144, 148, 150–51, 189–90, 262, 269– 70
Sall, Diawara, 168
Salleras, Bruno, 87 n.58, 124–25
Saltigi, 129, 161–63. *See also* Healers
Sarraut, Albert, 257
Santiaba (district of Dakar), 80, 95
Scapegoats, and bubonic plague, 130, 241–42, 261
Schmidt, Elizabeth, 183 n.99
Sebire, Father A., 145
Second World War in FWA, 237
Sen, Amartya, 12 n.19
Sène, Massène, 166–67
Sène, Moumar, 188
Senegal, 8, 9, 17, 22, 29, 44 n.90; electoral politics in, 32–36; medical crisis in, 22–26; post-colonial state, 261; war effort of, 74–75
Senegal Health Service, 9, 91, 109 n.6, 164, 167–74, 240–42
Senegal River valley, 119, 148, 199, 262
Senghor, Hélène, 49–50
Senghor, Léopold Sédar, 49, 238, 260– 61
Septicemic plague, 19
Sereer, 34, 36, 74, 122, 139, 160, 165; and bubonic plague, 160, 162–63, 171–74; disease etiology of, 160–61; funerals and, 129, 182 nn.86, 87, 183

n.93, 193–94; and plague zone, 141; religious beliefs of, 159–66
Sereer Léhar, 142
Sereer Ndut, 10, 139, 140–41, 154 n.16, 159, 161, 165; and bubonic plague, 163, 168–72; and plague zone, 142; religious affiliations of, 145–49, 160; territory of, 144–45; visions of bubonic plague, 152–53, 159–79
Sereer None, 142, 144; bubonic plague and, 147
Sereer Palor, 142
Sereer Safen, 142
Sergent, Jules, 34, 63, 189
SFIO (Section Française de l'Internationale Ouvrière), 238
Shaykh, 150, 152
SICAP (Société Immobilière du Cap-Vert), 260
Siin, Sereer of, 142, 144, 159, 161; and bubonic plague, 163, 167
Silla, Eric, 8, 242
Simond, Marc, 171
Simond, Paul-Louis, 20, 110 n.7
Sinou, Alain, 28
Sisters of the Immaculate Conception, 185
Smallpox, 7, 23–24, 32, 40 n.28, 92, 124, 162, 202, 256, 259
Snyder, Francis, 8
Social history of African health and disease, 5–8
Soninke, 119, 199
Sources, 8–9
South Africa, 4, 6
Sow, Fatou, 260
Statistics, demographic and epidemiological, 115–18, 184, 187, 189, 212, 215–18, 259, 260, 267–70
Streptomycin, 21, 249 n.84, 259
Sufi orders, 149–50
Sulfadiazine, 249 n. 84
Sulfa drugs, 11, 211, 226, 249 n.84, 259
Swanson, Maynard, 4, 7
Sy, Babacar, 151
Sy, Al-Hajj Malik, 128, 148–51

Synosternus pallidus (flea species), 233, 240. *See also* Fleas; *Xenopsylla astia*; *Xenopsylla cheopis*
Syphilis. *See* Venereal disease
Syrians, in Senegal, 99, 101, 112 n.57, 119, 185, 239

Taalibé, 239
Tall, Al-Hajj Umar, 148–49
Tall, Saidu Nuru, 149, 151, 157 n.61
Tanma, Lake, 36, 141–44
Tanzania, 6–7, 165
Tarabagans. *See* Rodents
Tatène (village of), 116, 121–22
Ternaux, Georges, 66–67
Thiam, Iba Der, 63–64, 66–67
Thiaroye (district of Dakar), 103, 113 n.64, 116, 238
Thiès, 10, 27–28, 36, 117, 119, 121–22, 132, 139–41, 144–46, 148– 49, 190, 217, 257, 269–70
Thiès-Bambara (district of Thiès), 188
Thiombane, Al-Hajj Serigne Malik, 160
Thiombane, Shaykh Serigne Alfa, 148, 168
Thiomboledj, village of, 116, 121
Thiroux, André, 91
at-Tijani, Ahmad, 148
Tijaniyya brotherhood, 10, 141, 147–52
Tirailleurs Sénégalais, 33, 60–61, 74, 80, 98, 119, 167–68, 188, 216
Tivaouane, 10, 28, 126, 139, 141, 145–46, 148–49, 152, 168, 190, 233, 256, 267, 269–70
Tiwigne, village of, 144, 146. *See also* Mont-Roland; Tiwigne Diassa, village of; Tiwigne Tangor
Tiwigne Diassa, village of, 145, 174
Tiwigne Tangor, 145
Touba, town of, 15
Toukar, village of, 163–64, 167–68
Tound (area of Dakar), 30
Trade unions, 260. *See also* CGT
Trypanosomiasis, 6–8, 141, 229, 257
Tuberculosis, 5–6, 40 n.23, 221, 259
Tukolor, 74, 148; and bubonic plague, 119, 122

Index

Tunisia, 7, 11 n.2, 150, 193, 203
Turshen, Meredeth, 3, 26, 165
Typhoid fever, 92, 259
Typhus, 7

Uganda, 134 n.41
Union Coloniale, 186,
United Nations, 213–14
United States Army Medical Corps in Senegal, 8, 10–11, 211–12, 225, 233–37
United States Consulate in Dakar, 214
United States Military Command in Senegal, 213–15
United States Navy in Senegal, 236
United States State Department, 233
Upper Volta, 201. *See also* Burkina Faso
Urbanization, 27, 184, 190–93, 260
Urban planning, 218–19

Van Heyningen, Elizabeth, 7
Vaucel, Dr., 257
Vaughan, Megan, 181 n.55, 262
Vector control, 106–8, 192, 227–33
Venereal disease, 221, 257
Veterinarians, 201
Vichy regime in FWA, 211, 213, 237
Vidal, Governor's Delegate M., 61–62, 109 n.6

Waalo, kingdom of, 148
Wallis, Charles Braithwaite (British Consul in Dakar), 69
Wangal, village of, 168, 181 n.60
Water supply in Dakar, 193
Western biomedicine, 6, 25–26, 132, 165, 193, 197

White, Luise, 86 n.41
Whittlesey, Derwent, 218–19, 244 n.10, 246 n.37
Wolof, 10, 139, 144, 147–48, 162, 165; and bubonic plague, 164; in plague zone, 141–43
Women, 165, 172, 183 nn. 98, 99, 190, 202, 218, 245 n.28, 256, 260; and funeral dirges, 174–79
Wondji, Christophe, 8
Wylie, Diana, 109 n.2

Xenopsylla astia (flea species), 18, 153 n.9. *See also* Fleas
Xenopsylla cheopis (flea species), 18, 142, 233, 253 n.137. *See also* Fleas
Xerus erythropus (palm rat), 18. *See also* Rodents

Ya el, 176–77
Yat, Dié, 161, 166–67, 173, 182 n.86
Yellow fever, 8, 17, 23, 30–31, 69, 92, 109, 124, 146, 225, 229, 261
Yembeul, village of, 120, 215
Yersin, Alexandre, 20, 110 n.7
Yersin's serum, 120
Yersinia pestis, 55, 93, 95, 106–7, 109, 118, 126, 129, 138, 142, 184–85, 215, 262, 265 n.41; description of, 17
Yoff (district of Dakar), 78, 116, 118, 214, 227, 235, 251 n.111; as a plague hecatomb, 97–98, 126
Young, T. Roy, Jr., 227, 234

Zawiya, 148–49
Zoonosis, 17, 261

ABOUT THE AUTHOR

MYRON ECHENBERG is an associate professor at McGill University, where he teaches African history. His *Colonial Conscripts: The Tirailleurs Sénégalais in French West Africa, 1857–1960* won the Herskovits Award of the African Studies Association for the outstanding original scholarly work published during 1991.